The Principles of Sahaj Marg

Set 1
(Containing Volumes 1 to 3)

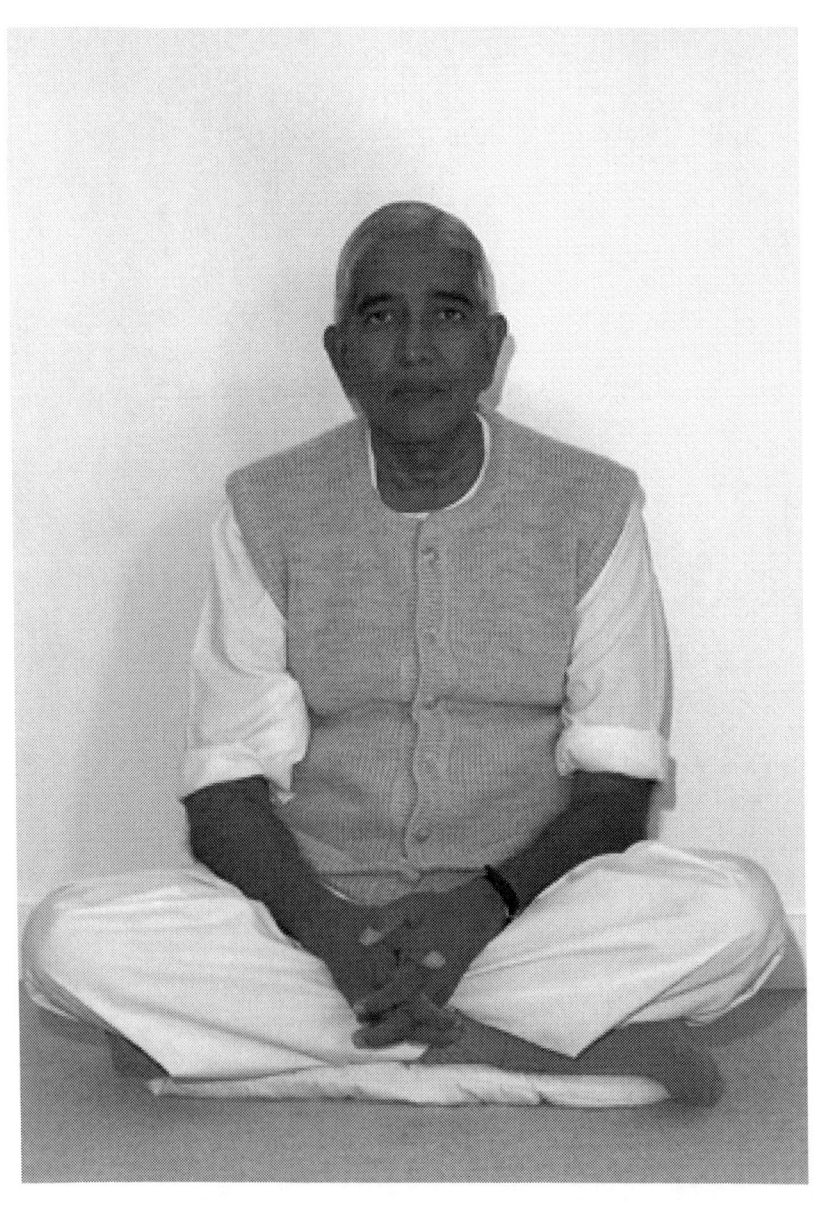

Shri Parthasarathi Rajagopalachariji
President
Shri Ram Chandra Mission

The Principles of Sahaj Marg

Set 1
(Containing Volumes 1 to 3)

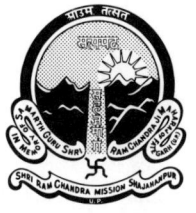

by
Shri P. Rajagopalachari

SHRI RAM CHANDRA MISSION
USA

Originally published as separate books:

The Principles of Sahaj Marg, Volume I
© 1986 by Shri Ram Chandra Mission, Shahjahanpur, U.P.
India

The Principles of Sahaj Marg, Volume II
© 1987 by Shri Ram Chandra Mission, Shahjahanpur, U.P.
India

The Principles of Sahaj Marg, Volume III
© 1987 by Shri Ram Chandra Mission, Shahjahanpur, U.P.
India

Shri Ram Chandra Mission
Post Office Box 269
Molena, GA 30258
U.S.A.
http://www.srcm.org

© 1999 by Shri Ram Chandra Mission (a non-profit California corporation). No part of this book may be reproduced in any form or by any means without permission in writing from Shri Ram Chandra Mission. "Shri Ram Chandra Mission", "Sahaj Marg" and the Mission's emblem are registered Service Marks and/or Trademarks of Shri Ram Chandra Mission.
All rights reserved.
Printed in United States of America

06 05 04 03 02 01 00 99   8 7 6 5 4 3 2 1

ISBN 0-945242-42-5

Contents

Preface viii

The Principles of Sahaj Marg, Volume 1

Lectures given on overseas tours in 1972 (Egypt, Europe, UK and USA), 1976 (Europe), 1977 (Malaysia, Singapore) and 1980 (Denmark, West Germany)

Religion and Spirituality in the Light of Sahaj Marg 3
Yoga as an Instrument of Human Evolution 12
Man and God 22
The Inner Needs of Man 25
Yoga and Sahaj Marg 35
Purification and Regulation of the Mind
        by Sahaj Marg Yoga 50
Need for Need 56
Prayer 65
Yoga as an Evolutionary Force 68
Cleanliness and Godliness 74
Religion and Spirituality 80
The Need for a Master 88
Love 96
What Should We Ask of God 103
The Two Ends of a Stick 107
Yoga as the Way of Experience 116
Sahaj Marg and Science 123
Morality 130

The Principles of Sahaj Marg, Volume 2

Articles written and published in various Mission publications 1969 to 1981

Sahaj Marg & the Problems of Personality 143

Superstition and Spirituality 149
Worship 153
Sadhana 157
Sahaj Marg and Formal Worship 161
The Goal of Spiritual Endeavour 167
Dvandvas or the Pairs of Opposites 171
The Disciple 177
What is Mine? 182
Father and Son 186
Karma Yoga or Work and its Reward 190
The River of Love 196
Yoga through Love 200
The Beauty of Sahaj Marg 211
Surrender and Freedom. 215
Work and Play 219
Idol Worship 223
Our Daily Bread 230
Craving, Reality and Adoration. 233
Serving the Master 238
Life and Liberation 242
The Friend Within. 245
True Abhyasi, Right Aspiration and Real Goal 249
Darshan 258

The Principles of Sahaj Marg, Volume 3

Talks and Messages given in India 1983 to 1985

Balanced Existence 263
The Purpose of Existence 276
Spiritual Growth and Development 286
Continuity of a Tradition 288
The Task Ahead 297
Call of Conscience 302
Revelations 316
Accept Him in His Essence 324
Interiorize Him 337
Discipline 349
Change and Discipline 364
As Above, So Below 369

Evolution, I	376
Evolution, II	382
Time	389
Reality Unveiled	396
Adhere to One Teaching, One Goal	403
Listen to the Heart	410
Glossary	425
Index	445

Preface

Since 1972, Shri Parthasarathi Rajagopalachari has been travelling throughout the world bringing the light of spirituality to men and women eager for spiritual growth. His formal presentation of Sahaj Marg, the 'natural path', began when he accompanied his beloved Master, Shri Ram Chandra of Shahjahanpur, on his first tour of the West. He gave several public talks about the need for spirituality in the modern world. Since assuming the mantle of spiritual master of the Shri Ram Chandra Mission in 1984, Chariji, as he is affectionately known, has spoken often and eloquently about Sahaj Marg and the need for inner change. He is constantly encouraging us to take an active interest in our own spiritual growth and, more importantly, showing us how to bring our lives into harmony with our highest aspirations.

Fortunately, Chariji's talks have been recorded and disseminated in numerous books, among them the several volumes of *The Principles of Sahaj Marg*, published in India since 1986. We are very pleased to re-release them now in a new series, beginning with this book, Set 1, comprising the first three *Principles* volumes.

The talks in Volume 1, delivered during four tours with his Master in Europe, the United States, Malaysia, and Singapore, were public addresses, intended to introduce Sahaj Marg to these countries for the very first time. Taken as a whole, they provide a clear and comprehensive introduction to the philosophy and practice of Sahaj Marg, explaining the practical elements of the system, its scientific basis, and the need for such a system in order to achieve balance in the modern world.

Volume 2 is unique among the *Principles* in that it contains articles written by Chariji during the 1970's, for publication in the *Sahaj Marg Patrika* (magazine) in India. In these works Chariji probes more deeply into the integration of Sahaj Marg in our lives and takes an in-depth look into the spiritual principles which underlie the practice. He brings to these works a sharp intelligence and a deep appreciation of the nuances of the system.

After Babuji's *mahasamadhi*, Chariji, as spiritual successor, undertook to travel throughout India, bringing Sahaj Marg to thousands of aspirants. Volume 3 presents the first series of talks in India; succeeding volumes contain further talks recorded in that country.

Over the years Chariji's talks have become increasingly penetrating, as he has explored every aspect of Sahaj Marg and its all-pervading influence in our lives. Chariji often uses examples from nature and society to encourage understanding of how to live a balanced existence, oriented towards the goal of oneness with the Highest. The simplicity of these observations can be deceiving: a little thought will reveal deep meaning and provide tips about practice. Chariji's works reveal to us a system of spiritual practice which includes all of existence, and he demonstrates how this existence is to be used for spiritual benefit. As he has said, "We are not here to run the world, we are here to use it for our evolution."

In these volumes he shows us how every instant of our lives may be used to do just that. May the whole world shine in the light of the selfless outpouring of his heart; and may we receive what He is constantly offering us with prayers for the upliftment of all beings everywhere.

The Publishers

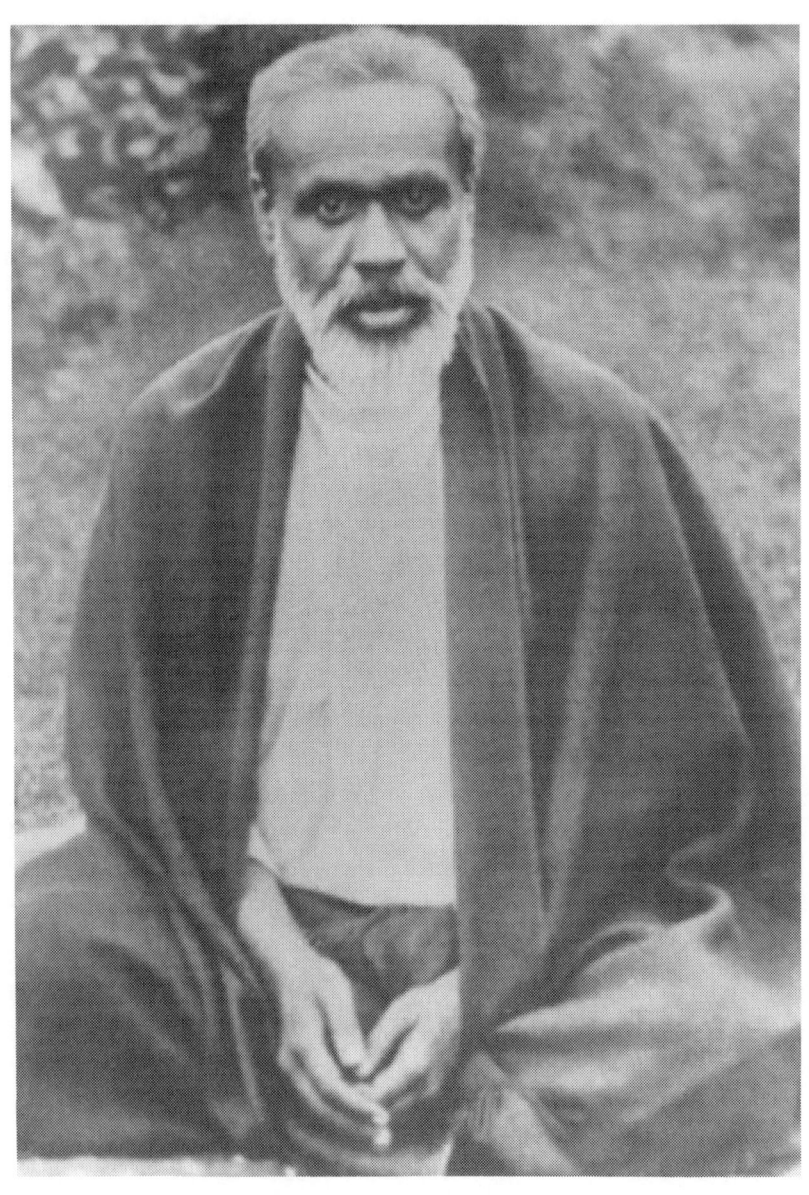

Samarth Guru Mahatma
Shri Ram Chandraji Maharaj
of
Fatehgarh

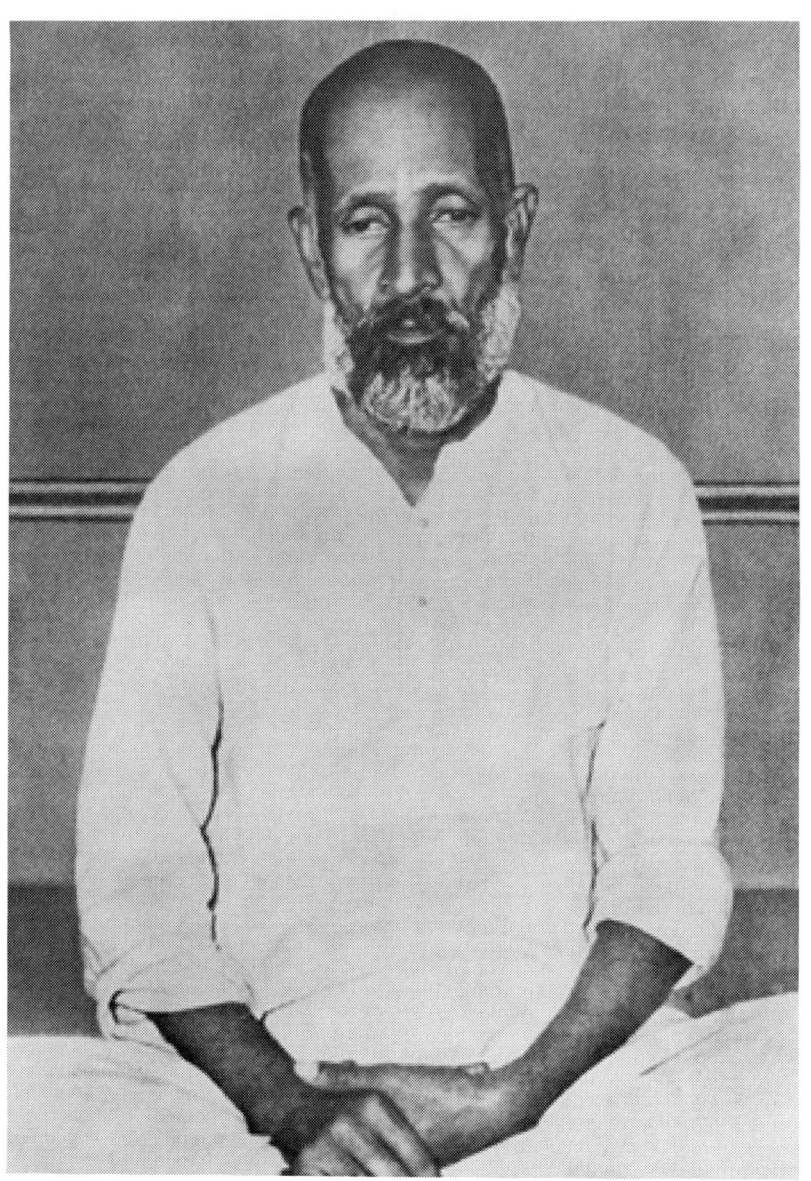

Shri Ram Chandraji Maharaj
of
Shahjahanpur

The Principles of Sahaj Marg

Volume 1

Religion and Spirituality
In the Light of Sahaj Marg

I have the honour to place before you some of the ideas that my Master, Shri Ram Chandraji Maharaj, has elucidated, particularly in respect of two terms–'religion' and 'spirituality'. We assume that these terms are understood by even the ordinary educated citizens. These terms are considered, quite erroneously, to be synonymous. Perhaps these two terms are most naturally misunderstood as far as their mutual identification in respect of meaning, systematic thinking and obedience to principles and practices are concerned.

The system of Sahaj Marg, which is a system of yoga perfected by my Master on the foundations of a new yoga created by his Master who bore his name, has set out to cast new light on the fundamental concepts of religion, philosophy, spirituality, yoga, and indeed through a whole spectrum of terminology associated with such practices, and also to establish a correct practice towards attaining the right goal of human life.

All of you are no doubt aware that religious feeling has always been one of the fundamental emotive aspects of a man's emotional make-up or psyche, and this is borne out amply by a study of anthropology from the earliest times of man's appearance on this planet. Of course, the expression given to the religious emotional content has varied from race to race and from time to time, but that hidden craving in man's heart which tended to seek an answer, or answers, to the questions which arose in him concerning the creation of the universe, the reasons for such creation and man's own place and part in it, has not varied. Expression depends on development of thought; thought stems from ideas; and ideas of course

---

Lecture given at the Accademia Del Mediterraneo, Rome, on Wednesday, 26 April 1972 at 8:30 P.M.

are governed by the development of various features of man's mental make-up, including such diverse factors as physiological, environmental and social.

A study of the history of ancient and modern religions, combined with a parallel study of anthropology, reveals that religious sentiment was almost simultaneous with man's own appearance. In the beginning, the religious sentiment expressed itself mentally in terms of fear and awe leading to the worship, at least in bygone times, of animal life, vegetable life, the phenomena of nature, etc. All these later became ritualized into general forms of worship where the object of worship was nature, fire in its various forms, and worship of the dead. This form of worship prevailed through most of early man's history, and was almost the only form of worship available and prevalent throughout the world up to the middle ages. Nevertheless, their very prevalence up to the emergence of higher forms of worship would appear to indicate that, in some measure at least, they had served to satisfy man's internal craving for some form of communion with what may be called his Maker or Nature or Universal Spirit, or whatever else it may be called.

Later, this religious sentiment turned its attention to somewhat more sophisticated objects of worship and, at this stage, we can see the commencement of the representation of God in terms of anthropomorphic forms, i.e., in terms of human figures which the human imagination enriched and endowed with higher powers than merely normal human powers by the addition of extra arms, extra heads, a higher stature, and diverse other similar embellishments. The craving was the same; the mode of expression of the emotive sentiment was the same; all that had changed was merely the object which was now worshipped in place of the earlier primitive ones.

Yet later in the history of humanity there arose even more purified religions where we find the beginning of what may be called ethical codes and laws being given to the people, often through a leader of the people themselves, who was proclaimed as a religious leader or the giver of the law, the revealer of the truth and so on. We have historical personalities such as Christ, Moses,

Mohammed, Buddha, Confucius, Krishna, etc., in the various religions as an illustration of this development. This stage of development in religions can roughly be stated to cover the past few millennia of human history.

Analyzing the religious content and the modes of religious approach of those coming under its fold, we find that all religions have heavily relied on two important instruments for regulating and controlling the behaviour of the flock under their control. These two instruments, by and large, have been fear and temptation. It is perhaps beyond any reasonable debate that this is an established fact. Religions have always held out to their devotees the temptation of redemption and a place in heaven, whether during the course of this life itself or after death. They have always tried to control and canalize man's behaviour in a desired direction by trying to induce him to accept this temptation for the fruits offered by the respective religions. This is one side of the picture. How to enforce a man's behaviour in the pursuit of the goal was the next question and here fear came in all too handy–the fear of punishment for swerving from the performance of religious rituals stipulated; the fear of punishment for not supporting the body of one's own religion in its continued existence; the fear of retribution for acts forbidden; and so on and so forth. Therefore, fear on one hand, and temptation on the other, would be a fair representation of religious activity, and religious control.

Modern psychologists will no doubt agree that an imposition on the human mind of two opposing forces of this nature could do nothing but create tension in the mind of the individual, and this tension cannot be eradicated by the practice of religion, because religion itself is the very force that created the tension in the first place. This would appear to indicate the necessity for a source outside religions to eradicate such tensions, and to normalize the human being at least in his mental make-up.

Perhaps the appearance of such diverse phenomena as the cult of hippyism, the associated habit of the taking of drugs and narcotics, the widespread and deeply penetrating discontent of the human being with his personal existence, which appears to pervade all sections of humanity at every stratum of social existence, all these would appear to be the results of such religious training which have not satisfied the real nature of man, nor given answers to his fundamental questions referred to earlier. You will pardon me if I therefore suggest that religions have not kept up with man's innermost needs and requirements of the soul. At this stage I may be permitted to add that it is not a failure in religion itself because, at the time when these great religions, whether Christianity, or Hinduism, or Buddhism, or Islam were founded, at that time the religious leaders who established them had moulded them into such shape, and given them such form as fulfilled the needs of humanity of those times.

It may also be noted that the founders of all great religions have preached love as being the only proper approach to the Creator, and this love, when properly cultivated by religious sentiment and religious practice, was expected to reflect in love for all that is contained in creation. How this has been forgotten, and religions have had to depend on temptation and fear, is the sorry story of religious decadence. Nevertheless, the fault can be attributed to lie in the fact that religions have become stultified, and to some extent petrified, and they have not altered or evolved in keeping with man's own evolution. I humbly suggest that the evolution of religion has lagged behind the evolution of man whom it is supposed or expected to serve for his vital inner spiritual needs.

This being the case as far as religion is concerned, what is it that spirituality has to offer? Now the term 'spirituality' has nothing to do with religion, as commonly understood. According to my Master, spirituality really begins where religion ends. While the basic education of man can be undertaken by religion, his further development when he has reached what may be termed adulthood can only be offered by spirituality. Spirituality is easily identifiable with mysticism in all its aspects. Religion enforces an externalization of the mind in man's search for God. Mysticism or spirituality internalizes the search and directs the mind to the heart of man where the search should really commence.

One of the great tenets or principles of all religions has been that at the heart of the human being God Himself resides. Of course this may be thought to be the mere doctrine of immanence; but it is true that God is immanent within us. When the search is externalized, the first thing man loses sight of, or touch with, is himself. The goal is taken to be far away, very often in some far distant sphere of existence not easily accessible to us. The search is therefore begun on the premise, often founded on solid theological doctrine, that the search will in almost all cases be futile and the goal inaccessible. The search is therefore begun and undertaken in a spirit of frustration and a foreboding of non-achievement of the goal. How can such a search ever help anybody? On the contrary spirituality focuses man's attention on the Divine effulgence radiating in one's own heart, which effulgence is created by the presence of the Creator Himself in the heart. This immediately presents the Divine in an altered light, and brings Him to a proximity with one's own person which can hardly come any nearer. Being within us such a Person is not only always accessible but readily reachable, and all that spirituality requires of us to achieve the sense of oneness with the Ultimate is to focus the mind inward upon the Person. Apparently, therefore, spirituality is by far the easier method of the two to achieve the goal of human life.

Again, religion concentrates heavily on ritual worship. Taking a parallel from the childhood development of the human being, toys may serve children but real living things alone can bring happiness to adults. Therefore, performance of ritualistic modes of worship may be given in the formative years of a human being's life but, after a certain stage, they cease to have meaning and, for a majority of human beings, degenerate into mere mockery. Spirituality on the other hand does not specify or advocate ritualistic approaches. In spirituality all that is required to be done is to sit comfortably in a comfortable room, close one's eyes, turn the attention from the external world into the heart, and meditate on the contents of that heart in the shape of Divine effulgence emanating from the Being seated therein. Here there is no mummery or any other form of bewilderment, or what can in some religions even be classed as trickery, but there is an honest approach to the search for the

Ultimate. Further, in the spiritual practice there are no associated threats or fears of retribution, nor are temptations held out to the seeker. All that is stated is that one's development depends solely and entirely on one's effort. If the practice is not indulged in, there is no benefit, and that is about all that there is to it.

Turning our attention once again to religion, it is a well-known fact that religions, while accepting or even arrogating to themselves the role of preservers of law and morality, have often signally failed in this duty for a very important but, at the same time, a very little noticed fact. I would like to emphasize this by inviting your attention to it, and it is this. Most religions while giving out their code of ethics or laws have only told their people what not to do. Therefore, these codes of behaviour can at best be termed negative codes or negative laws, because most of them do not tell man what should be done to attain a better life. I agree that we must know what not to do, but certainly this cannot be taken as more than negative wisdom, nor can strict adherence to such laws be taken as more than negative virtue. But all too often we come across people who ask, "Well, I know what not to do, but it does not help me in knowing what I should do," and this again creates not only confusion but a tension in their minds, leading again to mental distress and possible ultimate deterioration in character itself. Spiritual edicts, on the other hand, have mostly confined themselves to precise and simple sets of injunctions stating very understandably to the seeker what exactly he should do. It is my contention that once a man knows what he should do, whatever be the field of action, whether professional, moral, social, it at the same time excludes the entire field of activity which should not be indulged in. The contrary, unfortunately, is not true. To know what one should do it is not enough to know what not to do. This, to my mind, has been the greatest failure of religions throughout the world, and this was sought to be rectified by great spiritual Masters of the world.

It is common knowledge that religions have divided man from man, brother from brother, and often turned the father against the son, the husband against the wife, inciting much of humanity during history to violence against each other; because religions have their own separate gods of worship and the modes and rituals by which such gods should be worshipped. Religions, to hold their flock, have had to insist upon a strict adherence to their own religious paraphernalia while simultaneously forbidding even the thought of the gods of other religions. One of the paramount and deep-seated forces of hatred has been created by religion, and I believe this does not need any proof.

Spirituality on the other hand invokes no names, confers no attributes, demands no subservience to any such artificially created gods of the human mind, but focuses man's attention on the Infinite Ultimate Source of All Being Who, as aforesaid, is nameless, formless and attributeless. It is, I believe, a matter for easy agreement that such an approach to the Ultimate can serve as an integrating force and bring together human beings of all lands and all religions in oneness in the most fundamental aspect of human life, which is sadly lacking today. Spirituality, if widely practised in this spirit of a humble approach to the Ultimate, is perhaps the most potent force that can bring about such an integration.

Unfortunately, there have been no spiritual systems as such comparable in power to the great religious systems, and this is surely the fault of man himself, in that he has allowed himself to be guided by the nose and made to subscribe to established bodies and organizations without examining in detail either their make-up or his own. Nevertheless, spiritual teaching and instruction, even from the Middle Ages, has not been lacking. There have been great mystics and Masters of spiritual teaching in all lands at all times. You have had in the West such great figures as Jacob Boehme, St. John of the Cross, and in the Orient there have been great savants such as the great rishis of Hinduism, Buddha–the founder of Buddhism, Confucius and Lao Tse in China. Masters have therefore not been lacking, but the fear element in religion has successfully kept away aspirants from coming out of religions and embracing spirituality. So we find in yet one more way religions doing disservice to man by preventing his evolution.

I have taken the liberty of giving you a few of our thoughts on religion and spirituality. I think at this stage I must introduce my

Master's system of spirituality under the name 'Sahaj Marg'. The name Sahaj Marg means the natural way. In its basic teaching it offers what all other spiritual systems have offered. My Master does not lay any claim to originality in this system. It was, according to his own words, rediscovered by his Master, Shri Ram Chandra of Fatehgarh, a district town in U.P., India, and this word 'rediscovered' is important. My Master has said that this system of Sahaj Marg, no doubt under a different name, was prevalent thousands of years ago, but was lost and had to be rediscovered again.

While we do not lay claim to originality, there are however very important and unique features which set Sahaj Marg as a system of spirituality apart from all others. What are these differences? The most important one is that in this system alone, to our knowledge, we employ what is known as transmission. This transmission is something unique and enormously efficacious in its application. What is transmitted is the Master's own yogic or life energy, which is transmitted into the heart of one who begins the practice of meditation in this system. This transmission is not something ephemeral or merely put in words but something which is very tangible, and to the reception of which innumerable practicants all over India, and an increasing number of persons in the West, can personally testify. The transmission by the Master has very great importance because by receiving it the student is able to develop with such pace that it is incalculable. Therefore, the student's own shortcomings have in a sense ceased to have any relevance to the possibility of his development. In all other extant systems of yoga, to confine ourselves purely to yoga for the time being, the reliance is entirely on oneself, and we all know how much capacity or power the average human being of today has in the field of self-development, or for that matter even how much of inclination he has! Therefore, if an outside source of Divine energy is available to us, willing to infuse us with his own energy, to fill us with it, and thus make evolution possible to us beyond the reaches of the wildest imagination, how very fortunate should we not consider ourselves in having such a source available to us today?

It is my great privilege to introduce to you such a personality in the person of my Revered Master, Shri Ram Chandraji, who is before you all today. His services are available to one and all. In this system of Sahaj Marg there are no barriers of race, religion or sex. All are welcome to participate in the Divine experiment of self-evolution, and it is my earnest hope that all of you would like to undertake a trial to see for yourself whether this transmission exists or not, and to see what it can do for you.

I may assure you at this stage that there are no bondages implied or imposed upon you in any form. All that you are committed to do is to practise for a few months according to the principles set out by my Master and to test for yourself its efficacy, and if you are not happy with it, you are at liberty to bid goodbye to this system. Its principles do not in any way controvert or go against the individual's religious sentiments because the goal aimed at is the Infinite, Impersonal Almighty without form or attributes and is, therefore, a goal that must normally be acceptable to anyone, of whatever calling he may be. I therefore have pleasure in welcoming you all to this great system and I express the hope, with assurance, that there will certainly be great benefit from the practice of this system.

Yoga as an Instrument of Human Evolution

The facts of evolution may be said to be universally accepted not only by the scientists who have developed theories of evolution but also by the specialists in other fields of knowledge including religion and theology. Theories of evolution postulate the development of primitive forms of life into more and more complex forms culminating in the highest evolutionary type–man or *homo sapiens*. Scientific theories have proved, mainly by a study of palaeontology, that the earliest unicellular forms of life have developed through aeons of time, by the process known as natural selection, to more and more complex levels of existence assuming a multiplicity of forms. These theories indicate that the earliest physical forms at some stage of their evolution took on a mind. Today, evolution has reached a stage where future evolution has been stated by many eminent evolutionists and scholars such as Fr. Teilhard de Chardin, Professor Harris and others, to depend on the evolution of the mind, testifying almost to the fact that physical evolution has now culminated in a form where future physical evolution has very little importance or bearing on evolution itself. Fr. Teilhard has even postulated the existence of what he terms a *noosphere* and has predicted, on the basis of his scientific findings, the future evolutionary trend as being the mental evolution. Professor Harris, in his remarkable book, *The Foundation of Metaphysics in Science*, has reached what would appear to be a similar conclusion. Many other eminent scientists subscribe to this view.

Under the process of natural selection the evolution of one form into the next higher form takes millennia, and it is therefore an extremely slow process. Until the emergence of man with his thinking mind, the lower forms of life had no recourse but to subject themselves, albeit unknowingly, to this natural process because

---

Lecture at the Students Centre, Massachusetts Institute of Technology, Cambridge (Mass.) on Thursday, 25 May 1972.

they did not have the mental equipment to in any way interfere with, or guide the course of their own evolution. However, with the emergence of man there can be stated to be a drastic change in the evolutionary situation since, for the first time, a form of life which is evolving may be said to have acquired some degree of control over its own evolution. The modern marvels of the conquest of nature culminating in the beginnings of the conquest of space all testify to the basic validity of this view.

The ancient Hindu seers existing many thousands of years ago took it into their heads to study how best man could evolve to his highest nature, and achieve the highest goal open to him. Records of the ancient researches are unfortunately not available because these researches into the body and the mind of man *vis-à-vis* his environment were conducted and concluded at a period of history when the only means of communication was language, and the means of recording the findings of such research were still unavailable. The earliest Vedic and yogic knowledge based on such studies or researches is, however, fortunately available to us, having been passed on from master to disciple by word of mouth. The vast texts had to be memorized by mind, generation after generation and, thus preserved, they have come down to us today in their original pristine forms with very little change in the body of that knowledge.

Our concern is not with the religious or ritualistic texts or portions of the Veda which sought to preserve the religion and religious practices of Hinduism intact, known as the Karma Kanda. Our concern is with those texts relating to the techniques evolved, both physical and mental, which were created and destined for man's evolution. Some such texts are what may be called the yogic texts, and are included in the three great classes of texts, bodies of knowledge, the Brahma Sutras, the Bhagavad Gita and the Upanishads.

Yoga teaches that while natural evolution takes place over geological periods of time, man can undertake or participate in certain processes which condense the total possibilities of evolution into his own brief span of temporal existence.

What is yoga? As you are all no doubt aware, yoga comes from the Sanskrit root *yuj*, which means yoke or unite, and the term was applied to those sciences and arts which were created as a means of uniting man with his Ultimate Consciousness which may be called God, the Creator, the World Spirit, etc. Yoga today means many things to many people, and the original meaning of union with the Ultimate would appear to be mostly relegated to the background. Even in India there are a large number of so-called yogas such as *hatha yoga, karma yoga, laya yoga, mantra yoga* and so on. Most of these yogas deal with the physical system or organization of man, and have no relevance to the ultimate goal of human endeavour. For instance, hatha yoga is a purely physical system of yoga, with a gamut of exercises involving specialized postures and breathing exercises, the latter coming under the specialized name of *pranayama*. While some of the texts, even the original ones, postulate that such practices can lead to the ultimate goal, this is a questionable claim. No doubt some psychic values may be developed such as clairvoyance, clairaudience and so on, but it is a debatable point whether they can lead to spiritual growth culminating in Realisation. More or less the same is the case with *laya yoga* or *kundalini yoga*. These too are based on physical practices supposed to liberate certain powers in man. As far as *karma yoga* is concerned, it teaches that the proper performance of one's duties without regard to the fruits of labour can elevate man to the highest state. But as aforesaid, and as taught by my Master, it is very debatable whether physical practices, whatever be their name or classification, can lead to spiritual development.

At some stage in the history of yoga, the great sage Patanjali classified the then extant systems and created a consolidated yogic school of practice called the *Ashtanga Yoga* or the Yoga of the Eight Limbs. What this system would appear to have done was to consolidate the teachings of several schools, and to create a systematic body of organized knowledge pertaining to yoga.

In the West the practice of yoga has flourished, particularly during the last couple of decades, in various forms, but their practice has been restricted mainly to beautifying the body and making it more healthy. One of the claims of yoga is that the practitioner will become beautiful, his face will become clear, his voice must become musical, and so on. In the West yoga would appear to be restricted to these aims, with perhaps very few exceptions.

Raja yoga however is of a different plane altogether, since it deals with the mind of man. Most schools of yoga insist upon a prior practice of the physical parts or practices of *yama, niyama, asana, pranayama* and so on. Nevertheless Raja Yoga can be said to be a higher form of yoga as, at some stage, it comes into relationship with the mind which it seeks to develop and canalize in the direction of right thought and activity.

Raja yoga means the king of yogas, and rightly so. In raja yoga the main method of development is the art of meditation. Meditation may be defined as the continuous thinking of something, or about something. In a sense, therefore, anybody who is thinking continuously of something may be said to be involved in meditation. Ancient teachers, both in the East and the West, have taught that as one meditates so one becomes. It therefore follows that what we meditate upon we get or become and, inversing this formula, if we want to become something we must meditate upon **that** and nothing else. Therefore, if our aim is Realisation or the attainment of oneness with the Ultimate, the object of meditation must be that Ultimate, and nothing else. Raja yoga, in its purest form, excludes physical objects of meditation including the figures or forms of the various gods and goddesses of the Hindu pantheon. The object of meditation must be limited to the formless, attributeless, abstract Ultimate.

In Sahaj Marg, which my Master has developed as a purified form of raja yoga, and which system was rediscovered by his Master, Samarth Guru Shri Ram Chandraji of Fatehgarh, the correct way of meditation with the implicit and specified goal of Realisation is taught. In this system meditation is on this object, viz., the abstract Ultimate alone, because meditation on lesser objects can only lead to lesser achievements or accomplishments, falling short of the established goal.

In the Sahaj Marg system the student is asked to meditate on the heart. Ancient yoga systems teach meditation on the point of the nose, on the point between the eyebrows, on a point in the forehead, and so on. My Master has excluded such points and prescribed it on the heart for three important reasons. Firstly, the heart is the seat of life, and therefore when we meditate on this point we meditate on the source of life itself. Secondly, circulation commences from the heart and if the heart is purified, the purity extends throughout the human organization. Thirdly, all religions have stated and taught that in the human being it is in the heart that the Creator has His abode, and therefore this is the fitting point for meditation.

My Master recognizes that the abstract Ultimate as an object of meditation is a very difficult one for beginners. He therefore specifies light as the initial object, the method being to imagine that the heart is illuminated from inside by the presence of the Divine who resides therein. I must stress that this is only the beginning, and in fact we are advised not to meditate on light as a source of light, which would lead to wrong results. It is like the diving board in a swimming pool where the board enables the diver to get sufficient momentum to take off, and after the diver has taken off, the board has no further use for him until he dives again.

In our Sahaj Marg system all that you are asked to do is to sit comfortably, close your eyes, and do this meditation. My Master states that as one progresses in meditation the body acquires for itself a posture of repose and tranquillity which it can hold for the length of time necessary, and therefore *asana* becomes established in a natural manner. Similarly, as meditation progresses our experience testifies to the fact that breathing slows down and assumes a natural cycle, natural to that state of existence, and so *pranayama* becomes established. Under my Master's direction as the pupil progresses in meditation, purification of the heart proceeds automatically, and mental processes are purified which in turn results in pure action, and therefore *yama* and *niyama*, the first two stages of Patanjali's Yoga, also become naturally established. As yet another result of meditation, the mind becomes used to thinking about one fixed thing, and as the mind's capacity grows, the power of concentration becomes established, and this capacity grows so that it results finally in a stage where concentration becomes natural, and thus *pratyahara* and *dharana* aspects of yoga also become established. Thus, by commencing at the seventh stage of Patanjali's Ashtanga Yoga under the guidance of an able Master, the earlier six stages become naturally established without any undue physical or mental effort on the part of the practicant being necessary.

In our system of raja yoga we do not have much to do with the eighth stage called *samadhi*. Samadhi is a state where the human consciousness may be said to have lapsed into total quiescence, and a state of existence results in which the human being becomes almost a stone. My Master does not think such a samadhi to be a necessary state. A state of existence called *sahaj samadhi* or natural samadhi is offered, where, while the individual exists at a stage of consciousness which may be said to be superhuman, or non-human if you prefer it, the lower mind or the normal human mind also continues to be aware of all that is going on around it, but without being affected by the environment in any way. There is, therefore, no exclusion of the external world, but there is an all-enveloping samadhi which embraces everything in the world or universe, while being itself entirely absorbed in itself, and also simultaneously aware of the cosmic totality. My Master states that this is a higher stage of existence than the state of samadhi as traditionally taught.

The Sahaj Marg system is unique among Indian yogic systems as being a system specially developed for the average householder. My Master believes that the normalization of all functions leads to saintliness. Every faculty inbuilt in man has its legitimate function, and must be used in the performance of that function. Sahaj Marg therefore does not teach or prescribe celibacy but it does teach that a normalization of the generative function is essential. My Master teaches that it is in the world of the family that almost all of man's powers are perfected, including such diverse ones as the capacity for love, the capacity for renunciation, the capacity for taking on responsibility, the capacity for social function in a group, and so on. Therefore, this system does not recognize differences of race, differences of sex, or indeed any other differences between individuals, and all are qualified to practise this yoga, the sole qualification being willingness to participate in it.

Another feature of Sahaj Marg is that it does not impose any artificial and strict regimentation on the individual's life, though there are some basic and absolutely natural rules to be followed. There are no unnatural demands. My Master states very categorically that the purification of the human system must begin with the mind, and once the mind is purified the physical aspects of man's existence cannot help being purified because right thinking must lead to right conduct. Thus all the prescribed norms of human behaviour become not only possible but are naturally established in the individual's life. The conflicts and travails that normally attend on the practice of yoga under the earlier systems are therefore absent in the Sahaj Marg system.

The most unique feature about Sahaj Marg is what may be called transmission. Our Grand Master, Samarth Guru Shri Ram Chandraji of Fatehgarh, rediscovered the capacity for the transmission of yogic or life energy from his own centre of existence into the centre of existence of another individual. This art he has passed on to his disciple, my Master, who has perfected it. This transmission is something which is capable of being felt by anybody who takes the trouble of practising this system for a brief period. In fact it is the transmission which sets Sahaj Marg apart from other yogas, and from all other systems of human evolution. My Master says that when the transmission is made into the heart of the student, the student is filled with a force higher than himself, and therefore his evolution or progress becomes not only very much speedier but also becomes, in a sense, independent of his own capacity for progress. Therefore, the present condition of the individual has no bearing on what he sets out to be, and at one stroke all differences of present human situation are eradicated, because of the possibility of this transmission existing today.

In modern life most people would appear to have lost sight of the ultimate goal. The endeavour of most human beings is restricted to the attainment of a full material existence saturated with material comforts and sensual satisfaction. This has necessarily created a sense of loss of purpose in existence, and a bewilderment as to the purpose of life. The Sahaj Marg system of yoga, by its emphasis on right thinking, right conduct and right living, sets out to redefine the goals of human life, and thereby establish in the heart and mind of man the ultimate purpose of the individual's existence, and to establish in proper perspective the values of all the material and other affluences that surround him. According to my Master, everything in creation has a place and a purpose, but man must recognize precisely what the scheme of things relates to, and what his own part in the whole drama of creation is. When man understands his place in existence, understands his purpose and comes to realise his goal, it is possible for him to abstract from nature what he needs for his existence, forgetting all superfluities, throwing aside all unnecessary things, leaving behind all that has been spent and done with. He is thus made capable of proceeding on the evolutionary path untrammelled by the physical and mental drudgeries of today's existence.

My Master contends that by purifying the individual's mind alone can natural societies of human beings be created where the group's social aspiration becomes the sum total of individual aspirations, all geared to a common purpose of self-evolution with the goal of ultimate Realisation as the sole objective. Under such a scheme of things material existence falls into its proper place, as does every facet of existence. Material life can be pursued without mental obsessions, mental illnesses and other aspects detrimental to man's life, taking care that material goals do not become the predominant ones; and ensuring that material life is only indulged in as a ladder of evolution, because the embodied spirit has to use the body and its environment for the evolution of that spirit. My Master, as I have already stated, does not preach celibacy or asceticism for the simple reason that these reflect a swing in the opposite direction from materiality, and are therefore in some measure also perversions to that extent. I do not imply any disrespect when I say this, but anything which goes to one extreme is necessarily wrong for the individual whether it be asceticism or total immersion in a material existence.

The Sahaj Marg system has evolved an easily practicable yogic method designed for the average man whatever be his education, whatever be his racial antecedents, whatever be his profession, without differences of sex so that the ultimate goal is brought nearer to the whole of mankind. It is not restricted, as it was in the past, to a few members of the elite of society. My Master has stated that God is everywhere and in everything and must therefore be available to everybody. Any system which restricts its practice to a handful cannot, by the very nature of that exclusion, be right or in any way correct in its teaching. My Master also teaches that God is simple and the means to achieve Him must be simple, and I believe Sahaj Marg sets out to fulfil this.

Before concluding I would like to refer to an ancient Indian text which is called the *five ways* or *five methods*, which, according to eminent scholars, can apply as rationally to professional life or to army manoeuvres as to spiritual life. This text emphasizes that all human endeavour must conform to five principles if it is to succeed. These are:

- Acquire knowledge and understanding of the goal to be achieved.
- Select the right way or approach to achieve that goal.
- Correctly assess one's current state.
- Attract to oneself all favourable forces which will conduce to achievement of the goal.
- Repel or do away with all adverse factors standing in the way of the goal.

We believe that this text has much to offer in the wide scope of its coverage and the simple and succinct way that it puts it. The importance given to the goal is to be emphasized again and again, because one of the general aspects of our normal existence is that men and women indulge in a lot of activity without knowing precisely what that activity is for. This perhaps is the reason for the widespread frustration and disappointment in life that most of us feel, accompanied by the sense of non-fulfilment and aimless existence. All human endeavour should therefore start with a clear knowledge regarding our aim, and this applies to yoga as much as to anything else.

Man and God

We are assembled in a house of prayer and every such house of prayer is a house of God. All over the world where human beings exist there are such houses of God to which people can go and reconcile themselves with the Ultimate. We have the institution of the confessional which is aimed at ridding man of the burdens of his conscience for his actions in the past, and also to offer the facility of communing with God and making his peace. Whatever be the religion, and however civilized or primitive society may be, such houses of God are necessary for our existence and for our peace of mind.

Now, religions have a very vital part to play in the bringing up of the individual. We believe, as most religions believe, that when the soul takes human birth, it in some way suffers a fall or a descent from its lofty status and severs its connection with God. It is, therefore, necessary for religion, or it is the purpose of religion, to re-establish this lost connection with the Ultimate, and thereby make it possible for a connection with God to be established again. This is what religions are supposed to do and this is what religion means. The word 'religion' is derived from the Latin word *ligare*–to connect or bind, and *religare*–to reconnect. Therefore, religions start by taking the child into their fold and, by various rites such as baptism, communion, confirmation and so forth, they are supposed to train the individual until he reaches adulthood, by inculcating in him the idea of God, the idea of the need for God. Religions are thereafter expected to train him ethically and morally and to fit him into the social environment so that he emerges as an adult fully qualified to lead an ethical, moral and social life.

Talk given to a Catholic congregation assembled at the Rensselaer Newman Chapel at Troy, New York, USA, on Sunday 28 May 1972 at 10:30 A.M.

What comes after? This is the question. We believe that it is just where religion ends that this confusion of what to do further to strengthen this relationship with God comes in, and we find so much of the tragic lack of purpose in life, and the confusion of what life should mean or what life means, and what should be done about it. My Master teaches that it is precisely where religion ends that spirituality begins. All through religious training we are taught to worship the deity outside us, and to believe in the idea of His existence and to commune with Him as an entity external to ourselves. In India we believe—or at least in Hinduism we believe—that the Almighty God can manifest Himself primarily in three forms—the first one called the *Para* form where He is the Ultimate, and He is as He is, for Himself, in Himself. The second form we call the *Harda* or the *Antaryamin* meaning one who resides inside us, that is the spark of Divinity which exists in the heart of every created being, and of course in human beings, too. The third form is that with which we are all familiar, the *Archa*. It is the external form of the deity as we worship Him in temples, in churches, in mosques, and so on.

Now we teach, or at least our religion teaches, that by being trained to worship God outside us and reaching perfection in that form of worship, we must then advance to the next stage which we call spirituality, where we start worshipping God inside us, the immanent deity. This is mysticism, which we call yoga in the East. Therefore a transfer of worship of the deity from outside ourselves to inside our own heart, and seeking communion with Him within ourselves is what mysticism or yoga really means. This is what my Master is trying to teach. The only way possible to achieve this communion is meditation.

We find that at the base of all religions is the existence of God, and we also find that at the summit of all religions is the same God. It is in between that religions diverge and teach various ways of approach to the Ultimate; but the beginning and the end being the same, we should try to follow this mystic path and seek the deity within ourselves, and the way, as I have already stated, is meditation. That is, by closing our eyes and sitting comfortably and in a sense, if I may say so, of relaxation, we put our thought on the Ultimate within ourselves and try to commune with Him by constant thought of Him. Meditation literally means to think continuously of one thing, or to hold one thought continuously in the mind. This is meditation. What my Master teaches is precisely this, and we call it raja yoga in India, meaning the king of all yogas.

By practising this yoga we are able to slowly strengthen our association with the deity by constantly meditating on His presence inside our heart in the form of illumination. This is our system of yoga which we call Sahaj Marg or the natural way of realisation. We sit in a detached or a relaxed way, comfortably, and have the thought or try to hold in our mind this thought that the heart is illuminated from within by the presence of the spark of the Ultimate deity that is present within us. This, in brief, is what my Master teaches and I hope it will be possible for you all to practise this and derive such benefit as exists in it.

We believe that this is the only way to reach the Ultimate consciousness or what you may like to call the cosmic consciousness or the supercosmic consciousness. That is, we start with external worship of the deity, transfer Him ultimately within ourselves, and by practising this communion of the spirit with Him, we are able to at last realise what God is in Himself, for Himself, that is as He really exists and not as we would like to see him. Thank you.

The Inner Needs of Man

Man has been defined in various ways. He has been called a social animal, which he undoubtedly is. In a cosmic sense, he is a universe in himself when compared to an atom, and in turn is but an atom when compared to the universe. He is stated to stand midpoint between the atom and the universe. But a simple description could be that man is a complex of physical and emotional needs.

All living beings have needs which must be fulfilled if they are to survive. The basic needs are the very obvious ones such as food, shelter, protection from the environment, a mate, etc. When man existed at the level of the animal, the needs were basic to his existence and were comparatively easily fulfilled, even though his existence was, in what is usually called today, a primitive state. Nevertheless, primitive man would appear to have been a much happier and more contented person than modern man, perhaps for the very simple reason that there was no confusion in his appraisal of his needs, and therefore his approach to their satisfaction could be direct and immediate. Certainly primitive man did not have all the traumas, psychoses, neuroses and the whole gamut of psychological illnesses that appear to accompany human life throughout the span of its existence today.

How has it come about that simple primitive man could be happy in such adverse environmental conditions, while facing extreme conditions of life where every moment of survival was a victory over his environment and his foes, whereas modern man, with all the conveniences and appurtenances of life, a life which has been made so easy to live that very often the minimum of physical activity is all that is needed, and where almost everything that he needs is at hand, or can be easily acquired without much per-

Lecture at the Prince George Memorial County Library, Hyattsville (Md.), USA, on Saturday, 10 June 1972.

sonal effort or danger–how is it that in such an existence we find man unable to live in peace either with himself or with his surroundings? I do not think there is any question about this state of affairs particularly when we study the modern societies of the West. It is all too apparent that the more sophisticated and industrially advanced a society, the more the subconscious and repressed burdens members of that society appear to have to bear. Affluence indeed seems to have been accompanied by mental suffering, which in turn creates what are called psychosomatic illnesses. It is a moot point whether there are many free of the travails of such existence.

The aim of life, since the dawn of this century, appears to have become nothing less than an affluent existence made possible by the gigantic and incomparable advances in science, which in turn made possible revolutionary developments in technology. One of the great economists of the West has indeed termed modern society as the affluent society and paralleling this growth in affluence, we find a development below the surface of more misery than history would appear to indicate as prevalent in any past era. There were many dark periods in human history filled with much suffering arising out of lack of physical needs, strife, bigotry, but all these led or would appear to have led to nothing more than physical suffering. But the suffering today has been shifted in plane to the mental level, and the greatest suffering of the affluent is at this level. By comparison, the less developed societies of the Orient would appear to enjoy better mental health even today, though their physical levels of existence may very often appear shocking to the Western eye. What is the reason for this almost inexplicable state of affairs? I would venture to suggest that perhaps our needs and the way we approach the satisfaction of those needs is at least one factor contributing to the madness of modern existence.

My Master makes a significant differentiation between needs and wants. Needs are legitimate, and man can legitimately expect such needs to be satisfied. Wants, on the other hand, are creations of man from his knowledge of the external world. Needs arise from inside whereas wants arise from outside. If needs were all that are to be fulfilled, people and governments would have a very easy time doing so. But it is precisely the ever-increasing wants of today's society and individuals that are found to be difficult and often well-nigh impossible of satisfaction. Indeed it would be correct to go a step further and say that today's orientation in society is towards enlarging wants and even towards creating more and more wants to keep the wheels of industry spinning. Our society may therefore be termed a society dedicated primarily to the creation of wants which later it sets out to satisfy. Needs are limited, therefore easily satisfied, and once satisfied, man is at rest. Wants, on the other hand, have no limit, and each want satisfied gives rise to the next want based on the prior satisfaction of the earlier one. Therefore, it is a vicious spiral mounting in its demands, and developing in the individual and society a frenzied craving for its satisfaction, but the goal ever recedes from the grasp of the individual. This is one of the main reasons for the psychological condition of today's individual. Society is after all composed of individuals and can reflect nothing but the sum total of individual attitudes and aspirations.

Analyzing our needs, the most apparent one of course is the physical need for food and shelter. It would appear that these are comparatively easily satisfied provided only that degree of importance is given to them that they deserve. Primitive man did not indulge, until quite late in his own existence, in the art of cooking. Cooking is after all only the conversion of what nature provides into a form considered more acceptable to man himself. There is an art of embellishing what nature provides. It is a truism to state that very often cooking naturally available food, whether vegetarian or non-vegetarian, deprives it of much of its intrinsic value, adding perhaps something to its taste and appearance. I am sure there are numerous votaries of raw food who would be prepared to testify to the basic wholesomeness and palatability of raw foods. There are quite large communities of people who are able to subsist on them very happily and, what is more important, very healthily, too. When we proceed from cooking to the next stage of embellishment where it is dressed up merely to please the eye, we have already transferred the area of acceptability of food from the mouth and tongue to the eyes, nose, etc. That is, what should be examined from one level of the physical organization is now being examined from another. This undoubtedly is a perversion and is no doubt a contributory cause for much of the world's ill-health today in those societies where only the most highly dressed-up food is served. This shows us the importance of tackling each need from its own level in us, i.e., the physical must be treated purely from the physical, the mental from the mental, and so on.

Food must be such as will not only be palatable but will refresh and add strength to the body. This is, or should be, the primary consideration. Naturally, the body has to be strengthened by opposing it to external forces of nature, and the simplest way is physical exercise. Therefore, there are two aspects to physical existence, one is the provision of fuel for the inside, and the other is the pitting of the body against the external world to develop its strength, ability and other associated physical characteristics.

At the mental level, applying the same formula, what the mind needs is food for its existence, and solid effort in overcoming mental obstacles for its development. Man must devote adequate time to the study of such literature as will enrich his mind, and the literature should be of such quality and quantity as to make him throw his entire mental equipment into the study of such works. Unfortunately today we find that what most people read is the lowest type of literature such as the yellow journals, cheap romances, gory criminal fiction and so on. That such minds do not develop at all beyond the juvenile level is therefore no surprise. The curricula of most educational institutions do not appear to take this into adequate consideration from the point of view of the needs of the student.

Thirdly, coming to the emotional level of man, here again what emotional sustenance man receives is very often of the wrong type. Love is one of the fundamental aspects of man's existence, and in the fulfilment of this very vital emotional need such irrelevant media as romantic literature, cinemas and casual liaisons are indulged in, discovering too late that none of these can satisfy the pent up emotion where what is needed is a steady and canalized outlet for the emotional power of man which often does not need, or but rarely needs, physical expression. It is a well recognized fact that the physical expression of love must succeed the mental development of love or emotional development of love. But in modern society things are topsy-turvy, with very tragic consequences. The latest manifestation of such an unfulfilled need is the fast spreading drug habit combined with, or preceded by, a loose set of moral values.

Perhaps I may add that, as far as the emotional life of man is concerned, religions were expected, in a very fundamental measure, to make available an object of adoration or love which could elevate human emotional life to sublime levels far above the ordinary human level. The present day mental condition of most people would appear to indicate that religions, too, have not been able to play their part. Here again what man solidly needs is something which he can venerate and adore, but all that is offered in most religions is an idol or other representational form of the deity. And the only way he is taught of approaching such an object of adoration is the ritualistic way which is largely outmoded and which, to the mind of modern man, very often appears as mere child's play.

We all know that while the non-satisfaction of purely physical needs may at worst impair the physical organization in some way or the other, albeit not very seriously, the non-satisfaction of emotional needs is much more serious. In the field of emotion, love is dominant, supported by, and evoking in its turn, such sentiments as faith, hope, charity, courage, etc. If this basic emotional instinct is unfulfilled, such associated mental-physical complexes cannot manifest themselves. It is well known that where there is no love there can rarely be courage, and I would request you here not to confuse courage with sheer bravado or the front-line necessity to kill. Similarly, where there is no love, there can be no faith, charity or chastity and, therefore, existence devoid of love is an empty existence. Love must grow and embrace more and more within its orbit of expression. Love for one's wife must enlarge into a deep love for the family resulting from such love. Familial love must grow to include neighbours, for, after all, if a neighbour is sick, notwithstanding the marvels of modern medicine, we are likely to be the next victims; if the neighbour is poor, his poverty affects us; if he is the victim of gangsterism and hoodlum attacks, we are sure to feel the repercussions. So our neighbour's well-being is a matter of immediate concern to us. Thus, slowly, as love matures, it must widen in scope until ultimately it envelops the entire universe within its sublime embrace. My Master has said that the only way of approaching the Ultimate is through love.

What we all need is a god, or if you prefer to call it so, a Universal Power or anything like that, but what we need is such an entity as we can approach with love and reverence. This would appear to be a spiritual need, higher than the other needs. Even an atheist would agree that there are times in his life when he has, perhaps unconsciously, cried out to God for succour, only proving that the need for God is universal in its prevalence. When we negate such a need, we do so artificially without knowledge of the frightful consequences of such repudiation. The time has, therefore, come to re-establish in our minds the truth that God is necessary to us, whether He is visible or invisible. Whether He can manifest himself or not is not the point. What He is must ever remain a mystery because what is known has no mystery about it, and only the unknown is mysterious. As the old English proverb would have it, "Familiarity breeds contempt," and it is perhaps for this reason that God chooses to remain invisible and inaccessible! But this does not mean that God's existence and love cannot be experienced. As my Master has often remarked, God cannot be seen or known in the conventional sense, but His presence can be experienced if the approach is in the right way.

How to bring God into our lives is the question. The first need of course is to recognize that we need Him. The people of the West would particularly appear to suffer from some sort of complex that God is no longer necessary to them. I have come across such a statement in many discussions with my Western friends, particularly with those who are successful in material life, who ask incredulously, "But why do I need God when I have everything I want?" Such a question would never occur in the East where we believe that the foundation or the base of all existence is God himself, while also being its summit or crown. In the East we believe that God is in everything that we think, we do, we see and so on.

The Inner Needs of Man

That is, to us of the East there is nothing which is not of God and from God, and therefore this question of the need for God cannot arise at all to an Eastern mind. In the West, somehow man has become divorced from God, and according to my Master no health, whether of the body or the mind, can exist where this schism has been created between man and his Maker. This inner need is indeed paramount because even in the West we have innumerable aspirants who have recognized and accepted it and who, after a brief period of practice of our Sahaj Marg yoga, have testified conclusively that their existence has become filled in some mysterious manner.

This paramount inner need, a universal need in the minds of all men everywhere, is what my Master has set out to satisfy and fulfil. If God is not in us He must be put back into us, and Sahaj Marg, which is a form of raja yoga rediscovered by my Master's own Master who also bore his name, and was called Shri Ram Chandraji of Fatehgarh, claims to satisfy this vital need. I have told you that Sahaj Marg is a system of raja yoga. Raja yoga is of course yoga of the mind, the term meaning literally the king of yogas. You all know what yoga means or should mean–union. The union is the ultimate union of man and his Creator, and no lesser union is implied. In raja yoga the way is the way of the mind, and what is done is meditation. All this is very simple because no doubt all of you have come across various yoga systems and are familiar with all the concepts or the broad concepts and terminology of such systems of the East. But Sahaj Marg has something very unique which sets it apart from all other yogas.

What are these features which set Sahaj Marg apart from other systems? Firstly, you all know of the great rishi Patanjali's eightfold or eight-limbed yoga. It is said to incorporate the entire yogic learning in a practical form. Of the eight steps, the first two are devoted to eradicating negative factors from the human system, and to develop within the system the purity of mind and body necessary to go on to the third stage– asana, or postural yoga. Asanas are today very familiar to all, and have found ready acceptance over a wide section of the population. There are numerous schools of Indian yoga which teach nothing but *yogasanas*. There is another term under which this yoga goes, hatha yoga, which embraces within its practice, asana and the fourth stage, viz., *pranayama* or the art of right yogic breathing. According to my Master, these first four steps of yoga are really unnecessary and impracticable. He says that all men, even the evildoers, know right from wrong, but the problem is that this knowledge alone does not help, the will to act right being lacking. We must perhaps accept Master's statement that no man who knew right, and who had the opportunity of doing right, would deliberately do wrong.

I remember, in this connection, once there was some discussion about the efficacy of hatha yoga for realising the ultimate aim of yoga, which is union with the Ultimate. My Master categorically stated that hatha yoga by itself is valueless if that be the aim. When I asked him why it had become necessary for rishis to practise this, he gave me an explanation which I think you will all agree is very logical. The rishis of the ancient times used to sit in meditation continuously for days, weeks and, if legends be true, months and years too, without a break. They had, therefore, neither the opportunity nor, perhaps, the inclination for physical exercise. However, the body had to have a minimum tension imposed on it to keep it fit at least to a minimal extent. Therefore, the rishis devised a system of yoga postures which they could adopt one after the other while sitting in meditation or contemplation, and thus kill two birds, as it were, with one stone.

Sahaj Marg yoga also does not recognize the need for the next two steps in Patanjali's yoga, but it really starts at the seventh stage, *dhyana*, or meditation, leading to the final step or stage of mergence with the Ultimate. My Master's teaching indicates that when the highest activity is performed, i.e., when meditation is established, the body assumes the posture natural and convenient to it. Thus asana is established by itself, not in an artificial or contorted way, but according to the needs of the body of the individual. Similarly, when meditation is established the breathing slows down and assumes its own cycle, and pranayama is thus established. When the mind becomes purified by meditation, the first two steps of *yama* and *niyama* are also established naturally and automatically. A poor mind can think nothing but poor thoughts, and poor thoughts can lead to nothing but poor actions. But when the mind is purified and correctly directed, pure thoughts and pure action result. Therefore, when we commence with meditation and establish it firmly, all the other steps of the yoga of Patanjali become automatically established in us. This is an effortless and natural way of doing things. That is why Master's yoga is called 'Sahaj Marg' which literally means the natural way.

Secondly, there is the system of transmission, *pranahuti* as it is called in Sanskrit. If I may be permitted a short reference to the Upanishads, particularly the Kena Upanishad, a student asks his teacher by what does the eye see? By what does the nose smell? By what does the ear hear? And so on, and the teacher replies that it is not the eye that sees, but the eye of the eye. Similarly what hears is the ear of the ear, and what speaks is not the mouth but something behind the mouth, the real speaker. The rishi goes on to add that life itself lives only by the existence of the higher life which it contains, and this is called the *pranasya prana* or the life of life. My Master has maintained that while the body lives by the soul, the soul must in turn have that by which it exists, and this is the ultimate life force or *pranashakti*. In our transmission under the Sahaj Marg system, it is this that is transmitted into the heart of the student of yoga by the Divine power associated with my Master, and which power it has been possible for him to endow upon the preceptors, as they are called, who are vested with the responsibility of offering such transmission to students who come to them. This transmission is something which must be felt and which can be felt. You will agree that all life is transmission. In every action that we perform, or by which we receive, an act of transmission is involved, but in the transmission of Sahaj Marg it is the highest gift of life's life itself, and it is this that sets the Sahaj Marg system of raja yoga apart from all other extant systems of yoga.

We therefore believe that a hitherto largely unfulfilled need of man is now being satisfied by such transmission. While the other needs, the physical, the mental, the emotional, can be taken care of by man himself without recourse to much assistance or guidance from others, for this paramount spiritual need a Master is a must, because it is the Master who has this power of transmission, and without him it cannot be either given or received. Even the preceptors, to whom I have referred earlier, transmit only by virtue of the power that is opened up in them to do so. Without the Master there can be no preceptors.

I know that to Western minds the concept of a Master is very often repugnant and I have often wondered why it should be so. Do we not seek guidance even in trivial matters where our capacity falls below our need? Do we not seek the guidance and assistance of doctors, of launderers, of barbers, and in fact of innumerable other offerers of service? And we do so without losing our individuality or sacrificing our ego! Why should not such an attitude also include a Master of yoga for spiritual needs? After all, as my Master often says, when a man is in a serious physical condition he literally surrenders to a doctor, gets anaesthetized and loses all consciousness, and what is going on is unknown to him. This surrender to a doctor is purely on the basis of hearsay, on the basis of the doctor's reputation, or his degrees. Why it should not be possible for us to similarly surrender to a Master of yoga is something that passes comprehension. I am glad to note from our travels in the West that the Western mind seems to be changing, and is now willing to seek guidance in a sphere very vital to its existence. This change is something which must be fostered and allowed to develop and become universal.

I have given you some ideas inculcated in me by my Master. My Master sits before you, having travelled to the West solely to offer his services in making available the highest help in attaining oneness or identification with the Creator. I request all of you to participate in his programme and realise the benefit that his presence among you can confer.

Yoga and Sahaj Marg

We are very pleased to be here in the First Spiritual Science Church of Washington and my Master is particularly happy to be with you because the *summum bonum* of his existence is the propagation of spiritual training, spiritual practice supported–only supported–by the necessary degree of spiritual teaching–if I may call it that, because we do not believe that spirituality needs any teaching behind it. Our fundamental belief is that spirituality is a practice unnecessarily supported by theory except where our intellect demands stimulation, satisfaction and justification. In fact, one of my Master's cardinal teachings is that the simpler the mind the more, if I may use the word, rustic the mind–of the villager, ploughman–the more suited it is for spirituality; because in such minds there is that innate closeness to the Divine, to nature, to truth, which sophisticated living often robs us of very tragically. So we do not believe much in talking, but unfortunately some talking is necessary because people would like to hear what we have to say about it. The essence of his teaching is, practise and experience, read and enjoy. Reading can give enjoyment, practising can give experience. After all spirituality is a path of evolution, and evolution is progress which must be felt and experienced. That is one of the aspects of this training.

The other thing is, how to distinguish spirituality as such? Because we find in our travels all over these countries of the West that very often most people do not really know what spirituality means. For instance, we have heard people saying, "Oh, he has such a beautiful spiritual face," or "That lady is feeding so and so– she is such a spiritual lady," and remarks like these, remarks made with kindness, made with all charitable feeling and made with hu-

Lecture delivered at the First Spiritual Science Church of Washington, D.C. at 8 P.M. on Saturday, 10 June 1972.

man sympathy, but applying meanings to spirituality which are not covered by the performance of such people. My Master says spirituality has to deal with the soul and the soul alone. It has nothing to do with the body; it has nothing to do with the intellect; it has nothing to do with the mind and other paraphernalia of human existence. He alone is spiritual who seeks the Ultimate consciousness or the Godly consciousness in himself, and strives to unite his personal individual consciousness with that Ultimate consciousness. This is spirituality. And one who strives in such a way alone can be called a spiritual person. The rest are covered by religion. Ethics, morals, codes of behaviour, laws, these are all covered by religions. And as my Master has often said, religions divide, spirituality unites; because it is a fact that we have each our own religion, and each religion says that its god alone is the ultimate God and, "Thou shalt worship no God but me," and that sort of thing. Therefore, when we come to religions, they have always sought to divide man from man, brother from brother. Whatever be the reason, it is not the fault of religions themselves because religions never taught that. But the teachers of religion, the guardians behind the religions, these have always had this sort of conflict created between man and man. But when we identify the Ultimate as a nameless, formless and attributeless Divine, then we cannot identify my god or your god in a specific way, and differences are removed. So we believe that in spirituality, when we come to the spiritual practice, all men and women become brothers and sisters, and equal in the eyes of God, and not till then.

Another important lesson of my Master is that where religion ends there spirituality begins. I am sorry if I am upsetting some apple carts here, but this is his teaching and it is my business to tell you what he teaches. You have invited us to speak to you and I owe it to you to tell you what he really teaches. His teaching is, where religion ends, there alone spirituality begins. This is because religions play what we may call, for lack of a better term, a kindergarten role in man's evolution. They take up the baby, the human baby, at birth into their fold, baptize it, give it initiation and absorb that child, absorb that human soul, into the corpus of their own society so that it can be brought up with love, with devotion as is necessary to develop it into an adult. And in the course of this training they give it the ethical, the moral instruction that it needs to fit it into society as an acceptable member of that society, so that wittingly or unwittingly it does not transgress the laws of its particular society. However, we very often find peculiar, shall we say, opposition between the codes and laws of one religion and the codes and laws of other religions. One religion says, "Thou shalt not kill." Another says that on the feast day you must eat the meat of a freshly killed goat. Therefore, these laws are, by and large, environmental developments at an epoch in history when certain laws had to be created as needed at that time, in that place. We believe that such religious laws do not hold for all time, because as time changes, as societies change, as environment changes, we have to change with it and our laws have to change with it. For instance, as my Master says, in Islam there is a law which says if you waste water you shall have to pay for it, for the simple fact that Mohammed the prophet was born in Arabia which is a desert country, where water is perhaps more valuable than gold. Now it would be absurd to impose that law in the lake districts of your own country where water is plentiful. What I am trying to pinpoint is that religious laws are localized sets of values created for that society, for a specific epoch, for a specific place. They are not in any sense eternal. So religion develops in us these localized sets of behaviour patterns by imbuing us with those codes of conduct and those codes of behaviour, fitting us into society.

What happens when we come into adult state? And shall we say now we have to face God on our own? It is all right as a child to be led by the hand, to be taught. But there comes a time in our life when, as adults, we have to face the situation. We have to evolve, and we have to face the situation with our families, with our wives and with our children. My Master believes it is at that stage that spirituality takes over from where religion has left off.

In religion we are taught to worship a God outside us or external to us, what we call the theory of emanations. God is outside in his heaven, somewhere far off, unattainable, unachievable; the journey is very far; the travails are many; the renunciations called for are tremendous. This is the sort of worship that we are taught. From that external worship of Divinity which we put into forms of the Divine, we have now to transfer it to the concept that God is within us, too. If God is omnipotent and omnipresent there is no reason why God should not be in us, as He is in everything else. So religion leaves and says good-bye, and mysticism must now take over.

In mysticism we have the approach to the eternal presence of the Ultimate in our own heart as the spark which we call consciousness. This is the spark or the voice of God present in us. In most cases, unfortunately, that spark seems not to exist, for the simple reason that it has been covered over by ignorance, covered over with conduct which is not conducive to its development. Therefore, all that is necessary is to uncover it. Remove the covering of ignorance, of all conduct, and there the light begins to glow again. So spirituality means first the concept that God is in us, to be approached by the inward practice, so that our communion with the Ultimate should be an inner communion with Him by us, rather than an external communion or form of worship of a Divinity that exists outside us. Spirituality does not say that God does not exist outside us. But what spirituality says is, when He is inside you why take all the trouble and all the expense to go to all those places of worship when He is right inside you.

There have been times in history when churches have been razed to the ground, when mosques have been razed to the ground, and when temples have been demolished. Then where will we worship? We are not dependent on all those temples and churches for our worship. If that were the case, religion's case is indeed a very sad story. So there must be the Ultimate available to us as a ready reckoner, as a permanent reference, and He is inside us– this is what spirituality teaches us.

Now this science of spirituality which we call mysticism in the West, we call yoga in the East or, to be very precise, yoga in India. Yoga means the union of the individual consciousness, the individual human consciousness, with the Ultimate, cosmic, Divine consciousness. Really yoga does not mean anything else. Of course many yogas are taught these days, the yogas of the body, the hatha yoga, yoga of mantras or mantra yoga, laya yoga, kundalini yoga, and in fact a whole spectrum of yogas all trading under the name of yoga but not conforming to the original definition of yoga as propounded by the Vedic seers who coined that word. I am not criticizing this. It is the original Vedic seers who are criticizing this misuse of the word yoga, because we have to re-establish truth.

One of our Divine incarnations, avatars as we call them, Krishna, has very specifically stated that whenever there is disruption of *dharma*, of right conduct, of right living, and when society needs to be corrected, and right has to be re-established, "I come again and again." In Hindu religion we do not believe in a personality coming once and for all. I am not talking now of spirituality. We believe that as time demands, as the needs of the time develop, the Ultimate presence can descend on this planet of ours again and again at His choice. It is His choice to decide where He will descend, how He will descend, in what form He will descend. If the Ultimate is illimitable and unconditionable by us, surely He has the free will to decide where He will descend, in what form He will descend and at what time He will descend. And He does this precisely to re-establish truths which have become corrupted by the very establishments initially created for the propagation of those very truths.

All great men have taught great sciences of living, sciences of the soul; but when they disappeared and two or three generations of disciples handed on their tradition, corruption was inevitable, distortion was inevitable, in practice, in theory, in the very foundations of these practices. And it is not the fault of the disciples either, because when you talk you know how even a motor car accident can be misrepresented and misreported from one to the other, to the third person. It is human nature, and we are all human beings. We generally tend to magnify, we tend to personalize what we have seen or what we have heard, and transmit that personalized concept of what we have seen or heard or listened to, and therefore it happens not wantonly, not intentionally, but nevertheless inevitably. So teachers have to come again and again to re-establish in us the truth which was lost but which existed and prevailed once upon a time.

In our own system of Sahaj Marg we have this unique feature of the transmission by the guru or Master, of his personal yogic or spiritual energy–it is not psychic energy, it is spiritual energy–into the heart of the aspirant. We call this yoga Sahaj Marg, which means the natural way to Realisation, because my Master teaches that God is simple and, therefore, the way to reach him must be simple. As he puts it very tellingly in one of his books, if a pin falls on the ground you do not need a crane to lift it up, you stoop down and pick it up. And when people ask how to achieve this God, he says, turn your face away from yourself and there is God waiting for you. It is not as simple as that! But it implies a change in one's mental standpoint or outlook. Divert your attention from the external world and there you are in the internal. There are only two sides, the external and the internal. And when we divert our attention back inward where it belongs, that which resides inside must manifest itself, as everything outside us manifests itself to our vision when we turn our attention outwards. There is no logic which says that a similar thing should not happen when we turn our attention inside.

Just because people have taught us God is difficult to achieve, God is power-mad, He is crazy, He is waiting to punish people, so we are afraid of Him. Our approach to God is one of fear. All religions say that God is love. But in no religion is there a man who can approach his God with love. I know because there have been instances when people have had to spend a night in a church or inside a temple and they are aghast at the very idea of having to sleep inside a temple. They worship and offer prayer and sometimes make fantastic offerings of their wealth, but one night in a temple, I cannot yet find a person who will sleep there for one night. If your God is there who is almighty, all powerful, all love, who is our protector, what is this fear that makes us stay away from this place? We are, therefore, afraid of God, in all religions without exception. I often tease my friends and say, "Well, suppose the particular God to whom you are praying, whether it be Christ or

Krishna, or anybody else, suppose He were suddenly to manifest Himself in front of you and say, 'What do you want?' you will run scampering. There will be a massacre perhaps. But God is love!"

Spirituality tries to put the approach back in its right perspective that we must love God because He is inside us. He is not something external to us waiting with a rod in his hand to punish us for our transgressions. He is inside us and being inside us if He punishes us, He has to endure that punishment Himself whether He likes it or not. Because that which is inside must suffer as much as that which is outside does. When my skin suffers, my body suffers; when my tooth suffers I suffer with it, and I do not see how God can escape that suffering. So when we turn our mind inwards and approach Him with this love, then there is no question of suffering and there is no question of punishment. The Godly spirit, that spark of Divinity enshrined in our hearts, then begins to be fanned by the breeze of our love, and as it grows, the voice of conscience begins to develop again. We call this the flowering of the consciousness.

Conscience in our terminology, according to my Master, is nothing but the growth of a superior consciousness in ourselves. And when this real conscience develops, we find that true morality develops, true ethics develop, not because some church says so, or the police say so, or the government says so, but because my inside tells me, "This you shall do and this you shall not do." So, love breeds communion with the Ultimate, that communion makes Him grow in us. This breeds ethical and moral living, and we find that as we progress, increasingly higher states of consciousness become ours. It is difficult to say what these states of consciousness are because it is like a bank of clouds, the lowest one hiding the rest, and if you fly up in a plane and go above, then you find it is light above though it is dark below. But one has to fly to see this phenomenon. Even when it is darkest and it is raining, you go up above that and there is light, brilliant sunlight. So we have to pierce through this cloud, this cloud of ignorance, the first cloud which limits us as human beings, and prevents us from flying into the Divine realms which inherently are our birthright whatever be our race, colour or anything else.

God did not create Himself for any one race or any one country or any one set of people. He created everything and if He created everything, everything is His whether we like it or not. And in ourselves it is spirituality. We are only seeking to cease being our own and to become His. This is what surrender implies. Surrender says, "My Lord, I am no longer my own as I thought I was, I am now yours, do unto me as you will." This becomes possible when there is love, not when there is fear. When there is fear we cannot surrender. We may talk of surrendering. We can surrender only our arms, as one set of forces does to the victorious. So surrender in those terms means victory and defeat. Here, surrender of the soul to its Creator is only returning to Him what belongs to Him. There is no question of victory or defeat. On the contrary I would consider it our victory over Him, because we are able to persuade Him to take us back when all our life we have been trying to run away from Him, to negate His very existence. So in that sense every soul that can go back to its maker has won a victory over its own maker by persuading Him to take it back in spite of all transgressions, of misdeeds, in spite of saying that God does not exist. This is the general picture that emerges from my Master's teaching.

Now what about his particular teaching of yoga? It is based on the old system of raja yoga with which I have no doubt you are all familiar. Raja yoga has unfortunately been translated by many persons, eminent ones too, to mean the way of kings. It does not mean anything like that. It means king among yogas. That is, it is the kingly path, that which is at the highest level of practice. It is at the very summit of yogic practice. It is king among practices–that is raja yoga. Raja yoga deals with the mind. It has nothing to do with the rest of the human system, physical, anatomical, intellectual or otherwise. We believe, raja yoga believes, that it is in the mind that everything originates in the human body, whether it be behaviour or non-behaviour or anything like that. Intellect, body, emotion–everything is guided by the mind. My Master says that mind is what destroys us but mind alone is what can regenerate us into the spiritual welfare and spiritual well-being of communion with the Ultimate. So the mind must not be destroyed. It is the only means of communication with the Ultimate and also with the lower self so that the diversion of the mind again is what is necessary. Turn it from **here** to **there**. As the Hindu scriptures say, we are like the lotus with its bud pointing downwards and which, as it develops, turns up and opens up to receive the nectar of Divine Grace. This is very common symbolism with which I am sure you are all familiar. The turn from the downward pointing to the upward pointing is yoga, the ability to receive grace as it comes into us.

So, yoga is a diversion of tendencies of the mind, from the externalization of its action, its field of activity, to an internalization of at least a part of it to begin with. Now we are only externalized, or most of us are only externalized. In the beginning we seek to divert a little of it inside and by contact with what is inside us, the bliss that is inside us, we wean the mind away from the outside. Not by strict and rigid adherence to commandments which impose a tremendous strain on us, or renunciation which is almost impossible. True renunciation is impossible. We may give up our wealth, but when you have it in the thought it is almost as bad as having the wealth. And it has the complication that we have the feeling of having renounced, and then ego develops–"I have renounced." So egoism develops. Therefore, renunciation has no benefit when it is an imposed renunciation. But when the tendencies of the mind are slowly turned inwards, and the mind is itself attracted by what it finds inside, the outside world loses any charm that it has had up to now. And by the very loss of that, there is renunciation. That is, instead of our giving up the world, the world gives us up! Because now the mind is no longer externalized, it does not go out.

This then is what my Master teaches: first turn the mind inwards. Now what is the way to do this? Sit in meditation, because it is only in meditation that we turn the mind upon ourselves. When I say ourselves, I do not mean this self (the body) but the inner self. We do this in our system of Sahaj Marg which my Master has evolved as a very simplified technique of meditation. We do not meditate on the psychic points of the body, we meditate on the heart. He prescribes meditation on the heart. He says the heart is the seat of life. According to all religions it is in the heart that the

Divine resides. And physiologically, it is from the heart that circulation flows and everything else happens. If this point, the most important point in the human system, can be enriched and purified, then it must permeate to the rest of the whole system without our having to bother with the other parts, like the head, the muscles, the feet and so on. It is a radiant flow from the centre outward, from the centre to the whole system, whereas in traditional practices the external change is drastic, overnight. Shave the head, put on yellow robes and have some beads in the hand and we are yogis! But what about the internal change which is the real transformation of man? This is not transformation but only change of attire. I can appear in a white suit at one moment, and in a black suit the next, or in yellow robes within a few minutes. This is not transformation. It is acting. Like the actors on the stage who walk behind and change their dress suitable to the part they have to play. But many of these yogis, and I have spoken to many of them, will tell you that even after twenty years of violent faith, violent religious practices, violent renunciation, subdued lives, some of them do not even feel that they are ready for meditation. And this is tragic. It is no joke when you hear people talk like that. I have spoken to people who have worked in an infirmary for three years, then in a kitchen for three years cutting up vegetables and washing pots and pans, and then they go into the laundry for three years. They pass through this rigmarole of so-called preparation of the soul for meditation and before they know where they are, there is possibly no possibility left for meditation at all. So we asked Master what is needed, or what is the preparation needed for meditation? He said, "Sit and meditate, that is the only preparation." Meditation is a simple thing. It is something to do with the mind and does not need any violent exercise or preparation.

Unfortunately, there are systems which teach that it is necessary to prepare the mind, when meditation alone can prepare the mind. It is meditation which prepares the mind, but we believe that by external association with activities such as required charities, sympathy and love and devotion, we prepare the mind. But it is very often a funny thing that in them there comes a hatred for the very thing which they do. If you are made to nurse a person whom you cannot nurse, and you are put into a nursing capacity, I doubt if even one out of a thousand will come out of it as purified and clean in the soul as people pretend that they do. Whereas, when we purify the mind and shear it of all the superfluities of good and bad, the opposites as we call them in Hinduism, the *dvandvas* of existence—good and bad, virtue and vice, knowledge and ignorance—when the mind is shorn of these attributes of our day-to-day existence, then it knows neither opposite. It does not know what is good nor does it know what is bad. It instantly does the work which is necessary and gets back into itself.

By this training of yoga, we are therefore made capable of working without either attraction or repulsion. We are made capable of existing without love or desire, hatred or antagonism. Because we are in communion with what is inside ourselves, the Ultimate, that association alone becomes valuable to us, and the rest of the world ceases to have any meaning for us. Therefore, all tendencies, all attributes, all desires and hates, all these are struck off. And, as my Master says, this is real renunciation. Not the giving up of wealth or the writing of a cheque to some mission and ending it all. That is not renunciation. So when we develop by spiritual growth, we renounce without really knowing that we are renouncing. By enriching ourselves and coming closer and closer to the Ultimate within ourselves, we become more and more dependent on that inner self. We seek His guidance, we seek His advice, we obey His voice when He speaks to us; and as this dependence on Him increases and it becomes Ultimate, it becomes surrender. It is surrender without surrendering; it is renunciation without renouncing; it is truth without seeking it. So all this becomes possible through the simple act of meditation.

As I told you, we meditate on the heart imagining that inside the heart, by the presence of the Divine, the Ultimate, the heart is illuminated. We try to hold this thought for about thirty minutes initially when we sit in meditation. We close our eyes and sit comfortably so that the body does not interfere with the mind. That is all that is required. According to Patanjali himself, asana is something which is steady and comfortable. "S*thiram sukham asanam*," this is what Patanjali has written. So we sit comfortably as we normally sit, and allow the body to rest in itself so that the mind can act in its own way. Hold, or try to hold, this thought that there is illumination in the heart. If other thoughts come into the mind–as they surely will, because they are welling up from inside ourselves, they are not something which is imposed from outside, they are our own thoughts seeking to come out now that the mind is pegged onto something else–we allow them to go by not attending to them, by ignoring them. It is one of my Master's important techniques that if you do not attend to thoughts they have no power. It is our attention which gives to thoughts the power they hold over us. So we, in meditation, do not attend to these thoughts, we allow them to drop off by themselves. This is the technique of meditation that we are required to practice.

Now I come to the very important role of the Master in our meditation. There have been many masters and there will be many more masters. But most masters teach us theoretically. They show us what to do, but beyond that their assistance does not extend. In India we recognize three types of masters. One is like the hen which lays an egg and must sit on it to hatch it out. That is, physical contact between the Master and the disciple is necessary, without which they cannot interact on each other. The second type of master is like the fish which lays its eggs in the stream and goes round and round them, keeping away marauders. That is, there is visual contact. So without at least visual contact such masters cannot interact with their disciples. The third and highest is supposed to be like the tortoise which goes onto the bank, lays its eggs in a shallow pool, covers it up with sand, goes back into the river and mentally looks after it–by transmission or whatever you may call it. So we recognize basically three types of masters: the hen, the fish and the tortoise types. To which class a particular guru conforms is something that you can decide for yourself.

We believe that my Master has this capacity of transmission because we have all felt it ourselves. What he transmits is his own spiritual energy which he has got access to by virtue of his own yogic accomplishment under his own Master. It has opened up in him the possibility of transmission which was rediscovered by his Master after many many centuries of lost wisdom. It has been rediscovered that one human being can transmit to another this energy which is not limited in any way just because it comes from a human, but is really unlimited, because by virtue of its real nature it is connected with the Ultimate source of all energy. Therefore, this transmission has no boundaries, it has no limits, there is no end to the amount of transmission that can take place or, if you like, the quantum of transmission that can take place. It is, therefore, possible to transmit to one, or to a hundred, or to millions, there is no limit. Also he can transmit here or he can transmit to a person wherever he is.

By this transmission, the Master is able to put into our hearts his own energy. That is, now we have the possibility of growing by someone else's energy which is put into us. We are helped with a crutch. Instead of being dependent on ourselves, we have now become dependent on him. Because he gives that food for the soul which we need to quickly develop, quickly develop beyond what we believe to be the possibility for human beings hitherto, precisely because he is able to put his wealth into us. It is as if we get a million dollars, we become rich overnight. We do not have to work for it. If somebody gives me a million dollars, I am a millionaire. He makes us spiritual millionaires, as it were, by putting into us his own wealth of spiritual attainment. This is something which I hope you will all agree to experience because normally we talk a little and then we meditate for half an hour, during which my Master will be transmitting.

This transmission gives us the possibility of growing without limitations. Secondly, it erases by his power all past impressions which we have built up in our minds–impressions of good, impressions of bad, it does not matter which. Because impressions condition our behaviour, impressions condition our existence. In that sense the past is a burden on us. Every day we are adding more impressions, and therefore we are increasing the burdens on ourselves. Every day that lapses is one more day in the past. Thus we are adding to our burdens instead of decreasing them. My Master is able to decrease this, and often eradicate it completely, by his own power whereby he removes all impressions of the past from the mind. It is a liberation from the past assisted by his own transmission which infuses us with his spiritual energy for our own growth, and therefore the possibility of our development has no limits. My Master says that if there is an earnest practitioner it should not take more than seven months to reach the Ultimate goal of human life, and in any case it should not take more than three years. But I suppose it is a sad commentary on even his own disciples that there are many who have not done it after years and years of practice.

What he needs most is not our wealth or our physical energy or anything like that but a simple measure of co-operation, that we sit in meditation for the prescribed period and **allow** him to work on us with his transmission. And it is here the trouble comes, precisely because it appears so ridiculously easy for such an important and almost unachievable aim hitherto, that our mind cannot reconcile the easiness of the system with the difficulty of the attainment. We ask how is this possible? How can it be so, when all these centuries we have been told that it is so difficult? We can say nothing but sit down and try. And having said that I now request my Master to give you all his transmission because this is all that we can do, to sit down and try.

We do not ask for faith because my Master says faith is impossible in the beginning. Anybody who says, "Have faith in me and I will lead you to your goal," is saying something which is impossible, because faith can come only out of experience. But we do ask for a measure of trust in the beginning. Trust those who are associated with you, who talk to you about Him, and then your own experience will ripen that trust into faith and ripen faith into surrender. This is the way of surrender–trust, faith, surrender. If anybody says that he has faith in someone in the very beginning, he either does not know the meaning of faith or he is blatantly lying. Nor is the person who asks for faith in the beginning doing the right thing by the person from whom he is demanding it, because it cannot be done. This we believe. So we ask you to start with a little trust and if it ripens into faith and surrender, surely you will benefit by it. We will now sit in meditation for about thirty minutes and after that if there are any questions, we will be very pleased to answer them. Thank you.

Purification and Regulation of the Mind by Sahaj Marg Yoga

I don't know whether people in the West recognize that all the modern problems that the world faces, particularly in the developed nations–problems of pollution, problems of corruption, problems of health–originate in the mind, and through the mind in science, in technology. I raise this question because when we talk of yoga, people are generally inclined to say, "What is the value of yoga?" They wish to know what is the applicability of yoga to modern life. There is also a general tendency to belittle yoga as something which is not applicable to societies except primitive ones. The teachings of my Master are specially formulated to prove to the world that yoga is a **must** not only for primitive societies but even for the highest developed ones. The basis for this is the fact that everything originates in the human mind and, therefore, unless the mind is purified and regulated in its functioning, and has a definite orientation in which it should function, it may yet function efficiently, but not necessarily for the good of mankind.

We are all familiar with the use of power. You see power by itself is neither corrupt nor good. But the way in which power is used, whether it be physical power or mental power, is what determines the utility of that power to mankind. And when we recognize that everything begins with the mind, whether it is scientific discovery or philosophic speculation, whatever it may be, then we will understand that if we are to cure the ailments that are facing modern societies, it is with the mind we have to start working and not at the periphery of existence.

Now, right at this stage, I would like to clarify that yoga is very much misunderstood, particularly in the West. What people generally mean by yoga here in the West is hatha yoga which is

Public lecture at the Hotel Eisenreich, Munich, 14 May 1976.

good for the body, of course. I am specially mentioning this because at any level we function, the force that is used or the power that is applied can work only at that level. When we work at the physical level the effect can only be at the physical level. So, in our Sahaj Marg system of yoga, which is based on raja yoga, the culminating point of yogic systems, the emphasis is on the mind and the training of the mind by appropriate techniques. My Master says that when we start with the subtlest level of human functioning, then the effect of that purification or regulation automatically percolates into the rest of the system, into the grosser levels of the system. It is not only automatic, it is natural. But on the contrary if we start at the grosser level it need not affect the finer levels of functioning. In our system of Sahaj Marg we therefore start with the mind.

In this system there are two aspects of mental training. The most important one concerns the Master's own work. By continued thinking, by continued activity, we impress upon the mind certain impressions that we create and that are created in us. As habits are strengthened by repetition of the same act, similarly the mind also gets a tendency in a definite direction by the formation of such impressions. What my Master says is that the first step in yoga is to purify the mind and remove those impressions of the past. The essential step, the first step, is of course to accept his work and permit him to work on us. Having accepted his service, the second step in yoga is what we have to do ourselves. Master generally covers this in the single word 'co-operation'. Now co-operation is very easily understood but it is practised with considerable difficulty. To really co-operate we have to accept that his work will be successful; and secondly, we must follow the instructions and practices that he prescribes for us. We can call this second step the moulding of the person by his own effort to some extent. In that moulding, there are of course the practical aspects of yoga itself which we have to follow meticulously. Then there are the usual ethical and moral precepts that are laid down, and assuming that we are able to do all this, we are then in a position to begin the practice of yoga. So the system of Sahaj Marg, which is the name of the yoga system that we practise, accepts any individual human being, whatever may be his present condition or state of mind, because the past, the burden of the past, the Master removes, and the future we create by co-operation with him. The process of removal of the impressions is called 'cleaning'.

You will all appreciate that there is no use in removing the impressions of the past if we are going to continue creating further impressions by thoughts and actions. So our participation in this yogic teaching is to mould our lives in such a way that we do not create more impressions, and thus we avoid creating a further past for the future, because everything becomes the past. Today is the past for tomorrow. The next step is to take the forward step of practising the meditation, which makes the mind capable of becoming a real instrument of human endeavour. So our system is very simple. That is why it is called Sahaj Marg, which means the 'natural way' or the 'simple way'.

We are taught that we should sit in meditation for about an hour in the morning. Nowadays, Master specifies half an hour, but originally it used to be one hour. And about this meditation, we are often asked a question, "We are not able to concentrate. What should we do?" My Master has clarified that meditation is the process and the result is concentration. Now this concentration, by itself, is not of much value in our development because concentration is only the use of a power, and power, by itself, does not lead to evolution. But it has a positive advantage in our daily life because by meditation, when we are able to make the mind concentrate, we are able to exclude thoughts we don't require, or we don't wish to receive. Here I come to one of the most important teachings of my Master. When we have thoughts it is our attention, it is the power of our attention, that gives the power to the thought. A thought by itself has no power. It is the attention that we give it that gives the thought its power. By meditation if we are able to exclude such thoughts without fighting with them, without attending to them, then the mind achieves a state–a state of existence, a state of being–where a single thought alone can exist at a time. Thus, the process of meditation gives us the ability to concentrate, or makes the mind come into a state of concentration, which we in India call one-pointedness.

Meditation must always have a purpose because nothing is purposeless. Even without bringing yoga into the picture, we are almost always meditating on something or the other. When we are looking for a higher standard of living, or when we are keenly pursuing a better job, we are constantly thinking of it. I say this because the correct definition of meditation is to think constantly of something. When we bring yoga into the picture we get confused as to what meditation really means. The only sense in which yogic meditation differs from our normal meditation is in the aim of that meditation, the purpose of that meditation. Therefore, we have to meditate with a purpose in mind, and when we come into the field of yoga that purpose is evolution, or the fulfilment of human life to its highest perfect condition.

My Master often says that we are born as human beings but most of us die as animals. I was myself shocked the first time I heard him say this. So I would not be surprised if you are shocked now. But when we understand the psychology behind the Sahaj Marg system, we will ourselves appreciate that we have no choice in the matter, because our past existence, the impressions of the past existence, are definite and positive forces giving us a direction in this life. And unless we can find some power outside ourselves to eradicate those impressions of the past, we continue to be pushed in the same direction that we have laid down in the past. I say this because very often we are asked, "What is the need for a Master?" It is clear that without the help of an external force–you may call him a Master, or a Guru or anything you like–the removal of the burdens of the past is impossible by our own effort. Therefore, however well-intentioned we may be, our actions from now to the future are but a further superstructure on the foundation of the past. It is for this very important reason that all yogic systems, all mystic systems, have specified the need for a Master to help us. That is a brief outline of the system of yogic practice that we adopt, and on the need for a Master.

Now coming to the practice itself, we are advised to sit in mediation three times a day–morning, evening and bed-time. What we do is to sit comfortably without any botheration about *asanas* or things like that. I mention this point particularly, because people think that without adopting an asana, meditation cannot be done. Patanjali, the codifier of yogic systems, has himself said that any position which can be held comfortably for a length of time is an asana. Therefore it is not very important how we sit, or in what position we sit, so long as we can sit in that position for the length of time specified for our meditation. The only necessity is that the body should not disturb us during that period. So, having assumed a comfortable position, we close our eyes. Sometimes people ask us, "Can we not meditate with eyes open?" It is certainly possible when we reach higher levels of spirituality, but not at the earlier stages. It is the eye which receives most of the impressions from the external world. Obviously it is better not to receive further impressions, because we are trying to remove the old impressions. Therefore, we meditate with eyes closed.

In this particular system the meditation process is very specific because we have a specific aim, which is somewhat higher than what is normally specified in the West for yogic systems. As I said earlier, our purpose is to achieve the highest human possibilities. Now we meditate on the heart. What we meditate on is the heart. There are systems which meditate on other points, like the point between the eyebrows, the point of the nose, etc., but we meditate specifically on the heart for three very valid reasons, very important reasons.

The first point is that it is the heart which is the seat of life. The second point is that when we meditate on the heart the effect of that meditation spreads throughout the system. The third point is the most important, but often the least acceptable, and that is that the heart is the particular seat of whatever Divinity we possess.

Therefore, for these three important points or reasons, my Master specifies meditation on the heart. In the Sahaj Marg practice we meditate on the heart, imagining that there is effulgence or light in the heart. We don't try to see light or to project any light.

We begin with the idea that there is light in the heart, and if there are disturbing thoughts, as I told you earlier, we just ignore them, because it is our own attention which gives power to them to disturb us.

That now brings me to the most important and fundamental point in Sahaj Marg. In a sense we can think of Sahaj Marg as operating in three layers. The lowest is the cleaning of the past impressions by the Master's own power. The middle level is our own effort in meditation and avoiding such thoughts or such activities that can create further impressions. And at the apex we have the most important feature, and that is the system of transmission that is unique to this system.

When the vessel is cleaned, we must put something into it. When the human system is similarly purified and cleaned of all the past, it is emptied. Then starts the final process of yoga, which is final not in the sense of time, but final in the sense of culmination. Master starts filling us with his own self. This process is called *pranahuti* in Sanskrit, which means 'life offering' or 'offering of life'. So this is the most important aspect of Sahaj Marg. Once we start this yoga, the purification is done by the Master. Our co-operation is minimal in trying to live a better life, think better thoughts, perform better actions, avoiding the negatives. Then comes the most important part of Master's work. He puts His spiritual essence into us, thereby transforming us into Himself.

I think that I have said more or less everything I have to say about Sahaj Marg. If any of you would like to experience this transmission, my Master generally has a short session of transmission after the talk is over. So if you would like to sit for a few minutes in meditation, following the practice that I have just explained to you– I must emphasize there is no compulsion behind this–those who would like to remain and experience the transmission are welcome to do so. Thank you.

Need For Need

Sahaj Marg is a system of spiritual practice based on the ancient system of raja yoga, adequately modified to suit the conditions of today's existence. In its essence, it is an ancient system of spiritual discipline and practice. In the days of our distant forefathers yogic systems included many arduous and time-consuming practices, necessitating sacrifices often beyond human capacity to make. They were designed for the people of those days, but even then such practices were capable of being adopted only by a few members of the human family. Their rigid disciplines and austere demands excluded the large majority of humanity. In most extant systems too, this continues to be the case.

Shri Ram Chandra of Fatehgarh, our Grand Master as we call him, and my Master's Guru, recognized the need for a simple but effective system of spiritual practice which could be universally practised by any human being. Such a simple universal system should exclude no aspiring individual on any consideration whatsoever, whether it be of race, colour, religion, occupation or sex. Nor should the system make such enormous demands upon the individual as to make him shy away from the spiritual life, thus excluding him from its promise. The Grand Master's researches led him to rediscover a long-lost system of raja yoga which he remodeled and simplified, maintaining the spiritual essentials while discarding the practices and disciplines which few can adopt. This system he offered to the world. His successor and spiritual representative, my Master Shri Ram Chandra of Shahjahanpur, has further refined and developed this system of yoga to its present form in which it is practised by many all over the world today.

Yoga and yogic practice have been generally reserved for the celibate sannyasi, the 'monk' of the Hindu religion. Thus the large mass of humanity, in fact the whole of humanity with but few exceptions, has been denied what my Master emphasizes to be the natural birthright of every individual–the right to develop to the ultimate level of human perfection. My Master bases his spiritual teaching on the fundamental principle that every human being naturally aspires for self-improvement to the highest level possible. This is a universal aspiration. Any system of personal evolution must therefore be universally applicable, and not designed merely for the chosen elite, whatever may be the criteria involved in the selection of such an elite group. And where such factors, which have hitherto excluded a majority of mankind, seek to impose unnatural restrictions and prohibitions on human life, tremendous reactionary tensions are generated which can cause havoc in the individual's system.

The Sahaj Marg spiritual system is a universally applicable one, excluding no one who wishes to practise it. It is the system par-excellence for the normal householder with everyday duties and responsibilities to be performed and undertaken, but who cannot afford to devote long hours (and years too, if ancient traditions of *tapasya* or *askesis* are considered) but yet wishes to develop to the limits of perfection attainable in human existence.

The average human being of today gives a great deal of thought, and applies a great amount of energy, to attain high levels of material welfare. In this endeavour the people of the industrially advanced nations have been significantly successful. But notwithstanding this, there is yet much unhappiness, discontent and misery pervading their lives. Why is this? My Master says that it is the result of unbalanced application of effort. My Master teaches that human existence consists of two planes of existence, the material and spiritual, and that both these are important and essential for the harmonious well-being of the individual. Where one's efforts of thought and action involve only one of these spheres of existence, discontent, unhappiness, etc., are inevitable consequences of such unbalanced living. My Master says that as a bird needs two wings to fly with, so a human being needs the two wings of existence, the spiritual and the material, to lead a natural and harmonious life. If either is neglected for the other, such a life becomes unnatural, and the result cannot be what we desire it to be. Totally denying the material existence to pursue a spiritual path is therefore as unnatural, stultifying and goal-defying as total denial of the spiritual for the material life. Master teaches that to achieve one's full potential, the individual must apply himself equally and impartially to the material life and to the spiritual life. One's efforts must be applied simultaneously in both the spheres. Most spiritual systems have sought to bring about spiritual growth by negating the material existence and denying its necessity. Sahaj Marg corrects this distortion, by emphasizing the need for a proper and natural application of one's energies to both spheres of life. In this lies its universality!

The name of the system, Sahaj Marg, translated into English means the 'Natural Way'. This system offers, perhaps for the first time, a spiritual system of simple practice which makes possible the fulfilment of one's spiritual purpose in life while simultaneously making it possible to attain similar fulfilment in one's material life. All the faculties of a person are developed to perfection, and the perfect functioning of all one's faculties is what my Master calls saintliness.

The first step in spiritual practice is to recognize the fact that most human beings are human merely in the form that they possess. My Master has stated that, "Man is born man, but dies an animal." It is an intriguing statement, but with a wealth and depth of meaning lying hidden in its simplicity. What does it mean? It means that when we take human birth we are born with the promise of, and the potential for, growth and development to the state of human perfection where all our faculties perform perfectly. As we grow, we lose sight of this goal. Material life hems us in on all sides. Material ambitions become our sole ambitions. Material affluence and prosperity attract us more and more until they become obsessively compulsive. Sensory pleasures become the only pleasures that we seek, but such pleasures, by their very nature, egg us on to greater and greater effort in seeking yet more pleasures in an endeavour to find that satisfaction which they cannot give. Out of desire, only greater desire is born. Thus we fall into the whirlpool of an unfulfilled existence, sinking deeper and deeper into misery and wretchedness, knowing not where we missed the way to our goal.

We find that our life has lost any meaning that it might have had. Our successes are but empty shells. Our wealth is but a sham and a mockery, incapable of procuring for us the things we most ardently desire–peace, happiness and contentment. Pleasure it can buy for us, but not happiness! Satiation, but not contentment! Flatterers and sycophants, but not friends! We can buy luxury with it, but not ease! And so it goes, on and on, the catalogue of human misery brought about by unbalanced aspirations and the consequent unbalanced use of one's powers.

The first and most significant step one has to take is to understand that the life of the spirit cannot be ignored except at the peril of wasting one's life utterly. Incomplete human growth is unnatural. We have to develop and grow simultaneously in the twin realms of matter and spirit. When this understanding comes, the possibility of true and harmonious growth opens up for us. We begin to recognize that a partial existence, a life solely of matter divorced from the life of the spirit, is no more than the life of the beasts of the fields from which we have evolved. By living such a partial life we are negating the possibility of further growth and evolution opened up for us by the changed form of existence, the human form, which nature has endowed us with. We begin to understand that in effect we are yet but animals in human form, swayed by greed, lust and passion to such an extent that if thwarted in achieving our desires, few of us would hesitate to destroy anything that comes in our way. If such tendencies are allowed to prevail and to grow, then surely that which was born a human being does die an animal.

To humanize the animal-human being is then the first step in spiritual practice. As my Master states it, animal-man has to become human-man or man-man first, before he can think of further development to the perfect man. To do this the individual's tendencies have got to be corrected and oriented in the proper direction. The impressions of the past, engraved upon mind and memory, have to be erased. Such impressions are the source of present thoughts and actions. Therefore, so long as they persist, action along certain lines is compulsive. The cleaning of the system is thus of paramount importance. A bottle which contained oil can be cleaned comparatively easily to become a milk container. But how does one clean a scratched gramophone record? However much we may wipe it or clean it with detergents, it still continues to play the same jarring tune. Of such scratches and deep cuts is our life composed. Scratches of disappointment! Deeper grooves of degradation and corruption! Is it then any matter for wonder that the needles of our individual destinies run but in those same worn grooves, repeating everlastingly the same disappointments, the same failures and misery, and the same degradation and corruption? The cleaning here has to go deeper. It involves a remoulding of the system to re-create a new record capable of playing the sublime music that the Maker had originally impressed upon its unblemished surface.

Sahaj Marg lays the greatest emphasis upon the need for such cleaning. All impressions which lie in us, created by our past thoughts and actions, have to be cleaned out thoroughly. The Master does this by using his spiritual power to liberate us from our buried impressions. When this is done, we take new birth, as it were. We are spiritually reborn. Superficial physical cleanliness of the human system will not avail us. A deeper cleaning is essential to rid us of the burdens of the past, and these burdens of the past are nothing but the impressions that we have engraved upon ourselves by our own wrong thoughts and actions. Such cleaning is therefore liberation from the past in a very real sense. We enter into a present unconditioned by a past. Hitherto our present represented nothing but the inexorable culmination of tendencies and trends established in the past. And the future could be nothing but the further inexorable trend of the same tendencies continued beyond the present. We see therefore the effect of the past on the future! Once this cleaning is effectively undertaken by a Master of spiritual calibre, we enter into an unconditioned present–a present, therefore, which can be correctly used to control and achieve a predetermined future goal. And that goal is the goal of perfection.

In the practice of meditation as taught by my Master, this spiritual cleaning is a continuing process. All thoughts and actions create impressions. As they are created, they have to be cleaned off. In the beginning of spiritual practice this is more difficult because the past impressions lie deeply buried within us. But as the Master takes charge of the aspirant, he undertakes the cleaning of these deep impressions until we arrive at a stage where few past impressions, if any, exist. Such impressions as do still exist are superficial impressions, easily cleaned off.

At this stage, we have to realise the importance of conducting our lives in such a manner that our thoughts and actions no longer have the capacity to create impressions. This can only be done by creating an attitude which my Master calls "non-attachment attachment." He does not preach detachment. What he teaches us is to be attached while maintaining an attitude of non-attachment. As human beings, we have our duties and responsibilities. We must not ignore or discard them as it is all too easy to do so on the ascetic paths. Master says that having accepted duties and responsibilities, we have to fulfil those obligations while striving for our own growth. When this realisation comes, the sense of duty is what remains uppermost. We no longer work for personal satisfaction, or personal pleasures, or for personal success. We work because we have a duty to discharge, obligations to fulfil in respect of those whom we love and cherish–members of our family, friends, employers, etc. Because our work is no longer conditioned by our desires but is undertaken only out of a sense of duty and dedication, impressions cease to be created. The past has already been done away with. The cleaning process of the Sahaj Marg practice has seen to that. It is as if the past never was. We have entered a present where our thoughts and actions are no longer creating a past which will condition the unborn future. The present is eternal without a past to weigh it down. We have entered a life-dimension which the ancient seers of India, the rishis, called the 'eternal present'. Now begins the final approach to the realisation of our goal.

Yoga means union. Two things cannot unite when they are not fitted for each other. If one is imperfect to start with, it has to be corrected and remoulded and made perfect before it can have union with the perfect one. Therefore yoga, as union, is the culmination of spiritual practice, and not merely a practice itself, as commonly represented. The perfection of the imperfect is what has to be achieved before union is possible. This is achieved by the cleaning process under Sahaj Marg. Now the two have to merge to become one–yoga is yet to be achieved.

I have so far dealt with the Sahaj Marg philosophy and tried to explain the salient features of this system. I would now like to take a little more of your time and explain the practice of this system as it is to be adopted by one aspiring to the goal that Sahaj Marg indicates as the correct one. It is necessary to emphasize that one must have a correct appreciation of one's goal before a method can be selected. The only goal that Sahaj Marg proclaims is the goal of human perfection, implying, and embracing within itself, total perfection in every aspect or facet of human personality and functioning. We have seen that such a goal is all-embracing and includes within itself physical, mental, moral and spiritual perfection of the human person.

What the aspirant is taught to do is to sit in meditation in the morning at a suitable time, seated in a convenient posture. The process is to be repeated once again at bedtime and, in between, Master prescribes a cleaning process in which the aspirant has to clean out the daily accumulation of impressions which in Sanskrit we call samskara. In meditation the practicant is asked to imagine Divine light pervading his heart and to meditate on that. Meditation is a process of continuously thinking about a single idea and does not mean concentration which, my Master teaches, is the result of meditation. If during the process of meditation other thoughts interrupt or flow into the mind, we are advised to gently ignore those thoughts and become inattentive to them. An important aspect of my Master's teaching is that thoughts gain power solely by our attending to them. Thoughts draw the power to affect us from the mental power that we devote to them. If we ignore them they fall off and have no further power to disturb or to distract us. If this technique is meticulously followed, the aspirant will soon find himself arriving at periods of thoughtlessness during meditation, the thoughtlessness having been achieved almost effortlessly. It is important to remember during meditation that the process is entered into for the purpose of realising one's goal. This makes the process highly dynamic.

In the evening, after one's daily routine of life is completed, Master advises us to sit with eyes closed and to imagine that the Master's grace is flowing through us removing with it all the day's accumulation of impressions, thus wiping off the effect of the day's activities and thoughts. Meticulous practice of this technique ensures that the individual is not adding to the burdens of the past which the Master is quietly cleaning away by his own spiritual power. We are, therefore, able to progress unimpeded by fresh accumulation of impressions. The culminating process for the day is to sit in meditation for about ten to fifteen minutes before going to bed, meditating on the meaning of a short universal prayer which my Master has given to us. The prayer is:

> O, Master!
> Thou are the real goal of human life.
> We are yet but slaves of wishes,
> Putting bar to our advancement.
> Thou art the only God and Power
> To bring us up to that stage.

As soon as this is over we should go to bed.

It will be seen that starting with meditation in the morning we end the day in a meditative mood, meditating on the thoughts and ideas contained in the prayer, and when we go to bed in that contemplative mood a continuity of spiritual consciousness is established from the moment of sleep to the next morning's meditation. By practice it is possible to bring into existence this contemplative mood to pervade right through the day, and when such a state is reached the need for any further meditation automatically falls off.

Once such a state of spiritually elevated consciousness pervades the individual self, normal worldly life goes on while spiritual progress also follows hand in hand, thus bringing into play harmonious and balanced development of the human being in the twin fields of existence, finally culminating in our achieving our goal.

Prayer

Ours is a simple system. It has just three elements in its practice. These are prayer, meditation and cleaning. When a system is so simple as to have just two or three elements in it, then all the elements are essential to the system. If even one element is lacking or is discarded, the system will probably be ineffective in its functioning. In Sahaj Marg practice, we cannot afford to discard any of these elements if the efficacy of the system is not to be impaired.

I have found that here in Europe, and particularly in certain countries, there is a deep-rooted aversion to the use of prayer. Even in our own groups there is this aversion, and many abhyasis have refused to use the Mission prayer which Master himself has declared as having come to him from above! This aversion seems to arise because religions have advocated prayer, and people who have given up religion do not wish to follow anything that religion advocated. Now I wish to say something about this. Perhaps the use of the word "prayer" is unfortunate but, call it what you will, it remains what it is. I would not like to deceive people by calling it something else. It is prayer, and nothing else but prayer. But, I would like to tell you what I think prayer really means. To me it is a cry from inside, addressed to we know not whom, for the fulfilment of a need within. Take a tiny baby. It cries when it is hungry and its mother rushes to feed it. But does the baby know it is hungry, and that it should cry to express that hunger? Surely not! It is a cry of nature from within for the fulfilment of a need which it does not know, and nature in the form of its mother responds from outside to fill the need thus expressed inarticulately by the baby.

I would, therefore, define prayer as a call from nature within to nature outside for the fulfilment of a need of which the self is not consciously aware. But the inner nature recognizes the need and

Talk before abhyasis at Centre Azur, Sanary (France) on 28 May 1976.

gives utterance to it. If we view prayer in this light, then we find that the idea of asking or begging for something, generally associated with prayer, no longer exists. Master himself has said, "Prayer is begging," and it is an unfortunate fact that that has been the only attitude in prayer–to beg for something. But we should not misunderstand Master as saying that prayer has to be an act of begging. All that Master means is that through the religious history of mankind, prayer has rarely risen above this attitude of begging to anything higher.

Our Sahaj Marg prayer is profoundly different. It is different in content and in purpose. It is a mere statement of certain facts with no request attached to it. Master says that by uttering this prayer mentally just once, a connection with Him is created, and that is its only purpose. The flow of transmission commences thereafter. It is like a switch which, when activated, permits electricity to flow. It is, therefore, vital to our purpose. If the system we are following is to help us achieve our goal, the use of the prayer is of absolute importance. I would remind you that Master prescribes the mental recitation of prayer just once in the morning, before meditation is commenced. Now if the prayer is what connects the abhyasi to the Master, then if the prayer is not mentally repeated, the connection is not established. It is perhaps for this reason that many abhyasis show lack of progress! In our morning practice, it therefore works as a connecting switch.

The prayer is used a second time at bedtime. Master asks us to repeat the same prayer mentally a few times and then to meditate on its meaning. Now what is the function of prayer here? I believe the function is now of an entirely different order. By meditating on the meaning we are embedding the spiritual meaning of the prayer in our deeper consciousness, in the subconscious, to keep it alive there right through the period of sleep. In the morning, when we repeat the prayer just once, the spiritual consciousness is brought out into our waking consciousness again, and thus a twenty-four hour cycle of permanent, uninterrupted spiritual consciousness is maintained. It is like covering live burning coals over with ash at night before we retire to bed. The fire is not allowed to go out. In the morning all that we have to do is to blow away the ash, and the fire is there ready to be built up as we want it.

I wished to discuss these ideas with you because André and I had a long discussion on this very subject last night. He liked my explanation so much that he wanted me to tell it to you in my own words. I hope what I have said will convince you of the need for prayer and that you will no longer have any reservations in using it in your sadhana. Thank you.

Yoga as an Evolutionary Force

From what my brother Don has just told you, we see that there is a past, there is a present, and there is a future. When we talk of the past, the present and the future, we talk of a flow or evolution in time, from the past to the future through the present. Now all life is in the process of evolution. We find that life forms have been evolving to the present state of the human form. All human life has been evolving from its ancient forms to the present form, the human form, which we consider to be perfect. Well, everything was perfect in its own time. When the dinosaurs were present on this earth, they were considered to be the most powerful, the strongest things living. They were certainly the strongest physical things ever present. But nature seems to have decided that physical perfection, or physical size or physical power is not enough for the final goal destined for evolution. This is the assumption of most scientists and philosophers who say that because man has been reduced to his present size, it reflects nature's decision that physical power and size is not enough to fulfil nature's aim for the final goal of evolution.

Now when we come to the human being, medical scientists tell us that after conception the human foetus in the first few weeks goes through all the evolutionary forms until it culminates in the present human form. What really happens is that life starts at the original level, and the entire course of evolution is compressed into a few weeks until the foetus assumes the human form. The same thing is reflected in education. When we educate our children we compress all the achievements of the past and feed it to the child, so that our children learn everything that we have learnt, but learn it at a much earlier age than we ever learnt it. So in a sense education is mental evolution of the human being.

Public lecture at the Food and Agriculture Organisation, Rome, Italy on 4 June 1976.

When we come to the spiritual life of man, we again find that there have been systems developed to offer similar means of evolution of the human being to his goal. Now here comes the trouble or the problem. Where the physical and the mental planes are concerned, we are able to appreciate everything. Our intellect is sufficient to deal with those two spheres of existence. Even there we find that when we start with education, for example, it is the research scientist who represents the spearhead of evolution because where education is given and it stops at the general level already attained, then there is no further evolution. So, even in education we find that the bulk of humanity stops with the achievements of the past. If that is the case with such a mundane subject as education it is no surprise that in a highly abstract subject like spirituality there should be a lot of confusion, incomprehension, and even misunderstanding.

Now evolution has two forces. This is generally not appreciated by most people. There is a push from the back and there is a pull from the front. Because if there is an evolutionary goal already laid down in the very far past when creation was brought into existence, then the very first organism which was created had only the pull of evolution, and there was nothing to push it from behind. But as life forms advanced on the evolutionary path, they managed to create a large past for themselves, a historical past which is not so bad, but also a past of impressions which Don has already told you we call samskaras. Now it is precisely this past which, instead of pushing us from behind, manages to pull us back from behind. So the samskara is a very important thing because it acts in an anti-evolutionary way. Instead of having a push from the back and a pull from the front, we have a pull from the front and an opposing pull from the back so that we are held powerlessly in a situation which we cannot overcome. This pull from the back is precisely what we have to overcome, because the pull from the front is always acting on us. If the pull from the back is removed by a Master who can remove our impressions, then the attractive or the full power of the evolutionary goal already established acts on us without resistance from us. Therefore, the cleaning of the impressions of the past is of the highest importance in any system of yoga.

When that is done all that is necessary is to just feel free to allow the forward pull from the front to take us with it. That represents what we call in the philosophy of yoga 'surrender'.

So, when we look at surrender in this way, we find that it is clear of all the metaphysical implications attached to that word. In metaphysics they say so many things about surrender which frighten us. And unfortunately the use of the word surrender in other contexts, such as surrendering to the enemy in warfare, has given an unsavoury meaning to this word. But really and truly speaking, surrender is only sitting in a boat and allowing the current to take us with it. Now anybody who has struggled against the current in a river knows how much effort is necessary, and how little progress we really make. Whereas if you just sit back and allow the river to take you with it, it takes you to your destination, except of course in those unfortunate cases where our destination is backward in time, backward in evolution.

So far, I have tried to explain to you yoga in a very simple way, in an evolutionary way, so that the usual apprehensions associated with the word 'yoga' need not be felt by us.

In the past, it was the custom to deliberately obscure certain high teachings with the idea that only the true seeker would look for them. In a sense they dealt with us like research scientists who put a rat into a cage with a number of mazes and with a bit of cheese at the end. But my Master says that in nature there is nothing secret. So anything which obscures is wrong and against human evolution. My Master repeatedly says God is simple and any way of achieving Him must also be simple. That can almost be taken as the platform on which Sahaj Marg stands.

In speaking of evolution, I have so far dealt with two aspects, and that is what governs material evolution or physical evolution. But when we come to spiritual evolution there is a third force which is that the goal of evolution comes to us instead of our going to it. So, instead of there being just a goal pulling us to itself, our craving for the goal pulls the goal towards us. That is achieved in Sahaj Marg by transmission, called *pranahuti*. This the Master achieves by pouring Himself into us and therefore we become like Him in essence. As power can be transmitted, as thought can be transmitted, as speech can be transmitted, so also spirituality can be transmitted. This is something which is unique in the discovery of spiritual research, and even in India, the home of yoga, we find virtually no reference to it in the past. Therefore, all past systems have tried to force the human being to conform to certain systems, and by the very nature of force there is always a reaction. That is a law of nature. But when something comes and puts itself into us, our attitude is to receive it and not to throw it back. So the Master's transmission works without resistance because it is the power of love, if we may say that, which is reflected back in us as the power of love. Hate breeds hate. Similarly, when we are afraid we also breed fear in the other person. But when there is only love the reaction can only be love. So the only force in nature which, while obeying the law of nature, acts in our favour, is the power of love! In a sense all yoga is based on this creation of love, and this love manifests itself initially as a longing to reach our goal, or as a craving. So all that is necessary to begin the practice of yoga is to have this longing to reach our destination. I say this because people often ask us whether they are fit for yoga at all. My Master says our willingness is our only fitness. Nothing more is necessary. You see, that again is an inheritance from the past–that we have to be fit, that we have to qualify ourselves, ideas like that.

We now come to the practice of our system of meditation. It is a very simple system, but like all simple systems, it has features of practice which are essential for success. If you put two things together and they create a third thing you have to have both, otherwise the third thing cannot be produced. But if there are twenty factors involved, perhaps one or two could be omitted without much risk of our losing our destination.

In yoga there are two elements. There is the self and there is the goal. These two are absolutely essential because without us there is no goal and without the goal there is no need for yoga. This is represented in our system by the Master and the disciple. The third thing which is necessary is a way to achieve our goal, and that is what the system offers. We sit in meditation. Meditation means just to think constantly about something. Meditation is another word which has been much abused by being considerably obscured but that has all been unnecessary, because meditation only means to think constantly about something. What we think about is what we want to achieve. That is the normal human way. So also in evolution, we have to think about what we are going to achieve. So it is only a small change from thinking of what we want, to thinking of what we have to become. My Master calls this "diverting the tendencies of the mind to the right direction." So, much effort is not necessary because the power of thought is already in us.

In our daily meditation we utilize the power of thought which is already in us, to think about the goal which the Master offers. This is the goal of evolution to the highest state of perfection. Now this abstract goal is difficult to meditate upon. It is like the number zero which has no value, but without zero there can be no mathematics. Similarly, we have a goal in our heart which it is difficult to imagine until we achieve it. To make this possible my Master gives us an object of meditation, though it is really not an object, and that is light inside the heart. We sit comfortably imagining the heart to be filled with this light, and if there are other thoughts which disturb us, we gently avoid or ignore those thoughts. We are told to ignore them because if we apply power to reject them then there is the reaction about which I spoke earlier, and that is the power of that thought to interfere in our meditation. So this is all that we do. The rest, as I have told you, is the third factor in evolution, the Master's transmission to us. That is his business and we leave it to him.

Even though in the past gurus tried to hold the power of yoga in their own hands, my Master says that no people should be dependent on a distant country or a distant guru for the attainment of their goal. My Master has been able to bring this system right to your doorstep by creating what we call preceptors who are ordinary people like you and me. Any one of us can be a preceptor. These preceptors are able to do this work for him, for the benefit of mankind in the various countries of the world. So it is no longer necessary, at least in this system, to read Sanskrit or to go to India to find a guru.

My Master has broken the past tradition of secrecy, by opening what he calls "the mysteries of nature" to the public mind, to the mind of humanity. This he has done because, as I said earlier, he says there is nothing secret in nature. Now these preceptors work in exactly the same way as he does, and we, wherever we may be, are offered his services to us without having to undertake expensive and difficult travel, as in the past. It is as if a shop was being thrown open and we are told to take as much as we can of what he offers! And it is not just one shop, it is shops all over the world which we are allowed, if I may use the word, to loot. This statement my Master is able to make because the power at his command is infinite. It has no limitation because anything in contact with the infinite must have the infinite as its resource.

I have tried to explain to you at some length some fundamentals about the system. Those who wish to know more about it are welcome to come and see Mr. Saravanamuttu or any of our preceptors in Rome. Master is here until the 10th of this month and we are all at your service to give you sittings, or transmission as we call it, or to answer questions, to discuss matters as you like. We generally have a transmission from the Master at the end of our talks. I hope you will all be willing to sit in meditation and receive it.

Cleanliness and Godliness

I don't know what my sister Antonietta has been telling you, but I propose to give you a short introduction to the Sahaj Marg system of raja yoga. It has been said for ages that cleanliness is next to Godliness, but it is a commentary on human understanding that, as with everything else, we have given a very superficial interpretation to this statement. Through generations of human life, we find that civilizations have concentrated exclusively on the physical cleanliness of our living conditions. And in most nations of the world, we have made considerable progress in this direction, although in countries like mine, and all over the East, we are still living under very dirty living conditions. At least the impression of the Easterner when he comes to the West is one of absolute cleanliness, and when the Westerner goes to the East it is the contrary opinion of absolute filth. Superficially, these personal impressions or opinions are correct. In my travels through Europe during the last twenty-five years, I have found that conditions of cleanliness have been increasing day by day, year by year, till today in the very advanced nations of the world, the cleanliness inside the house is almost clinically sterile. Of course much effort goes into maintaining it that way.

There is a surprising comment I have heard often, that in the East we employ a lot of servants to keep our houses clean. I have often tried to explain that when we use vacuum cleaners, detergents, electric appliances for cooking, etc., the energy that we use is nothing but the consolidation of the services of a vast army of servants. Now the use of servants, human servants, has some definite advantages. First, it provides employment for people who badly need it and, secondly and more importantly, it does not pollute the atmosphere and our surroundings. The most important advantage

Public lecture at Latina, Italy, on 5 June 1976.

is the conservation of scarce energy resources. But of course human effort can only be limited to the number of people available for service. So we find a peculiar inversion that in the Eastern countries there is a lot of dirt around our life but we do not have pollution of our rivers, of our lakes, of our atmosphere, while here in the West we have clinical conditions of life inside the house, whereas in the lakes and the seas the fish are unable to live, and a stage is slowly coming when we will be unable to breathe the atmosphere we live in. I have not talked about cleanliness to make criticism of our ways of life, either of yours or of mine. I have tried to show you that when there is no balance between the outside and the inside, something has to suffer in consequence.

So far I have talked to you about the outside and the inside of our homes. There is a more important association of two sides within the human system itself. As we have an outside, we also have an inside which is within us. Here again, there is a big hiatus between the people of the East and the people of the West. My Master has often remarked that in the East, where people are so dirty outside, they seem to have an inner spiritual cleanliness which seems to be lacking in people of the advanced nations who are very clean outside but have a lot of grossness inside. I have deliberately used the word grossness because grossness is not uncleanliness *per se*. Now it is this inner grossness that is a bar to our advancement on the spiritual path. Hitherto, this subject of inner cleanliness has been largely neglected. Even advanced yogic systems, such as the hatha yoga and other systems, have restricted their efforts more to the perfection of the physical system than to the perfection of the inner life of man. I think it is one of the unique features of my Master's system of Sahaj Marg that the greatest importance is given to the cleaning of the inner system, the spiritual system, of man.

This grossness, my Master teaches, is an accumulation of the impressions of the past. Every time we think of something, and we become attached to what we think about, an impression is formed in the mind. That impression which the thought creates becomes the parent of an action or of an activity. And when the activity is indulged in, when the activity is undertaken, the impression becomes deeper. And as the impressions become deeper in this way, we enter into what we may call a repetitive cycle of existence. It is perhaps in this fashion that habits are formed. For the superficial habits like smoking or drinking we know the reason, but we do not inquire deep enough to understand the fact that a person's whole personality is a reflection of such patterns of impressions in his mind.

So when we talk of personality, we are talking of the grossness inside resulting from actions and thoughts, and as these impressions become deeper and deeper, they solidify. At that stage, we find that we are in a very real sense captives or prisoners of our own past. It is, therefore, an unfortunate fact that in reality we have no free will which we think we have. If each one of us would examine his life without bias or orientation to himself, we would find that we have been repeating our thoughts and our actions in very specific predetermined patterns, in very definite patterns too. But because we are unwilling to face the truth about ourselves we always think that we are original in everything that we do.

Now when we come to practise the Sahaj Marg system of yoga, the first thing that the Master impresses upon us, which is at the same time the most important, is that these past impressions must be removed from our mind. Now it is natural that if we had known how to do it, we would have already done it ourselves. But while we have absolute freedom and control over the creation of impressions, we are helpless when it comes to their removal. This is precisely why we need an outside force, or assistance from an external source, to help us. We call such a person who can do this for us a guru or a master. So the first thing is to find a master who can do this for us. Without a guru there can be no yoga at all. You see this is something that has to be understood very definitely, that there can be no yoga without a guru.

There are, I think, people who have tried to do it by themselves but in most cases the results have been disastrous because, as in everything else, we need somebody to guide us. We need a guide to help us. Now, when we call a person a guru or a master, there seems to be some feeling that we have become helpless and therefore we need a guru. In Sanskrit, from which the word guru comes, guru only means one who is great, and his greatness is in a particular sphere, as there are great people in other spheres: doctors of philosophy, doctors of medicine, and so on. Now when we need medical assistance, we do not consider it a sign of weakness or helplessness to go to a doctor. Why should we consider that it is something demeaning to go to a guru? In a very definite sense, a guru is a doctor of the inside. When I say 'the inside', I don't just mean the inside of the body, I mean the inside of the inside! Because if the doctor is the doctor of our body, a capable guru is the doctor of the soul. So first of all we find a guru, and we accept his services in removing all of our accumulated grossness from us. That is the first step in yoga.

The second step is that we have to practise meditation. Meditation is a very simple thing. It means to think continuously about something. Unfortunately, here again there is a great deal of misrepresentation of this term, because most systems treat meditation as concentration. Now, meditation has nothing to do with concentration, at least not in the process. My Master says that meditation is the process that leads to the result which is concentration. The successful practice of meditation leads to concentration. In fact, what we achieve by meditation is a state of mind where the mind can be said to be concentrated. That is, we do not concentrate but our mind is in a state of concentration. You see it is very similar to happiness. I do not 'do' happiness, I am happy, isn't it? So similarly concentration is also a state. "I am concentrated," or "I am in a state of concentration," is the correct thing. When I say, "I concentrate," it is not correct. So, the practice of meditation enables us to achieve finally that state in which we can say the mind is in a state of concentration.

Now in meditation, as I said earlier, we think continuously of something. Meditation is such a universal activity that it is surprising there is so much misunderstanding about it. Because without realising it we are meditating all the time on something or other. A man who is obsessed with the idea of becoming rich is meditating on the idea of wealth. Another person who is obsessed with the idea of being successful in business is similarly meditating on success. But unfortunately, because meditation has been used only in a spiritual context, we do not understand that it is a very commonplace human action, upon which unnecessary esoteric connotations have been brought to bear. Now all that we do in spiritual meditation is simply to change the object from a material object to a spiritual object. And we find that it is very simple and very easy to practise.

It is very necessary to realise that meditation is not something foreign to our nature, in which we have to be trained, because meditation is something we are naturally doing all our lives. Only what we have to meditate upon is what we have to achieve. So it is simply a diversion of the mind from its normal activity not even involving a change of direction, but merely a change of the goal that we have to gain. The spiritual goal that my Master offers in this system is the goal of perfection that we can attain. This perfect state is something that is abstract. We do not know what it is until we have achieved it. So my Master has specified for us a simpler goal, a simpler object of meditation which, while serving the purpose of being an object, yet approximates closest to our goal. And that is what we meditate on: light in the heart. My Master says light is the closest to the Ultimate, and therefore it is the most beneficial and effective object on which we should meditate. So this covers the second activity. The first was the cleaning, which I have told you about, the second is the meditation.

Now, when you have cleaned something, something has to be put into it. We can clean a bottle but only with the object of replacing the dirt with something clean. What Master now puts into our cleaned purified system is Himself, or His spiritual essence, in the form of what we call transmission. This transmission is done by Him in a highly spiritual fashion and it does not involve any physical contact, or any mental contact, or anything like that. Therefore, it is possible that He can transmit from wherever He is to a person on the other side of the world, if not on the moon itself. Now, we are all familiar with wireless transmission where there is no physical contact between the transmitting station and the receiving station. It should therefore not be difficult for modern man to accept the possibility of such a transmission. And in any case, it is easy to prove because no instrumentation or receiver is necessary. Here is a transmission from one human person to another human person which both feel, and by which both benefit. In fact, the proof of his system is that the people receive his transmission and testify to it.

So, these are the three major components of Sahaj Marg Yoga: the cleaning, the meditation and the transmission. Master generally offers this transmission to people that come to attend our meetings, and it is for that reason that my Master comes personally to these meetings. He rarely delivers lectures in public, his purpose being to serve humanity in a much higher spiritual fashion by transmission.

Religion and Spirituality

This is the second visit my Master has undertaken to Europe for the purpose of teaching his method of meditation called Sahaj Marg. On these two visits, Master has met thousands of people, and one question which seems to crop up from almost everybody is the question, "We have given up religion, what should we do now? What shall we do having abandoned religion?" Now in the East, this question is phrased the other way round, "How can we meditate without giving up religion?" In the West they ask, "What to do having given up religion?" So we find two diametrically opposed approaches to the same subject. Now even though these questions have been coming to my Master only on these last two visits to Europe, long ago, I think at least forty years ago, he had formulated and given to the world a truth which we can almost call a slogan of Sahaj Marg. And that is that spirituality begins only where religion ends. He puts this into a very definite formula which, in his own words, says, where religion ends spirituality begins. Where spirituality ends Reality begins, and where Reality ends, then commences that stage of the ultimate existence which for the lack of a better word, he calls Bliss. Now, it is clear from this that religion has to have a definite end in the pursuit of our goal.

Master has often said that religion is like the kindergarten school which has a very definite purpose but also a very limited purpose. The purpose of religion is to put a developing child into an environment where ethics, moral living, truth, all these things are taught and where, in addition, some idea of God is given to the developing child. Now the trouble begins when we start becoming attached to these religions, whatever religions they may be. It is immaterial whether it is Christianity or Hinduism or Islam, because all religions are but the foundations upon which we have to build a life of

Public lecture at the Food and Agriculture Organisation, Rome on 9 June 1976.

spirituality. It is a somewhat intriguing factor common to all religions that each religion proclaims that there is only one God and that there cannot be a second God; but at the same time each religion tries to exclude the God of one religion from the other. If we would only treat this subject rationally rather than emotionally, we would appreciate that the gods of all these religions can only be but one God, called in different religions by different names. And if the truth is that infinity can only be one, they must be the same. If infinity can only be one then *ipso facto* there can only be one God, and the confusion arises only out of sentimental or emotional attachment to the names and forms that we attach to them in each religion.

Now here we have, Master says, one of the great truths of life, that religions have always done a great disservice to humanity–not intentionally, not knowingly, but nevertheless it has been done. It has happened that religions have always divided man from man. History contains ample justification for this statement, for this truth, which Master has stated. Now when we come to spirituality, which has also been called by the name mysticism, we find that highly developed persons have come out of all those religions, the mystics of those religions. For instance, we have had the mystics of Christianity like Eckhart and Boehme, and the great Sufi mystics of Islam. We have also had the rishis of Hinduism. They have all been able to escape or graduate out of their religions.

If we read the literature that these great mystics have left behind, we find that except for the language in which they have been written, the values of the truths that they have established are almost identical. It is an interesting fact that long before we started speaking about this, these mystics have themselves criticized religious rituals and religious formalities. Literature will testify to the fact that many mystics have even spoken outright about the need to burn down or destroy the places of worship, because they said these things imprison man. They have themselves stated that religious bondage should be broken; emotional attachment to forms must be broken; intellectual slavery to teachings must be broken; and some have gone to the extreme by preaching that all external forms symbolizing religion should be destroyed if mankind is to be liberated from the thraldom or servitude to religion. So we find that mystical teachers have themselves stated this.

Now what is it that happens when we come to the level of the mystic? All the difference is that instead of worshipping external forms by using external formalities or rituals they turn their approach, their attention, to the Divinity that is inside. It is said that God manifests primarily in three forms: the Ultimate form where he is nameless, formless, attributeless. Then we have the closest to that manifestation which, in Sanskrit, we call the *Antaryamin*, meaning 'one who resides within'. The third form is that in which he is worshipped in external idols, icons, pictures, etc. The way of development is to start with the external worship at a young age when we are not able to conceive of some more abstract forms. And when religion has served its purpose by giving us some idea of God, giving us some piety, morals, ethics, then the search has to be turned from the outside to the inside. That is precisely where spirituality begins.

What we do in spiritual meditation is to try to approach this Ultimate, and the easiest way is to approach it through ourselves, because He resides right here, inside us. For this approach we don't need to undertake travels; we don't need to go outside; we don't have to go to places of worship; we don't have to incur any expense whatsoever. It is unnecessary to know about God from philosophy, or theology, because we have now come to a stage where we are not worrying about the attributes and the forms that He possesses; but we are trying to penetrate to the very essence where all the descriptive terminologies and philosophies will no longer serve us.

Suppose I say that this lady is called Antonietta Bernardi; well it conveys something to me. But to know the real person I have to go into something deeper, some deeper form of association. So some form of approach which goes beyond the name is first necessary. Then we come to the personality, the personality of this lady. Even that has to drop off if we are to really know what she is inside, what is her heart, what are her qualities. So even in interpersonal human relationships, we go from the name to the form, and then to the content. It is exactly the same approach that we adopt in spirituality. We start with the names and forms of the deity. Then we read all the extolling or the descriptive literature praising God, giving His attributes, His powers. Then after that we have to go beyond that to the essence from which these attributes and names are derived. So, in a sense it is a reversal of the process of creation. In creation the essence comes down to manifest in the material. Here in spirituality, we go from the material backwards to the essence. So what my Master says is that there is no difference except that we have to turn the mind from the outside to the inside. In effect there is only a change of direction, not even enhancement of effort. Now we have to think about this turnabout, and for this Master says we have to use the power of the mind.

We have the mind, we have its powers and we see that they function in various spheres; but we do not appreciate that it can do many more things, many higher things, than what we normally do with the mind. For instance, we find in every religion that at the beginning of creation God said, "Let there be light," or God said, "Let creation begin," or some such thing. Now I would much prefer to say "God thought, 'Let there be light,'" because there was nobody to speak to, there was nobody to give an order to. It must have been a thought. So, in the very beginning we find that thought was what was used even in effecting the creation of something as big as this universe. Now we all have thoughts, but we do not put power behind those thoughts. In Sanskrit there is a word called *sankalpa* which means the power of the will applied to a specific thought. So when we think, we are only thinking, but when we make a sankalpa, we are putting our will behind that thought. So the power which is there in the mind is the motive force, while the thought gives the direction in which that power is to function. What meditation teaches us is to develop this power. It makes possible an approach by using the mind to strengthen itself to achieve a state of concentration where the entire mental power of the human being, which we call will power, can be focussed in a particular direction. Even mundane people like psychologists have said that the human being, that even a brilliant human being, uses but a fraction of his mental powers. Now yoga is setting out to achieve a means of utilizing the unutilized part of the mind, the mental power, to achieve a stage where the spiritually developed person can use the total powers of his mind in a specified direction. Then we achieve what can be called an indomitable will, an indomitable purpose, in life.

People often ask how the mind can be used to strengthen itself. A simple example from our life will show that in every case we use the same thing to develop itself. Even to develop the body or muscles we start by lifting small weights to develop the muscles, then lift bigger weights until we come to the limit of our capacity. So each function or each organ of the body has to be used to strengthen itself. And the mind is no different from the rest, except for a very important difference that whereas the others are limited in their capacities the mind has no limits. In fact my Master often says that even time does not exist for the mind. He does not give us any metaphysical explanation for this statement, but he uses a very simple example to illustrate this truth by saying, "Suppose you think you are in London, you are there at that very moment. So thought takes you wherever you want to be without any lapse of time." Therefore, he says, for the mind, time does not exist. It is merely an illusion, or it is a subjective experience which is imposed upon us by our environment, by our surroundings. Anyway, that is a departure from the topic, so I won't go into it here.

Coming back to the mind and the strengthening of the mind to a stage where we can utilize it fully to achieve all our purposes, Master teaches us a method whereby the mind can be regulated. The mind is not controlled but regulated. The first step is the practice of meditation where the mind is put upon a specified exercise. I call it an exercise because the mind is brought to bear upon a single subject, and all intruding or disturbing thoughts are allowed to drop off by non-attention. Non-attention is the greatest weapon to fight thoughts because, my Master says, thoughts without our attention have no power. So, at a single stroke in meditation, "by throwing one stone we get two fruits." We train the mind to hold one thought while simultaneously excluding all unnecessary thoughts. Even the very first sitting will give us some taste of that experience naturally. In innumerable cases people have come to

Master and have voluntarily given the information that not only did they feel peaceful and calm, but at the same time they had much fewer thoughts than they normally have in the same interval of time.

When we enter into this practice, we imagine that there is light in the heart, which is the subject of our meditation. There must be some subject, as I have told you, to divert our mind towards a specified channel. The subject is light in the heart. This is the specified approach. And we train the mind by excluding thoughts. My Master says that even with a few months' practice a stage of sufficient concentration is achieved, which we prove in our own experience by achieving moments of almost thoughtless existence. Now a thoughtless state means that there are no disturbing thoughts too because there can be no disturbance without thoughts. This initial achievement makes it possible for us to proceed with greater vigour in our meditation until we come to a final stage, where not only in the state of meditation but even in our normal waking state, we find that we are capable of being thoughtless for quite substantial lengths of time. Now there are two states of thoughtlessness—one in which we are aware that we are thoughtless, and the second state in which we are not even aware that we are thoughtless. In the latter state something suddenly makes us aware that we have been without a thought for a long time. So this state of thoughtlessness, this state of concentration, we achieve by the practice of a very simple system and with very little effort except to sit in meditation.

What is most important is that we do not use techniques of force, compulsion, or control which inevitably breed an opposing reaction in the mind. All that we do is to adopt an attitude of non-attention. And if it is a truth that action and reaction are equal and opposite, then non-attention can only bring about non-attention in whatever we are applying it to. So there can be no resistance from inside ourselves. My Master says that is why systems which have focussed their attention primarily on concentration, generally create more problems for the practicant than any definite development or progress. In such an attitude of forced concentration, we are fighting with everything that is trying to come into us, and therefore there is a resistance from what we are trying to overcome or exclude. And as we apply greater and greater power to overcome that resistance, the resistance is also increasing in power. In this system that sort of thing is avoided. Master carefully avoids this problem and makes it very easy for us to come to a state of concentration without any effort on our part.

Now at that stage where the mind becomes one-pointed, in a sense, spirituality really begins, because it is now that the full power of the mind is being applied to the subject on which we are meditating–light in the heart. The preceding practice was but a foundation for this stage. From there we have to proceed further and further, but the process is always the same. For general interest I can say I asked Master a question, "How can the same technique take us to higher and higher stages?" "How can the same technique or the same method of practice take us higher and higher to the highest stage?" Master answered in a simple way, "When you put a seed into the ground you water it. When it comes out as a small shoot you water it. When it becomes a plant you still water it. And all that you give to it is water, and it goes on growing."

In a similar way we find that in human development too the food that we eat, except in the first few weeks of babyhood, is no different. And now, what is it that our Master gives us that is like food to the human system? He gives us the very great and Divine assistance of transmitting his spiritual self into us. I deliberately use the word 'self' because the Sanskrit word *pranahuti* means 'offering of the self'. When can we offer something again and again to as many people as we meet, without any loss to the giver himself? Only when our resources are infinite! So, as Master says, we have to get hold of a guru or a master, whatever you like to call him who, by virtue of his own connection with the infinite, can make that infinity available to us. Spirituality is not a progress, or a search or travel in time. It is travel in eternity. So, as we continue to progress, we continue to need this transmission in greater and greater measure, and as we rise higher and higher, his assistance becomes more and more necessary until, at the final level or stage, we can do nothing without his assistance.

Now this is a very important difference between Sahaj Marg and all other systems. In other systems they say when you have practised for so many years, "Now you are on your own." In Sahaj Marg we are on our own when we come in but then, progressively, we become more and more dependent on the Master. It is a dependence not involving loss of freedom, but a dependence which makes the infinite resources of Infinity available to us. In a sense, Master acts as a transformer giving us the power of the Ultimate in graduated doses. And by giving us those graduated doses he develops in us the capacity to receive higher and higher doses until, at the final level, we become capable of receiving Infinity itself into ourselves, without any limitations! This he calls the state of merger with the Absolute. Now, since there cannot be two infinities, the receiver, the Master who gives him what he is receiving, and the infinity which he is transmitting to us, all become one. So the goal, the seeker and the way all merge into one Divine entity. And that represents the culmination of our search.

The Need For a Master

I think my brothers and sisters who preceded me have told you almost everything there is to say about the Sahaj Marg system; so I am in somewhat of a predicament as to what to say because the subject is limited, being a very simple subject. All that we can stress when talking about Sahaj Marg is the absolute simplicity of the system, the absolute simplicity of the practice and, what is most surprising, the absolute simplicity of the very goal that we are striving for in life–our perfection.

All through human history we have had people all over the world trying to practise some system of yoga, some system of meditation, some system of evolution by which they could rise to the highest potentials of human growth, of human development. And the mystic, religious and yogic literature of the world is full of such experiments, some successful, and many naturally unsuccessful too. All this literature emphasizes that there are normally three factors in the process of yoga. The first factor is of course the aspirant, the student who is beginning to develop himself to reach his goal. He is the very first factor. The second is the goal that he sets before himself as something which he wants to achieve in his lifetime. The third is the thing which connects these two, the beginner and the goal, and that is the way by which the aspirant goes to his goal. But I believe that through the ages the fourth and most important factor has been forgotten, and that is the need for a Master who can take us on the way.

Knowing that a way does exist is not enough, because on the way many things can happen. As Jackie Sabourin just told you, we can stumble, as there are pitfalls. So our need is not just for a way, but for somebody that can take us on that way. For this, yogic lit-

Public lecture at the Kunstakadamiet, Copenhagen on 13 June 1976.

The Need For a Master

erature specifies a guru, what we call a Master, as a factor which I consider to be of paramount importance.

Now, if I were to grade these four factors in order of importance, I would give the goal, the way and the Master about equal importance, and the seeker himself the least importance because he is the one who is trying to raise himself to the Ultimate. So in the beginning he is perhaps the least important but, because he is personally involved in his own evolution, to himself he becomes the most important. The other things lose significance. So the aspirant thinks he is himself the most important factor in this pursuit of yoga. But here comes the problem, that when I think of myself as the most important thing, and my evolution as the most important thing, it is but human nature to tend to downgrade the value and the importance of the way and the one who is leading us on the way and, all too unfortunately, the importance of the goal itself.

Now it is a sad fact, a sad commentary, that the word yoga is used too loosely nowadays to imply all sorts of achievements, physical and mental, but very rarely indeed the spiritual attainment to which the word yoga should properly be applied. According to the Sanskrit literature from which the word yoga originates, yoga means union with the Ultimate. It does not mean union with anything else, or anything less than That. So even the goal itself has been downgraded because the self has been upgraded too much in the process of seeking one's evolution. This, in ordinary parlance, we call egoism. We are so filled with ego, our own importance, that we tend to give lesser importance to the goal, lesser importance to the way, and lesser importance to the guide who is to take us on that way, than we give to ourselves. Now, if we should ascribe the proper or relative degrees of importance to these factors, then the first thing that comes in us, or descends into us, is a feeling of humility because, after all, it is I who am so low that I have to raise myself up to evolve by some means to a specified goal. When that humility comes into us then we automatically know that we, by ourselves, are perhaps not strong enough to follow a way successfully. Until this feeling comes, people tend to reject the need for a Master. People often ask, "Why do I need a Master? We have a way, we have a goal. Why do we need a Master?" I will explain this at the end of this talk, or rather the explanation will come by itself.

First, we have to establish what is our goal. And if the goal falls something short of what we should truly aspire for, then it very often happens that our search ends unsatisfactorily. It does not satisfy us, and we cannot reach the real goal because we have reduced the goal in our own eyes. People who shoot with rifles know that when you shoot at a distant target you have to raise the sights. Similarly, for an examination, if you want to come first, you try to be first in the country or something like that. You see, you have to set your sights higher than the goal which you have to achieve. If we start out by lowering the goal itself then our achievement will fall short not only of the actual goal but even of the lowered goal that we have set for ourselves. So the first and most important thing is to determine our goal.

The second thing is to find the appropriate way. I won't say the correct way because, technically speaking, there is no wrong way. It is only a mismatching the way to the goal that brings in this concept of wrongness or rightness. Therefore the word 'appropriate' is more suitable, and we have to find the appropriate way for us to reach our destination, our goal of evolution. Now there are too many ways available, there have always been too many ways available. But here comes, I think, the wisdom and the grace of Nature that it endowed us with an intellect which we are expected to use in assessing not merely our needs, but in seeking a correct way of raising ourselves up to our own goal. So the intellect is there to help us. We have to study available systems. We have to seek a guide. And when the intellect has evaluated or assessed perhaps two or three systems of practice, then we have to come to a final judgement regarding one of them, before we commence the practice of that system and see what it can offer us. Even though to achieve the goal may take a long time, to know whether a car will move does not take much time. You just have to sit in it and start it and see whether it will go at all. If it does not go we reject it straightaway. So the movement of the abhyasi in the vehicle which he chooses for his evolution can be evaluated from the very outset. It does not need much effort, it does not need much time. But we in the modern world, being too intellectual, always try to get proof first instead of just getting into the thing and trying to prove it for ourselves.

Now that we have the goal and the way, I come to the third thing, the Master. To me, the need for the Master is definitely a paramount one because without a Master I don't think we can achieve anything. Why? Because even when the roads are most carefully mapped, there can be disasters which have happened since the maps were printed. There can be changes. I remember an amusing incident when we were in the United States four years back. A young lady, who is here with us today, was driving us from one place to another. She had a road map spread out on her knee. We had almost come to our destination. We were just about ten miles short, when we found that what was marked on the map as one of those express highways did not exist. It just was not there. We had travelled 160 miles to find that the last stage, the last ten miles of the road, did not exist any longer. The lady who was driving us then called a policeman to ask about the right way. The policeman said, "Well, you are referring to an old map. You should have got a new one." So as ways change, maps change; and as ways of evolution change, as people change, the ways have to change themselves.

So what was held to be something which was practicable, which was demonstrably practicable two thousand years ago, need not necessarily be practicable today. I am not saying it is not, but it need not be. So we have to prove for ourselves the efficacy of existing systems which were there in the past. They generally enjoy the privilege and the prestige of being of hoary tradition. We tend to value yogic systems as we value antiques! In yoga there is no antiquity; it is not of antique value; it is not something we can exhibit in our cupboards and say, "I paid so much for this." That can be true of material possessions. Old age means something in material possessions. Unfortunately, in people it does not seem to have much value. In today's society old people are not looked up to. So we value age in some things, but in other things we don't value it at all. This idea of value we should attach to yogic systems, too. Just because a thing is three thousand years old, or five thousand years old, it does not mean that it is therefore a practical system, something which will work today.

Here comes the need for a Master to guide us, because tradition says, people have testified to this, that Masters come mainly to modify ways to suit present conditions of civilization, present conditions of life and, most important of all, to make or remake systems to suit the conditions of living that exist today. For instance, if you take certain yogic practices which demand practice over hours, days, months, and years, sometimes, obviously, it is not practicable for today's human being to follow these systems where every minute of the twenty-four hours of the day has to be bestowed upon the practice. That does not mean the goal becomes something denied to us because Nature never denies goals. Nature keeps the goal in view; Nature modifies us to reach that goal, and simultaneously Nature offers to us better methods, easier methods, simpler methods of reaching the goal. To make this available to us, Nature sends the Master to us. So in this context, the Master is of the greatest importance because he redesigns past systems, past methods of approach, to suit our own conditions of life today. This is the first and most important need for a Master.

The second thing is, he is one who has already gone over the path several times. Not only did he do it when he first set out to evolve himself under the guidance of his own guru, subsequently he has got the job of taking people up to that destination. Now a person who goes again and again on the same path becomes an adept. In spirituality, in mysticism, we call such people adepts. So a Master is an adept because he has travelled the same road many times. And what would take us much effort, much time, and perhaps much anguish in finding out for ourselves, he does for us very simply. That is the second thing.

The third factor is what in Sahaj Marg we speak very specifically about–the process of cleaning which refers to the impressions of the past which are buried in us as samskaras, as they are called in Sanskrit. In a sense it is these samskaras which become the burden tying us down to this existence, being worked upon by gravity, let us say. Now when he cleans us, Master refers to what

The Need For a Master

he calls a vacuumization of the inside of our own system, so that something new can be put into it. When you remove something from the system a space is created inside into which he pours his transmission. That is the fourth aspect of the Master's work.

Restricting myself for the time being to this cleaning–I have always wondered why so many sincere, extraordinarily sincere, people who practised yogic systems in the past with almost fanatic zeal, subduing every human instinct they had, yet fell short of achieving the goal. Thinking over the past so many years about this, it was only two days ago, while I was myself sitting in meditation, that the answer came to me. Every one of those aspirants had in some way cleaned himself and created a vacuum. But what is it that is going to fill this vacuum? Please note, when a vacuum is created, unless it is attached to a source from which the vacuum chamber can itself be filled up with the appropriate thing, it is only going to attract everything that is outside itself!

Now we have vacuum cleaners in our houses and even though they are vacuumized they only pick up the dirt and the dust from the carpets on which we expose them. In a chemical plant, if you want something to flow from one chamber to another, you vacuumize it and connect it to that precise chamber from which you want something to be fed into it. If not, it will only take in the surrounding air and the dust. It is like the rather euphemistic instrument that you have in cars for fresh air. You open it and all that you get inside is the polluted atmosphere of the outside. There is nothing fresh about it except the inscription 'fresh'. This is what happens to a very serious and very practical abhyasi who, without guidance, without connection to the goal, by great effort over very long years of time, vacuumizes himself, and finds that everything he is throwing out is coming back into himself. I think this is a matter of simple logic.

In those cases where people have had Masters, and have been deeply connected to them by love, by devotion, by emotional attachment of a spiritual nature, all that they could draw from their Master was what the Master himself had within him. If the Master had physical progress, they got physical progress. If he had knowledge, they got knowledge. If he had wisdom, they got wisdom. If he was psychic, they became psychic. Therefore, it becomes an absolutely important thing that when we connect ourselves to a Master, the Master must be of that order who can take us to the Ultimate stage of our evolution. Because, what he does not have in himself he cannot give to us, however powerful the vacuum inside us may be. If I am attached to the wrong source, the greater the vacuum, the more dust, the more unwanted things I am sucking into myself. So it has been a tragedy of past yogic practice that by mis-connection the most serious aspirants, the most sincere aspirants, have ruined their spiritual life by wrong connections with wrong people, with wrong systems.

Now here is what my Master says in one of his books, "If you cannot find the right guru, it is better to be without a guru. There can be no substitute for the right guru." We cannot substitute a lesser goal for the highest goal. Therefore, if anyone is aspiring for the highest goal, it is better that he waits, even if it is necessary to wait a hundred lifetimes, until he finds a proper Master who can take him to his goal. If an aspirant indulges in makeshift or make-do arrangements with lesser things, they cannot raise him but will probably lower him in his evolution. I think this is the most important aspect of the Sahaj Marg teaching, that to have no guru at all is better than having an unevolved or inappropriate guru. When we connect ourselves to the wrong source, the very process of vacuumizing ourselves can lead to our degradation–I don't mean in moral values, I mean in the sense of evolutionary degradation– rather than to the uplift that we are so earnestly trying for.

It thus becomes obvious that by connection with a Master who has in himself the highest ability, the highest achievement, the highest goal that he has achieved for himself by such a connection, the Master can, by the mere and very simple process of emptying my inside, pour himself into me without any effort on my part. This is possible because he cleans my system, he creates a vacuum in me, and by creating this vacuum in me, his Self flows naturally into me. He offers Himself. We call this *pranahuti,* or offering of the life principle into life.

The Need For a Master

So when we realise that the Master is the cleaner, the Master is the vacuumizer, the Master is the one who comes into me and thus makes me like Himself in every way, we find that He is the goal, we find that He is the way, and we also find that He is the Master who is going to take me through the way to the goal. So in the proper perspective, and with the proper approach to spirituality, these three things–the way, the goal and the guide–all merge into one entity. And only where such a triumvirate merging into one exists, does the possibility of myself too merging into that, and becoming one with that, exist.

I therefore wish to emphasize that it is of the greatest importance that we seek the proper Master, one who has this ultimate connection, who has the ability to clean our insides, to vacuumize our insides. And if this is done, there is no question of time, there is no question of effort, there is no question of space. Achievement becomes instantaneous, evolution becomes instantaneous. We just jump, as it were, from our present mundane existence into the highest realms of spiritual existence.

Love

Our brother H.G. just mentioned that we are a family, and we are a family as he rightly said. A family requires parents and children and, in a family, they are all united very naturally by the bonds of blood. It is a blood connection. We call ourselves blood brothers, blood sisters, things like that. In human society, in human life, the blood connection has enjoyed very considerable support and strength. But of late blood ties are weakening, and we find that families are breaking up, relationships are disintegrating, and the old adage that "Blood is thicker than water," doesn't seem to hold any longer. Today water seems to be stronger than blood because people are crossing the water all the time to go elsewhere! So that is as far as blood relationship goes. And what has proved through history a very strong link keeping together people of a family, of a community, is disintegrating to a great extent.

Perhaps spirituality has come as a substitute to bring into our lives a firmer basis for unification not merely of members of a family in the smaller sense of blood relationship, but to create such a bond, such an impregnable bond which can never be broken and which will unite all humanity into one single family. So the aim of all of us should be to find a bond that does not disintegrate after uniting us.

I say this because again and again we have come across such cases of disintegration. Master has been meeting people practically every day where the tragedy is either that relationships are broken or, like the chemical bond where we have multivalent elements, you find one man with four connections or vice versa. How are we to normalize such connections and bring back into the family a sense of intimacy, a sense of love, a sense of affection, a sense of belonging, a sense of togetherness–while at the same time making

A talk before abhyasis in Denmark on 19 June 1976.

such a unity possible within a larger community of persons, whether a village or a nation or the world itself? This is to be examined. There is only one way! Love has to be personalized, while at the same time it has also to be universalized.

We normally think of love as a merely personal thing, something uniting two, perhaps three, sometimes four persons. But here is a concept in Sahaj Marg in which, as I said in the beginning, we have to replace blood by love, and this love is both personal and universal at the same time. It is as if the two extremes of a magnet are brought together to meet in the centre and produce what in science they say is impossible–a unipole! Such a love is directed towards one, and simultaneously towards all. In other words, such a love is a unity and also a multiplicity. In a sense, this is also the definition of God–that he is one and he is many; that he is the creator both within his creation and also outside his creation!

How something can be inside and outside the same object is something which defeats our imagination, but the coexistence of such extreme opposites is only possible in a spiritual pursuit. It is only in a spiritual family that we can have love united with discipline; where we can have love with arguments; where we can have love with differences between ourselves; where we can have love uniting people of many races, many tongues, many professions, because there is the silk thread of love that runs through us and holds us together! In the Gita, one of the descriptions that God gives of himself is that he is the thread that goes through the string of pearls and keeps all the pearls together without falling off! The human beings, or the family of human beings, need something which will bind each and every one of them together to form a grand necklace around the neck of God himself, if that is possible. According to Master this can be done only by love.

Now in love we have many things. It is not merely an emotion as psychologists say. It is not merely ecstasy as lovers feel. It is not merely something to talk about as philosophers talk about or speculate. In its true form, in its ultimate form, love is something which embraces some very fundamental principles. This is founded on old Indian philosophy which says that unless certain things come together love cannot exist. The first is purity. Purity means not merely purity of the body or of the mind, but purity in every aspect of our being, in every aspect of our existence. Purity of thought, purity of action, purity in our interpersonal relationships, purity of the house not at the cost of the environment but while keeping the environment also pure, all this is necessary. So we have to balance this purity between the inside and the outside. What H.G. said is very vital here, that the inner cleaning and the outer cleaning should go side by side. That brings us to the first step which is essential–a very vital and all-embracing concept that this purity has to pervade every form, every aspect of our life, every function of our life.

Then we come to possessions and things like that. We should not desire something which is somebody else's, whether it be material possessions or human possessions. And if we respect this, then much of the calamitous conditions of modern society would cease to exist. Taking away something does not refer merely to material possessions. It is easy to take away a brother from a brother, a sister from a sister, a wife from a husband, a husband from a wife. All this is taking away.

Yesterday Master was telling me the story of a saint in India who pretended to be very friendly with everybody. Following the Indian custom he would embrace anyone he met. When he embraced someone he would take away the spiritual attainments of the other person and hoard it for himself. One day Lalaji met this old man when he was going to his office and embraced him. Immediately everything the other person had went into Lalaji. In a sense that was a punishment of Nature. You cannot take what belongs to somebody and expect to keep it for yourself. So we have to be very clear that what is ours is ours, and that what is somebody else's belongs to that person.

Then we have the ancient concept of *brahmacharya*, which has been rather loosely and inappropriately translated to mean celibacy. Of course celibacy is one of its meanings but what it really means is pursuing the Ultimate. One who pursues the Ultimate is a *brahmachari*. So here we have to tie down the word to both its worldly or material meaning of celibacy, and to its ultimate meaning, namely the pursuit of the Ultimate itself. It embraces the whole spectrum between these two extremes. When we think of these concepts, then we find that the thread of love, the thread of purity, goes through all this.

We know that in a family where a father tries to control his children merely through authority or punishment, the family disintegrates very fast, because when his sons grow up and are as big as the father or bigger, they say, "Okay, let us have it out, let us see who is stronger." In fact in Tamil we have a saying that when your son grows beyond your shoulder, he is your friend, he is no longer your son! So we find that we develop from a level of obedience, a level of automatic obedience, automatic love, to a conscious level where we have now to consciously obey, consciously love; and this conscious obedience of principles of ethics, of moral ways of living, can only come out of love. It cannot come out of enforcement. If the son really loves the father, then he is prepared to sacrifice many things for the sake of the father. He cannot do something which the father would not approve of or tolerate. So the self is no longer the important thing, it is the other to whom we have given our heart who becomes the most important person. Love makes this obedience possible. Love makes the achievement of our aim possible, because the son wants to achieve what his father wants him to achieve. Therefore his co-operation is available. He knows that his father would not desire for him something that is bad, something which would not satisfy him.

We in our immaturity might think we are denied so many things. How are we to reconcile this with the ultimate freedom that Sahaj Marg promises us? This conflict of ideas between what is promised and what is given immediately arises merely out of immaturity, and because we focus our eyes not on the goal itself but on the lesser milestones which are approaching us as we proceed. Even on a motor trip, if you are going a thousand miles, it is easy to get disheartened at the twenty-fifth mile and say, "By Jove, let's go back. It's too far away. It is unattainable." Until you cross four or five hundred miles it can be quite irksome to proceed. But after that you feel that having come so far you might as well go the rest of the distance. Even then it is only something which is not accepted with the heart but accepted as something enforced upon us. When we reach our goal then finally we are happy and say, "Well it was worth it. I really did it even though I never expected that I would be able to do it."

Now love alone can make this possible. If you know somebody is waiting for you at the other end who desires you very much, not only you but your well-being, your spiritual uplift, your total well-being in all aspects of your existence, that makes the journey worthwhile whatever be the troubles on the way. So love makes morality possible. Love makes ethical living possible. Love makes pursuit of the goal possible–notwithstanding all the problems that we have to face on the way, the so-called privations that we face, the deprivations that we suffer.

In Sahaj Marg it is important to realise all this. We are the sons of one father but not because we are related to him by blood or by race or by anything. None of us is related to him in any way except that he is a human being and we are human beings, too. How then is he able to generate and hold our affection and our love with such a strong bond? It is the common pursuit of a goal, of an aim that he offers to us. This goal has such a magnificently enchanting aspect in our imagination that it holds us all together. It is so enticing that we are prepared to make every sacrifice. And each one by virtue of his attachment to Master becomes attached to the others who are attached to him. It is like the tree and branches and the leaves of a tree. Each leaf is connected to a particular twig, and each twig is connected to a branch, and the branch is connected to the main trunk. Therefore, the leaves belong to the tree, though the direct connection is only between the leaf and a twig.

So this family can be held together not merely by thinking that we belong to each other, but by bringing into our existence the sense of belonging, the absolute essence of that belonging. We are one because we are going to be one! We are all following one Master! Our aim is one! Our goal is one! Therefore, like a caravan moving on the streets, we are held together not because we are emotionally attached or communally attached, but because we are all going on the same pilgrimage to the same place. So we stick together until we reach our destination.

We must remember very clearly that the single aspect of love makes everything else possible, and love should not be narrowed down in its sense to mean personal or romantic love as we commonly understand it. The very love which can make and unite us, can also break and disintegrate us unless the understanding of that word is correct; unless the practice of that feeling is correct; unless the appreciation of that emotion is correct; and unless, in our lives, in our performance of every single function, we bring to this idea of love a totality of concept or conceptual meaning which alone can make love possible, enduring and meaningful.

So I would request all of you to bear in mind that love, very loosely used, can be a shattering force, a distracting force drawing us away from our purpose, from our goal, and very often ruining our lives in the bargain. It should be correctly understood as a total universe-embracing concept which, within itself, binds together every other single force in the universe and which, as Master often says, is the only thing which can produce love again. You give love, you get love. Here we have a function or a system which, while obeying the laws of science that action and reaction are equal and opposite, gives us back what we give which is what we need most.

I am grateful to H.G. for elaborating on this idea of the family. It is good that people from all over Europe are able to meet and exchange ideas. As H.G. very beautifully pointed out, we don't belong to a country, we come from a country. As Master says, even this whole world is not ours. We are here by accident, the accident of samskara, the accident of previous rights and wrongs, previous right and wrong thoughts, previous right and wrong actions. These have pushed us down into what saints call the ultimate hell of existence.

H.G. was asking Master today, "Where is hell?" I think Master wisely refrained from answering it because hell is right here. There is no hell other than this hell, but the human mind is so capable of making mischief with itself that it is easy to persuade ourselves that we are in heaven! When we persuade ourselves that this is heaven, we lose sight of the real heaven. So any illusion in life or any fantasy in life is our own creation. We miss the main thing because we are looking at something within us, and trying to fool ourselves into thinking that it is the thing that we most desire.

We often find people asking, "If I embrace Sahaj Marg will I be able to enjoy life?" Enjoy life in what sense? You are enjoying life in the evening, but the next morning you have a headache. Or you enjoy one day and then for a week you suffer. You go for a holiday for a month and then for the rest of the year you have to save money to pay for it! So enjoyment cannot be had without paying for it in some way. It has got to be paid for. We don't realise this. This is a very shortsighted view and if, as Master says, we balance or we bring into our life the balance that is the essence of Sahaj Marg, balance the inside and the outside, balance activity and non-activity, balance thinking and non-thinking, when all these are there, enjoyment loses its meaning and non-enjoyment also loses its meaning.

In striving for this balance, we have also got to see that people from different places and of different temperaments, are all coming together. And the tolerance that H.G. referred to is nothing but the sense of balance that while I am at one extreme, the other man is perhaps at the other extreme, and we must balance each other. Tolerance is nothing but balance.

So, when we are able to bring, by this total appreciation of love, this concept of balance, of balanced existence, into our lives, it will be easily fulfilling Master's goal for us, the goal of liberation! Further beyond that is realisation. Further beyond that is reality and then bliss. And beyond bliss is the stage that Master calls the incoming of God or Godliness! It is a long way to our goal and it is a great distance we have all to travel together. We need cooperation between ourselves. We need tolerance. We need faith in ourselves and in the Master. And all this is possible when love pervades our life.

What Should We Ask of God?

It is a somewhat unique and rare privilege to be invited to speak within the sacred precincts of a temple. This is perhaps the first such occasion afforded to us.

It has been a delight to hear the lovely bhajans the devotees have been singing for the past one hour. One bhajan was very impressive, and particularly the phrase, *pachtaayegaa pachtaayegaa ye janam nahin paayegaa*! ("You will regret it, you will regret it; you will not get this life!") On the face of it, it seems to have no meaning. What does it mean by saying that we will not get this life? Have we not already got it? Then where is the need for this warning that we will regret it? What is it that we will not get, and not getting which will be a cause for regret?

We are here in this human existence which is said to be the highest existence. What I think the phrase means is, if we do not use this life properly, then we will deeply regret it because we may not get this human life again. This, I think, is what the phrase really means. This bhajan highlights and emphasizes the fact, albeit indirectly, that the human life is one very difficult to get. Having got it, we should ensure that we do not waste it in flippant pursuits. We should mould our lives in such a way that we don't have to regret any thought or action of ours later.

Now, what is the correct way to lead this life? Obviously we must try to reach our goal in this life itself. And that goal is the goal of realisation. What we have to achieve is God realisation. My Master, seated here before you, says it can be realised in even part of a lifetime if one's efforts are properly directed, and if one can secure the services of a realised guru to help him. A life devoted to this pursuit is the only one that can be said to have been used cor-

Lecture given on 10 April 1977 at Laxminarayana Mandir of Sanatana Dharma Sabha, Kuala Lumpur.

rectly, and in such a life there will be no question of regrets later. My Master says that, contrary to so many things that have been said about realisation, it is really an easy thing. And the simplest possible method is meditation on one's heart, imagining the Divine light to be present in it.

A second bhajan sung by the devotees contained a very important statement, which we should all try to ponder over and understand correctly. That part of the bhajan to which I am referring says, *yogi hrdyaana gamyam*. One of the meanings of this, as indicated extensively in our ancient literature is, "I am seated in the heart of the yogi and my presence can be experienced by meditation," or, "I enter into the heart of one who does yogic sadhana." According to my Master, what it means is that by the practice of *dhyana* one is able to bring the Almighty Lord into his own heart and enshrine Him there. Thus, by right yoga one becomes a yogi. In this sense, only one who has the Lord in his heart can be rightly called a yogi. Now, since the seat of the Lord is in the heart, my Master says that the Lord should be sought for in one's own heart. The Bhagavad Gita also confirms this. *"Hrdi sannivishtah,"* says Lord Krishna–"I am seated in the heart of all as the inner controller." And, of course, that famous Vedic hymn, the *Purusha Sukta,* which has the unique distinction of finding a place in all the Vedas, puts it very clearly without any ambiguity. It describes the heart very elaborately, and goes on to locate the *paramatman* therein very very precisely, in beautiful language.

Now, we all seek God. At least we all think that we do! But even those of us who do seek Him, seek Him for very divergent reasons. We are all praying for so many things, to achieve so many aims. Which is the right one? What should a devotee really ask of God? I seek your permission to recite a short story from the Mahabharata which, I think, answers this question beautifully and categorically.

The great war between the Pandavas and the Kauravas was due to begin. Arjuna, having pondered deeply, decided to go to Lord Krishna and ask him for his help. He went to the Lord's residence and found him asleep. He stood respectfully at his lotus feet, with folded hands and head bowed in reverence. Duryodhana, of the Kauravas, had the same idea of asking for Shri Krishna's help. He too came and, finding the Lord asleep, sat proudly and arrogantly in a chair placed at the head of the Lord's bed.

In due course the Lord woke up. Arjuna, being at his feet, was the first person he naturally saw. As he turned to get up, the Lord's eyes fell upon Duryodhana. To him to whom everything is known, the purpose of their visit too was known. However, he smiled lovingly at both of them, greeted them, and asked them what he could do for them. Arjuna and Duryodhana both answered that they had come to him to request his assistance in the ensuing war. The Lord smiled again. He said that they had placed him in a difficult predicament by asking for the same thing. He said he could not deny either of them. He could solve this problem in only one way. He would offer himself, alone, without armies to one of them, and to the other he would offer all his armed forces completely. Shri Krishna smiled again and added that since his eyes had fallen on Arjuna first, Arjuna should have first choice in the matter.

Duryodhana was anxious and jittery, afraid that Arjuna might choose Shri Krishna's armies. Arjuna was, however, no fool. He promptly prayed to Shri Krishna that he should go over, alone, to the side of the Pandavas, assigning his armies to Duryodhana and the Kauravas. Duryodhana heaved a sigh of relief when he heard this. He smiled sardonically and requested Shri Krishna for all his forces. The Lord smilingly agreed to their requests.

I don't have to continue this story further. You all know who emerged victorious, and to whom fell defeat. What is the moral behind this story? **We should ask for Him, not ask for things He can give us.** If the Lord gives us everything in the universe but withholds Himself from us, we gain nothing. But if we seek Him for Himself alone, we get not merely Him but all that is His, too! This is the lesson, perhaps the greatest lesson, that the Mahabharata contains.

Within the brief period of ten minutes allotted to me, I have tried to tell you what the correct approach should be, and how to approach Him through meditation. Those of you who wish to know more about my Master and his system, called Sahaj Marg, may please contact Shri Reddy. I am grateful to the Sanatana Dharma Sabha for affording us this opportunity of being with you all today. Thank you!

The Two Ends of a Stick

There is an ancient Chinese saying which says, "Every stick has two ends." I first came across this saying many years ago, long before I came to my Master. I could not understand it then. To me it seemed to be too simple, a mere statement of a visible fact which all can see. Who can, after all, deny that a stick has two ends? I wondered why an ancient Chinese philosopher had felt it necessary to make this statement at all. It appeared too superficial a truth to have merited any philosopher's attention. Many years later, after I came to my Master, I began to understand something of its meaning. And that was only after I had become somewhat familiar with my Master's thoughts and teaching. Even then, I think only the superficial layers of meaning were revealed to me. I perhaps understand it a bit more deeply today, and I realise what a profundity of meaning is hidden within those five words of that long forgotten philosopher.

The most basic truth that my Master has revealed is that our existence has two aspects, two areas, to it. They are the material and the spiritual realms of existence. When I first read this somewhere in our Sahaj Marg literature, I immediately remembered the matter of the stick and its two ends. "Here it is at last," I thought. But all that I had found was a correspondence. The deeper significance did not strike me. As I pursued this method of spiritual practice which my Master trains us in, and which he is offering to you all, I learnt a second lesson. There are not merely two sides to existence. The two sides have to be 'balanced' if one is to lead a full and productive existence. All of us live, but few lives have real content, real worth in them. The bulk of humanity leads an animal existence motivated by lusts, inspired by fear and driven by lower

Lecture given on 21 April 1977 at Kg Glam Community Centre, Singapore.

urges and appetites unworthy of being called even remotely human. So balance has to be brought into our lives. As Master says, a bird flies on two wings. Cut off one, and the bird will crash to the earth. It is immaterial how strong the wings are. No bird can fly on one wing alone!

What my Master offers in the form of a simple analogy is one of his most profound thoughts. When we, in our ignorance or in our one-sided approach to life, neglect either half of it, we are surely headed for disaster. It is immaterial whether we neglect the spiritual half, or whether we neglect the material half of life. Both are equally necessary, in fact vital, to our full existence. Without either of them, our lives are incomplete and such a life can end in nothing but the frustration and despair of an incomplete situation. Our ancient forefathers neglected the material existence, negating it almost totally. We modern ones today tend to ignore the spiritual life almost as completely. The pendulum seems to have swung from one extreme to the other with a vengeance. Our forefathers and we ourselves have both suffered in the bargain by leading incomplete, truncated lives, while all the while thinking we are following the correct way of life. All that we are doing is to do the exact opposite of what our progenitors did. And that is certainly not a wise way of finding a solution to the ills besetting humanity! It is therefore necessary to understand that it is not important which side of life we neglect. Neglect of either is wrong and will give us incomplete and unproductive lives. Such a life will be one of dissatisfaction, misery, insecurity and frustration, giving one a feeling that one has lost the way somewhere when walking on the road of life. This is true of all human beings, whether male or female, rich or poor, sick or healthy, and whether conventionally a success or not.

Let us examine this analogy of the stick, for it is no more than an analogy, a little more deeply. While a stick has two ends, it also has a mid-point. If the stick is symmetrical then one can balance it at its mid-point. Then the two halves will be identical.

A	X	B

Let us call the two ends A and B, and the mid-point X. If we now look upon life as a long, very long stick, then we can think of AX as the material half and BX as the spiritual half of that life.

I would like to remind you that it is not only a long stick which has two ends. Even a very short one still has two ends. In fact those of you who would like to try an experiment can try to cut a stick as short as you can by slicing off cuts from one end. You will find that even when you have come to a mere paper-thin slice, it still has two ends, or two sides. If we try to cut the slice any finer, we will probably end up by cutting off our thumbs or forefingers, perhaps even both!

While this appears humourous when we speak about it, it is unfortunately no laughing matter. It is precisely what numerous persons have done to themselves all over the world, in trying to cut the stick of their lives shorter and shorter. The thumb is supposed to indicate will power, and the forefinger is one which we use to indicate direction. Is it then any wonder that persons devoid of thumb and forefinger lack direction in their lives, and have no will to act responsibly? The enormous number of mental patients, suicides, society drop-outs and the like will testify to the fact that where this chopping of the stick of life has been carried too far, one ends up by seriously maiming oneself in body, or mind, tragically often both.

I would like to share with you a few further thoughts this analogy of the stick has given me. Suppose a person decides to be a great success in material life, and therefore devotes all his time and energy only to the perfection of his material life. It leads him to neglect his spiritual life, probably a little in the beginning, but increasingly so as he goes on. As he becomes more and more engrossed in the material life, material success, wealth, the neglect of the spiritual life increases. So, in terms of the stick, we now have a new one, A^1B^1, where A^1X is longer than B^1X. The material content A^1X of his life has increased while B^1X the spiritual content has been depleted.

A^1 X^1 X B^1

Now we meet an interesting, and an unconquerable, problem here. The mid-point of the stick is no longer at X as it originally was, but has naturally shifted to X^1 the new and natural centre of the stick! When this analytical reasoning first came into my mind one evening during meditation, it came as a revelation to me. What is it that has happened in this situation? In trying to cut off the spiritual part of his life so as to be able to extend his material existence, all that the person has achieved is to corrupt his spiritual life. The stick must have a centre, and the two sides, too, cannot be denied. What has really happened is that an automatic adjustment has taken place. Nature does not tolerate or permit imbalances. So X^1B^1 is still the spiritual half of life, but X^1X represents the corruption that has crept into it from the material half, solidifying it, making it gross, so that it has become tainted, impure.

As this process goes on and on, B^1X becomes shorter and shorter while A^1X becomes correspondingly longer and longer. In an extremely materialistic life, B^1X may be almost zero while almost the whole stick represents the material life. I must emphasize that the spiritual half of life has not dropped off. The centre-point X^1 still exists. But alas! B^1X^1, the spiritual half, has become so gross and solid, and corrupted by materialistic tendencies, that the spiritual life has become petrified.

If, fortunately, X has not merged with B^1, a tiny tip of spiritual aspiration may yet remain, but this manifests itself in nothing more than an occasional twinge of the conscience, and in gross and perverted approaches to Reality. In such an extreme situation the bird is indeed attempting to fly on one wing. Such a life is one of gross imbalance. Therefore, it is one fraught with fears of failure, feelings of insecurity and terrors of disaster. If these fears and feelings persist, they may very well lead to despair and consequent illness of body and mind which he can no longer cope with. Is it any wonder, then, that in the modern materialistic world of today, with all its glamour and glitter of material opulence and luxury, of which your city of Singapore has quite a share, there is so much mental and physical misery, so many suicides, and such high crime rates? I don't think that anyone who gives these matters proper thought can ever wonder at the situation. Such things, such ghastly and inhuman things, must positively and necessarily exist, given this gross materialistic orientation to life.

What is it that we must do to find happiness, contentment, fulfilment? My Master says that we must change our ways of life. We must balance our efforts in both directions. We must pay equal attention to our material and our spiritual welfare, neglecting neither of them for the other. If our forefathers neglected the material life, they paid the penalty of living in poverty, and in sickness that Nature vengefully poured upon them. But at least that is all that they had to put up with. When we, in our knowledge-saturated ignorance, ignored the spiritual life, we seem to have let loose upon ourselves all the horrors of man-made disease and viciousness for which Nature can no longer be blamed. Our sufferings are our own creation. By our allegiance to vice, corruption, and violence we have let loose upon this world horrors and possibilities of devastation which our grandfathers could not have dreamt of, even in their weirdest nightmares. So, to correct this sorry state of affairs we have to bring back balance into our lives.

Now, material life has very definite limits to it. One can, after all, only eat so much, and drink so much. Much of what we painstakingly accumulate is never used by us. It is only avarice that makes us do it. A normal, level-headed, self-confident person would never indulge in such frenzied laying-up of worldly treasures. It is not necessary. Therefore, given proper and sustained effort, our material needs are easily satisfied. Then it is time to think of the spiritual life. In this dimension, the possibility of extension is truly infinite. At the same time, my Master says, "Extension or growth in the spiritual life needs less time and effort–merely an hour or so per day!"

Now let us take another look at our normal stick AXB. As we extend the spiritual existence XB, without in any way neglecting our material life AX, we find that XB can be extended to XB^1.

```
A         X    X¹         B         B¹    B²    B³
```
── ── ── ── ── ── ── ── ── ── ── ── ── ── ── ── ── · · · · · · · ·

The mid-point will now naturally have shifted to X^1. And here we have another revelation. By extending the spiritual life, we have, **automatically and effortlessly**, extended the material life too! For now AX is the material life, and B^1X^1 the spiritual life. The life-content, or total substance of our life, has also become enhanced.

As I said earlier, Nature tolerates no imbalance, and so the new balance has been effortlessly and harmoniously established, often without our even being aware of it! Not only that. The area XX^1 which belongs to the material life in the new configuration, is really an intrusion from the spiritual life–the original XB! What we have here is a wonderful phenomenon. The material life is becoming spiritualized too! If we consider the mid-point as the base of existence, then X^1B^1 is wholly spiritual, from base to top, while the material life X^1A is having its base spiritualized. So spirituality has been introduced into the very base, the very foundation, of both aspects of our existence.

As we extend the spiritual life more and more towards infinity, all the time taking diligent care not to neglect the necessary and vital material existence, a time comes when the stick AB has extended to infinite length, say AB^3. Now the material life AX with which we started our spiritual pursuit and which we have diligently preserved as a vehicle for our existence, will be but the merest tip of the stick, though the total material life extends halfway along the stick. But the truly material part, the skin of our total existence as it were, is only the original AX. The rest has been spiritualized. We have achieved a life where it is almost totally spiritualized, leaving a tiny tip of materiality anchoring us to this world till our time to depart from here into the higher spiritual existence should come.

Great spiritual saints are the visible evidence, the proof, that such an existence is possible and practicable. In them we see the finest tip of spiritualized-materiality, a merest fraction of an im-

The Two Ends of a Stick

mensely, infinitely large whole! The normal human sees only the visible physical person, the exposed tip. Developed persons see beyond it. Only those who have learnt to 'see' beyond the physical realms of existence can see this reality.

In the case of persons who have devoted themselves entirely to the material life, we found that their spiritual lives became tainted with materiality. This tendency increased until the spiritual life became totally petrified. Yet, the spiritual half of life remains, as remain it must. In what forms does such a petrified spiritual state manifest itself? Perhaps it is hidden in the innermost recesses of the heart as faint glimmerings of higher aspirations; perhaps as the feeble stirrings of a long subdued conscience; perhaps as vague longing for higher values of life. But all this is covered over by the rock-like hardness of gross material coverings the person has encased himself in. All this notwithstanding, they are given expression to in gross approaches to higher realities.

We all know that most millionaires tend to give away their millions in later life. They establish charitable foundations, build hospitals, erect homes for the poor, build temples, churches or mosques and so on. I used to wonder why people who have worked so feverishly all their lives to accumulate wealth should, as feverishly, try to throw it all away later on in their lives. I think part of the answer is in the feelings of guilt–but it is only a part of the answer. I think the repressed finer feelings and nobler aspirations–the hallmarks of a truly human being–hidden deep in the heart, one day build up so much pressure that, in a moment of weakness, they explode. The result of any explosion is the same. All overburden is blasted off! The result of such an explosion in the human heart is to throw away precisely all the overburden of material life that one had accumulated during his lifetime. But since his spiritual feelings are petrified, and lack refinement, all that the release of the long locked-up finer feelings and nobler sentiments is able to achieve is to build in stone, concrete, or steel monuments to his personal failure. At this stage a person's spiritual inclination can find no higher expression. Only this rather negative expression is available. To be able to give proper expression to it, cleaning of all past impressions is essential. Such past impressions are the mental footpaths and highways on which we proceed. Until they are erased, we remain their slaves. This is an important, perhaps the most important, duty of the Master.

We therefore see the imperative need of giving a due share of our time and effort to our spiritual life. There is no need for me to emphasize that the material life should not be neglected. It should get its due share, but no more than that.

Now, when our spiritual aspirations open up, we have seen that they can go into gross channels of approach to Reality. The cleaning of impressions, which I referred to a moment ago, can alone guarantee that newly awakened spiritual impulses go in the right channel or approach. So here we meet with the second imperative, the imperative need of a Master. Who can be a Master? My Master says, "Look for one who can guide you to the highest. Don't be satisfied with anything less than that." Such a guide alone knows the way, having travelled the whole way himself. You may call him Master, Yogi, Saint, or anything else, but he remains a guide, whatever else he may be to us, and for himself. After cleaning our system of past impressions and thus, in a very real sense, lightening us, he takes us on the road which leads us to our goal. The more we trust him and the more we obey him in following his principles and practice, the quicker will be our success. If, fortunately, we can achieve that acme of faith-cum-discipline which goes by the name of surrender, then our goal is capable of being achieved here and now!

I now come to one final, but at the same time unique, feature of this system of Sahaj Marg. The Master, by virtue of his own spiritual attainments, is able to transmit the spiritual essence of himself into the heart of his students. We call this, rather prosaically, transmission. It is so simple to speak about that its very simplicity hides the infinitude of blessings that it can confer upon us. Imagine being left a million dollars by a rich relative, so that you become a millionaire overnight without lifting your little finger to achieve it. Multiply that by billions of times, and that is the benefit that this spiritual transmission of the Master confers upon us. This is a unique feature of this system. After my talk is over, my Master will transmit to all of us, and give you an opportunity of receiving it into your hearts.

Now, some of you will probably ask me the question which I was asked again and again during such lectures in Malaysia. What happens when the Master goes back to India? What do we do then? Well, it is a vital question. The answer is that in this system there is yet another unique feature. That is the system of training and permitting persons, like you and me, to do the work of the Master here. Such persons can do the cleaning and the transmission in exactly the same way that the Master himself does. They are called preceptors. So, when Master leaves for India, those of you who take up this system will not be left high and dry without guidance. Mr. Tan Kee Leng of this city is one such person selected by Master. There will be another preceptor, too. Both of them are at your service in all matters spiritual. My brother Mr. Reddy, Secretary General of the Asian Youth Council, seated to my left, resides in Kuala Lumpur but will visit you all as often as possible for further guidance.

I think I have explained, in some detail, the salient features of Sahaj Marg. I request brother Reddy to now explain the process of meditation to you, after which we shall all sit in meditation for about twenty minutes and receive my Master's transmission.

Yoga as the Way of Experience

Before coming to the main subject of yoga, I would like to correct an impression that this talk will be followed by a yoga demonstration. I find that it has been announced to the public in that way. In raja yoga, which concerns the mind, it can be only inner activity. So any demonstration can be at best an internal one only. All we do is to sit in meditation. That is all that is visible. So please don't be disappointed if you don't see any demonstrations of yoga exercises on the stage at the end of my talk. That is not what my Master teaches. Here the demonstration will be a silent one, or rather one of silence. We will sit with eyes closed, and I hope you will all participate. It will not be so much a demonstration as a participation by all of you in what the Master is trying to do.

Coming to what my Master teaches, I would like to say that all human endeavour and achievement rests in the two broad fields of knowledge and experience. I would hazard the opinion that experience precedes knowledge, at least if you think of it in terms of original beginnings. When the human being emerged from lower animal life, he gained his knowledge by experience of the world around him. If we go back to the origins of fire, we are told that man saw fire, perhaps for the first time, in jungles where trees struck by lightning had caught fire. By going near it he would have felt warmer. As he went nearer he felt hotter. And perhaps when, out of curiosity, he touched the burning wood, he got burnt. He then learnt that this thing in the wood could burn him. So knowledge came later, experience was its foundation. As I said, this is true if we think of the origin of things. At the base of knowledge lies experience. Subsequent generations naturally start with knowledge which the earlier generations have gathered. Perhaps many of you feel

Lecture given on 23 April 1977 at St. Patrick's High School, Singapore that knowledge comes first. But there are adequate, indeed overriding reasons why we should give first place to experience.

Our own generation has a great wealth of knowledge behind it. That constitutes our intellectual heritage, scientific heritage and artistic heritage. All this knowledge is acquired by us by learning from books and other sources of preserved knowledge. Why is it necessary to preserve knowledge at all? If you think a little deeply over this, you will understand that knowledge is preserved only to liberate us from the necessity of going through all the experiences which our forebears went through. In other words, knowledge is merely the experience of others who have recorded their experiences for us. In essence, therefore, knowledge is but fossilized experience. At least, that is our way of looking at it.

One difficulty with knowledge, or learning, is that it tends to go on and on. Twenty or thirty years back when we were in schools ourselves, what we had to learn of the various subjects was much less, in terms of quantity, than what children in schools learn today. This is true of all disciplines. We were not taught less because our understanding was limited, or anything like that. We were taught less because that was all there was to teach. Today the sheer bulk is so frightening that when we think twenty years ahead from now, one can easily see that it will be impossible for any individual to know much about even one subject. A hundred years ago one could, with diligent study, know everything about the world. Fifty years ago, one could perhaps master one or two disciplines only. Today we have specialization to such an extent that one can master only one part of one discipline. What of the future? The world as a whole may acquire more and more knowledge. The sum total of knowledge in the world will go on increasing, but what an individual knows, or can know, can never keep pace with the growth of total knowledge-content of the world.

One redeeming feature is that we need not know much. It is not necessary for us to know everything that exists. In one sense, such knowledge as we acquire is more in the nature of a survival kit to help us exist. We, each one of us, learn something so as to enable us to lead a productive life which can ensure our physical and worldly well-being. Even then we find that in all educational courses some practical courses are included. This is done to facilitate our verifying the knowledge offered to us. So the original experimenters developed a body of knowledge. We start with that knowledge and verify it by experience, and build upon that body of accumulated knowledge, increasing it, widening it, as we go on. This is all for the good of humanity.

When we came to yoga, or to put it another way, when we come to spirituality, there is very little that can be taught, in the sense that knowledge is passed on. Much of it, if not all of it, concerns the deeper levels of existence where only experience is possible. For instance, even such a mundane thing as happiness cannot be taught. I may be happy under a particular set of circumstances. But this does not mean that another person will be happy under the same set of circumstances. Nor can one person teach another what happiness is. Happiness can only be felt, can only be experienced. So inner feelings, emotions, states of being, are not amenable to methods or systems of education, but they can be experienced by each one. It is perhaps for this reason that one of the old systems of yoga called *gnana* yoga, or union through the way of knowledge, is not much heard of these days. While we hear and read a lot about hatha yoga, kundalini yoga, etc., we hardly ever hear about gnana yoga. Can one teach love? But when we love someone very dearly, we know what love is without being able to teach what love is. So here we have knowledge which we can't impart by the traditional means of education.

Yogic knowledge goes deeper than all these levels of knowledge. In fact it goes to the ultimate level of loving God, which is only another way of saying that we know God. We really know only that which we love. So love would appear to be an absolute precondition to true knowledge, to enduring and deep knowledge of the object sought to be known. It is for this reason that yogic systems, based upon association with a personal, living guru are more efficacious, provided such a guru is in contact with the Ultimate which we are seeking.

Now while experience may support and validate knowledge as in experimental modes, it is not necessary that experience should be supported by knowledge. Even today there are things about which nothing is known. When we first experience the thrill of coming into contact, through experience, with such things, that is absolutely unique for us. Many things are known about aircraft. But for each one of us the first plane journey is a unique thing. So even where knowledge exists experience is necessary. A single experience of any activity is enough to prove to us the value and validity of that action. Therefore, the experimental mode of approach is not only simple, it is easy and direct and instantly answer-oriented. Also, in such an approach, all can participate. Prior knowledge is unnecessary. When my Master says practise meditation and the stated or promised results will follow, practise alone can prove what he says is correct.

So, this is one great advantage that experimental systems have—that they do not take a great deal of time and effort to satisfy us whether the system can be accepted, at least for a trial. If you are asked to eat something and say whether that thing is good or not, one spoonful is enough. We don't have to eat the whole dish. We have a saying in my mother tongue, Tamil, that if you are cooking a pot of rice, it is enough to test one grain of rice to see whether the pot of rice has been cooked or not. You don't have to go through the whole pot.

In substance, this rather lengthy analysis shows us how knowledge, as a totality, is something which is almost impossible to acquire, except to the extent necessary for our livelihood. When we take up the question of the development of the Self in the higher spiritual sense, it is easier and quicker to participate in an experimental technique or system. This is precisely what raja yoga teaches. In our system of Sahaj Marg, which is based upon raja yoga, we start with the mind.

It is one of my Master's basic teachings that everything originates in the mind. Nothing originates from the physical system. What is born in the mind as an idea becomes a thought; what emerges as a thought goes further to end in activity. Activity gives us feedback information and the whole process is repeated again and again. So raja yoga directs work upon the point of origin, the mind.

Sahaj Marg is a system of meditation based upon raja yoga, but refined and greatly simplified to suit our time and the condition we live in. It is so simple that it can be practised effectively by any human being. It is, therefore, a universal system. A universal system should be applicable to all humans, without considerations of race, religion, sex, or occupation coming into the picture. My Master affirms that this is a system without any such barriers or limitations. No system of self-realisation can be denied to even one section of humanity, however small, for any reason whatsoever.

This system is very simple, requiring no more than an hour a day, divided into three sessions. What is done in those three sessions is set out in the literature that has already been issued to you. You may ask, what is realisation? Whatever it may mean, one thing that can be said is that it is a state of being. As such, it cannot be known except by experience. It is a state of being which cannot be known in the sense in which we know about things. The only manner in which we can test the validity, the applicability or the efficacy of this system of meditation is to participate in its practice and try out what he says. We will then be able to feel whether there is developing in us a sense of peace, an awareness of higher faculties opening up in us, both of which give promise of further growth and expansion in the direction of ultimate realisation.

Coming to the practical aspect, there are three, and only three, important techniques in the system. The first is meditation. Meditation means to think continuously of one thing. So there is an object upon which we meditate. It is said that "as we meditate, so we become." Hence the object which is used for meditation must be the correct one to lead us to our goal. My Master says that any object which has grossness or solidity is itself under a limitation. Objects which have inherent limitations cannot be adopted as objects for meditation where the goal is the subtlest one of realisation. In this system we meditate upon light in the heart. It is light in an abstract sense, not concretized as light from bulbs or even the sun. He calls the light that we meditate upon as light without luminosity. It is light but has no luminosity!

The technique is to sit quietly, in a comfortable pose, with eyes closed, having the suggestion in the mind that the heart is internally illuminated by the higher presence. We must try to hold this thought continuously. If disturbing thoughts intrude, we are taught to ignore them as something unwanted. Thoughts have no power of their own. They draw power from the attention we give them. So when we ignore unwanted thoughts they fall off. Should the mind wander from the thought that there is light in the heart, gently bring it back to this thought. Don't use force, for where force is used, a reaction is inevitable. Force creates opposing force. This is the first technique of Sahaj Marg.

The second one refers to cleaning of the inner system. The Master and his preceptors are largely active in this, but we have to practise it daily as a measure of co-operation. By this technique all the impressions we have engraved upon ourselves by our past thoughts and actions are erased. Such impressions have to be removed. Otherwise they form the channels for our future thought and activity. Such impressions therefore hold us in bondage. To get freedom, they have got to be removed. When we start our lives we are already following a particular path determined by such impressions of the past. They are strengthened by following the same pattern, over and over again. We do things in a certain way, think in a certain way, not because we want to do so but because we are following a pattern already engraved upon us by past impressions. We have, in a very real sense, very little freedom. It is only when cleaning is effective and impressions are removed that the element of freedom enters our life and we become capable of guiding our lives in a chosen direction. Master is able to do this cleaning for us by the use of his own spiritual powers, and we participate in it, assist in it, by following the technique outlined for us, and by trying to live in such a way that our thoughts and actions don't create further impressions. In this technique, both we and the Master are active participants.

The third technique is one in which the Master alone participates. We have nothing to do. This is a unique technique which my Master has developed. He is able to transmit his own spiritual accomplishments, his spiritual state or condition, into our hearts. This is something unique, but at the same time something which all of us can feel, even at the very first meditation sitting. All that we have to do to feel it is to be receptive to it. I must add that whether we feel it or not, it is yet there, working upon us from inside. But to be sensitive to it hastens our progress considerably. This transmission makes it possible for us to receive his accomplishments into our very being, and therefore, in a large sense, liberates us from our effort. We are able to acquire a state of being by receiving this transmission, which would otherwise take years and years of arduous practice for us to cultivate by our own efforts. The whole process towards realisation is greatly accelerated by the cleaning process which eradicates the tendencies created by past impressions. We are being purified, while being simultaneously filled with that which should be in us, for us to be spiritual persons.

A final item of practice is meditation upon a short prayer for a few minutes before going to bed. This ends our day's schedule of practice under this system.

Now somebody asked me as we entered this hall what happens to students of this system after Master leaves Singapore? Who will guide them? Will they have to come to India? This brings me to a final feature of this system. Master is able to prepare persons who can do the work that he does in exactly the same way. Such persons are called preceptors. Before Master leaves there will be two such preceptors to train and guide students of this system here in Singapore.

Sahaj Marg and Science

Master has been saying for the last few days that Sahaj Marg should be correctly understood and practised not only by our generation of abhyasis but also by future generations to come. Master is more concerned about the future generations of abhyasis. As far as the present generation is concerned, there is personal contact between the Master and his abhyasis. Because we have this advantage of direct personal contact with the Master, we have to consider ourselves as trustees of the system, holding it in trust for future generations to come. Master is, therefore, anxious that the present generation of abhyasis, that is all of us, should practise this system exactly as it is taught and prescribed; understand the Sahaj Marg system precisely as it should be understood; and thus preserve for our children, and for the children of our children, and their children, this unique system–this absolutely only system of attaining Reality which we have the privilege of having received direct from our Master.

So we have a double responsibility. It operates in two ways. We have to achieve the goal for ourselves, in our own lifetime; and we have to make the achievement of this same goal possible for future generations of mankind. That is, we have to consider ourselves as plants which not only produce grain or fruit for immediate consumption, but which also produce great quantities of seeds for planting acres and acres of the same crop for the future, again and again.

Master has emphasized in his message yesterday, that there is only one way; that there is only one goal; and that there is only one Master to lead us to that goal. Most of us have understood the fact that there is only one Master because we have physical contact with him, and it is patent that there is only one Shri Ram Chandraji

Lecture given at Munich on 22 May 1980.

of Shahjahanpur. It is, therefore, fairly easy for us to appreciate that physically there is only one Master. Still, sometimes, we tend to forget that the spiritual Master is also only one. We make the mistake of bringing in other sources of knowledge; other systems of practice; other systems of theology, etc., and thus dilute, and possibly entirely corrupt, our system. It is important to understand that though there may have been past Masters and past systems, they are not in the present and, therefore, are of no concern to us. Out of curiosity we may study their literature, etc., but if we practise any of those systems, the result can possibly be disastrous. It has specifically been stated that at any moment of time there can only be one such Master, not only here but in the whole universe. If we accept this statement, it follows that our Master is the only Master for the whole universe, in this particular epoch at least. It follows automatically that his way is the only way. It follows as a third point that his goal is our only goal. This leads to the inevitable conclusion that at any time there is only one Master, one goal and one way!

During our travels there has been much speculation as to whether there can be scientific approaches to Sahaj Marg. Science may have been a single discipline centuries ago; but today it is a hodgepodge, a mixture of multifarious disciplines, that goes by the name of science. All these disciplines have developed fantastically during the past fifty years or so. We have had intellectual giants who have penetrated into the mysteries of nature and of the universe in various disciplines. We have had great minds in the field of geology as also the biological and botanical sciences, all trying to penetrate into the secrets of the physical universe. We have had geniuses trying to probe beyond, far beyond, into the outer reaches of the universe–the astronomers! Quite recently some have tried to penetrate into the very heart of matter itself. These achievements in the material sphere are recorded and available to posterity; but in such records there is no mention of any spiritual achievements by these men of great genius that the past and the present generations have produced. We have also had the world of art–great painters, great sculptors–and if I have read their biographies correctly, many of them have led miserable existences, and have had no less miserable ends to their lives.

The field of scientific and artistic endeavour is one of gravity. The physical gravity of this earth holds us down here inexorably. There are other gravities equally dangerous. There are theologies and philosophies which similarly tend to hold us down, and prevent our rise to our spiritual goal. Please do not imagine for one moment that I am trying to decry even the smallest of the achievements in the fields of science, art, and philosophy. I have had some small familiarity with these disciplines, sufficient to give me an appreciation of the tremendous and truly magnificent achievements that human beings have made in these disciplines. At the same time, I have to say that I have not found anything of spiritual value in them. It is only during the last sixteen years of my association with my Master that I have been taught what spirituality is. Before I came to my Master, I had also practised very sincerely for some years, the various steps of hatha yoga – asanas, pranayama, mantra, meditation, etc. – but I only succeeded in making a psychic mess of my life. But for my Master's grace, I could very well have ended up in a mental home. It is his grace that he was able to extricate me from the shackles of my own foolish adventures into those dangerous fields.

It is my conclusion that no amount of research into the field of material science, whatever be the discipline, can ever lead one to spirituality. If somehow we can understand this, and we accept it in our understanding, then we are able to practise our system with this understanding embedded in us; then our acceptance of the Master and his method will be complete.

So I would request all of you not only to understand this properly, but to carry this understanding with you wherever you go. It is the duty, the most important duty, of our preceptors to see that this system is not diluted in any manner. If an abhyasi plays around with it, experimenting with it, well, he is jeopardizing only his personal spiritual welfare and his future. But if a preceptor plays about with the system, he plays not only with his own spiritual future but with the future of all the abhyasis given to his charge.

Preceptors are, in a very real way, the link between the Master and his abhyasis. Please note that I say **his** abhyasis. The abhyasis are his, not ours! This link is a very important link, because it must not interfere in any way with the transmission of Master's teachings and with the transmission of Master's transmission. Nor must there be any interference in the possibility of achieving the goal which Master offers to his abhyasis.

In accepting his own responsibility for the spiritual welfare of humanity, Master has taken upon himself tremendous burdens which we cannot even dream of. From the message he has given to us at Delhi, it is clear that preceptors have done very little to assist him in his work. Perhaps there is very little that they **can** do to assist him. But when we study what has been going on all around us, indeed is yet going on all around us–the dilution sought to be made in the system; the changes sought to be introduced; the teachings sought to be excluded on this or that consideration–it is very clear that much can be done by us to hamper his work and impede our own progress. It seems that our power to stop progress is much greater than our power to promote progress. I have always been concerned that the power to spread evil, the power to spread disease, the power to spread ignorance, this power seems to be so much more powerful than the power to do good. I asked Master about this once. Master smiled and said, "There is no such power, I mean evil power or power to do bad things. Our power acts in such ways because of the tendencies which guide the use of these powers. The tendencies are nothing but the working of our samskaras. It is, therefore, our own creation." This emphasizes the necessity for our own cleaning, both by ourselves in our daily routine as well as in cleaning sessions with preceptors.

We can understand very clearly that our grossness consists not merely of the impressions of past actions and past thoughts, but also of present actions and present thoughts; and much more importantly by the attachments we create for ourselves. I see that an engineer is **only** an engineer; a scientist is **only** a scientist; a psychologist is **only** a psychologist, and so on. These are also grossnesses. To put it very clearly in Master's own words, so long as we are not what we ought to be, there is always grossness. In Sahaj Marg the grossness of an engineer is no better than that of a chemist! The grossness of one who discharges his duties in a merely worldly sense is no better than the grossness of one who fails in his duties and obligations. Grossness is grossness. There is no such thing as good grossness and bad grossness. The nature of the grossness may decide the nature of our futures. But in Sahaj Marg, **the true future is the futureless future!** Social and educational conditioning makes us think that one who is educated is better than one who is not educated; that one who is higher up on the social ladder is therefore better than his social inferior. This makes us look up to educated people, cultured people, socially higher people as better people than those to whom these things have been denied. In Sahaj Marg, there is no such difference because every individual human being is a potential realiser of Reality. Master told me fourteen years ago, that it is easier for him to liberate a simple, uneducated person than a highly intellectual person, because the intellectual person has created for himself so many blocks.

Intellectuality demands research. We all do research in one way or the other. But the only correct way of research in spirituality is Master's way of research. Master often emphasizes this. In Sahaj Marg after one has achieved high stages of achievement, research is possible. Now the abhyasi knows what he has achieved, how it has been achieved, and so on. So he can do research. This is impossible at the lower levels. Master emphasizes this often.

In considering research, it is easy to make the mistake that experimentation will teach us everything. This is wrong. Master says that everything has its origin in the **mind** of the human being. We think; we brood deeply over what interests us, and then arrive at certain theories. Theories come first. It was by using his tremendous mental powers that Einstein evolved his brilliant theories of general and special relativity. Subsequent experimentation confirmed the truth and applicability of these theories. The experiments came **after** the theories had been formulated. Whatever be the nature of our achievement, they always originate in the mind. This is true whatever be the field of achievement. It is true of the arts as much as of the sciences, and no less true of spirituality. In fact in spirituality it is of paramount importance to realise this. It is wrong to think that the scientists are achieving what they achieve in a way different from achievements in spirituality. Both the scientist and the Sahaj Marg abhyasi work with the same instrument– the mind. The only difference is that the mind is turned towards a different field of endeavour. There is no difference between a road which goes from here to Frankfurt and a road which goes from here to Vienna. The difference is only in the direction one takes. If you think of the mind as a road, only the direction determines the destination or the goal we reach. It all depends on the direction.

It is for this reason that our Master has said that there is only one instrument available to us, whether it be for our annihilation or for our evolution to the Highest, and that is the mind. The mind is the sole instrument available to us. Master smiles and adds that liberation, realisation, all these things are so easy to achieve. "Just turn your mind from this to that," he says, "that is all that is necessary for this purpose." But from the way we are all struggling, it appears that it is not so easy. Why? Because we refuse to give up our attachments to our own personal ideas and disciplines. A doctor feels that he has spent so much money on educating himself to be a doctor. Another thinks that he has spent so many years working as an engineer. "How to give up all this?" is what they ask. Some people also ask, "Why cannot I accept Sahaj Marg and also hold on to all those other things?" Master says, "Well, I am telling you, if the powers of the mind are divided into many channels, no channel will get the full power. In each channel there will only flow a fraction of the power. So success cannot come, I mean complete success, in any of these fields. So what is the use? Select one and stick to that one. That may be anything, but it must be only one." This is the way of wisdom taught to me by my Master.

I am not at all suggesting that a Sahaj Marg abhyasi should not be an engineer, or a doctor or an artist. It is necessary for us to earn an honest living. However, the idea, the belief, that we can reach the goal through these scientific or artistic disciplines, **that idea must definitely be given up**. If our attachment to these material fields is given up, then, in a sense, our work in these fields becomes automatic. Master gives us the example of a sleeping person scratching himself without being aware either of the stimulus or of the response to it. A great advantage of this is that the idea of 'doer' is removed. One cannot say, "I did it," when we are not aware of having done it. Only requisite effort is used. There is no unnecessary waste of effort. Living adjusts itself. Sufficient energy is devoted to earning one's livelihood. One does not get obsessed with being a doctor, or an engineer or an intellectual. They fall into place in the overall scheme of things. To use Master's excellent example, we no longer use a crane to pick up a fallen needle! So we see that the canalization of the powers of the mind is of the utmost importance. The giving of a proper direction to the powers so canalized is of paramount importance. If these two are done, then the goal is at hand. Thank you.

Morality

Master's tour of Europe is coming to an end. As you all know, he is leaving tomorrow afternoon at three o'clock for India. On this trip, he has not been able to visit all the countries of Europe. Those of you who remember him from the last eight or nine years know that in 1972 he visited Egypt and then he travelled all over Europe. After that he went to England and then covered a small bit of the United States, after which he came back to Denmark for a second visit. He then travelled to some parts of Europe again and then fell sick in Germany. He was more sick in Italy and was almost on the point of collapse before finally returning to India. That was in 1972, and his tour then was of three months' duration.

In 1976 he came only to Europe. There were no visits in America. He did not visit England; nor was Cairo included. That trip lasted only six weeks. On that occasion Master came straight to Denmark. Then he went all over Europe and finally came back to Denmark. In between he fell ill in Switzerland, and this almost necessitated cancellation of all his travel plans. Then he staged a miraculous recovery, completed his trip and then returned to India.

His third tour abroad was to Malaysia and Singapore for a period of four weeks. That was in 1977. After about eighteen days in Petaling Jaya, a suburb of Kuala Lumpur, he had a minor accident and dislocated his left shoulder. He had to be in bed for three days. Once again we were on the verge of cancelling the tour and going home. However, he had a quick recovery and went on to fulfil his engagements before returning to India.

This is his fourth tour outside India, and this time it is only for one month. He has been able to visit only two centres in Europe this time—Copenhagen and Munich. As we all know, his condition

Lecture given on 4 June 1980 at Copenhagen.

has been such as to cause us all a certain amount of anxiety. But this morning he has staged a miraculous recovery, as usual, and is going back home tomorrow evening.

On all these four travels of his, he has been emphasizing that Sahaj Marg is a community where people come together, all over the world, with the sole purpose of spiritual growth and spiritual evolution. This emphasis was not felt so much in 1972 because it was an introductory tour and perhaps he did not want to emphasize too much those things which might be considered as major sacrifices by the people of the West. He just sort of skimmed over the surface, and let it go at that. In 1976, the advices he gave to the abhyasis were more pointed, the conditions for sadhana were a little more stringent. He introduced principles governing our normal daily life such as the need to obey at least some of the Ten Maxims; the essential need for good behaviour; the essential need for good-brotherliness and sisterliness among the abhyasis; not to harm or hurt others by our talk or by our deeds–things like that, which come under the norms of behaviour and ethical principles.

Now for the last three years he has been emphasizing very much the need for morality–including the prohibition of alcoholic drinks too. Some of our American brothers asked me the other day when we had a meeting, "Chari, how is it that he did not tell us these things in 1972? Why is he talking all of a sudden in 1980 about these things?" The only answer to this question is that when we bring up children, we give them a great deal of love and a great deal of freedom when they are young. But as they grow up they are expected to conform to more and more discipline and slowly come up to the norms of adult behaviour. They have to behave like adults. They have been given facilities to acquire knowledge and training and are therefore expected to behave in conformity with the principles laid down for adults. They are expected to know better than children. So we in Sahaj Marg have been treated by the Master in 1972, and the years before that, very much as children in the school of yoga, and he has given us all his love without much of these rules and regulations, obedience to which could not be expected from us at that time. You don't make such demands of children!

When a child becomes a youth of say sixteen years, there is still a great deal of freedom, but not as much of it as one had when one was six years old. But when one touches forty, one is expected to be fully mature, to know what he is doing–what is good for him, what is bad for him–and what his responsibilities are. He has now to participate in the building up of a society of which he is a part. Ours is such a society. Now we have wisdom; we have knowledge; and we have ability. It is now that there is the greatest possibility of doing good–or bad. At that stage if we go bad, well, as the English proverb says, "There is no fool like an old fool." When we are young it is expected that we will do some foolish things. But when we grow up, we are no longer expected to be foolish in our ways. We in Sahaj Marg, at least here in Europe, are quite young. No one here has been in Sahaj Marg for more than ten years. We can be considered to be entering the stage of youth in yogic life. This is the stage when we have to enter that stage of life when we have to be educated, disciplined, trained in following the ethical rules, the commandments of morality and last, but not least, we have to be trained to know what is good for us and what is bad for us.

It is for this reason that I think Master is slowly introducing us to these concepts of ethics, moral behaviour, etc., which, after all, are nothing new. They have been shouted from the mountain tops all over the world, literally and figuratively, for thousands of years. When we rebel against them, it is only because we have been flouting them for so long. Now when we are re-exposed to them, it is as if one is suddenly plunged into a pool of cold water. There is a shock! But every one of us knows inside that these principles are very important and very necessary.

Most of you would have read some philosophy. You will remember the Kantian ethic concerning the dilemma whether a particular thing should be done or not. Kant ways when in doubt, one should universalize the proposed activity. If everybody in the world did it, would it be good for humanity? It if is, then do it; if not, don't! Now why I am giving this preamble, showing Master's step-by-step development in his approach to us, is to show you that his teachings have not changed over the years. If you study his teachings clearly, all these points are already there in his books, his articles, his speeches, his messages, etc. The only thing that he is now doing is that he is shifting the emphasis from the lower level to the higher levels. I am very glad about this. I am also very proud about it because it shows that we here, in Europe, are growing to a level where he can give us the higher teachings that he has so far **withheld** from us. It is a sign of growth–our growth–when more demands are made upon us; when more discipline is imposed upon us; when more is expected from us as individuals, as individual Sahaj Margis, if I may use that term! It only shows that he sees in us that growth which now enables him to ask from us these things.

A father doesn't ask his little child for money! After all it is the father who is paying for the child's food, clothing and education. But when the son starts earning himself, and the father asks him for some money, the son may not like it. He may say, "Well! The old man never asked me for any money before this. All of a sudden he is asking me for some now." The son may resent such demands from the father. Most sons do! But the father asks precisely because he is now sure that his son has now come to a stage where he can give what is asked of him. Our father here is asking from his sons for more things. Now such an asking is not an imposition upon us. Please understand this very clearly. They are not impositions; they are not regulations; they are not restrictions upon our freedom. But they are things which a spiritual father is entitled to ask from those whom he considers his youthful, grown-up children. And I am sure that this tendency to expect more and more of and from us will grow in future years.

In his latest message at Delhi he has emphasized that he has been working alone single-handed ever since he started this spiritual work of his. There is a cry of pain in his heart that there is nobody who has developed to a level where he can help him in his work.

Now, it is not unwise on his part, or unusual on his part, to expect that every one of us would rise to his level. After all that is his work. Many of you are teachers. You don't expect only one child in your class to pass the examinations! One would be ashamed of such a teacher. More than that, we should be ashamed of such a school, and the school authorities should be ashamed of such a teacher. Isn't it? So the teacher is entitled to seek of every student in the class that he should rise to that level of expectation which the boards of education demand; for which the teacher is teaching them; and for which after all, the student has enrolled himself in the school.

We have joined Sahaj Marg not to be childish, not to be flippant, not to have that freedom which is license–mistaken freedom– but we have come here for spiritual growth which presupposes external changes in behaviour, in ethical and moral living, etc. The excuse is all too often advanced that our society is made that way; so how can we change? But if you look back sixty years, your society was not as it is today. If you go back a few hundred years, you will find that a Victorian code of ethics and morality prevailed– it was much more stringent. How does society change? Society does change, as we have seen. It changes because one individual enforces that change, and makes the change possible. Those were changes in a small, restricted society, applying possibly to a few hundred thousand people or to a few million people. But what our Master is seeking to do today with our co-operation is to change the world itself. It is not only for the Victorians, or the Danes and the French. It is a total change for the whole of humanity. It is a total change of humanity that he is seeking. If the change is piecemeal, we get a society which is like bad toast, raw bread on one side and burnt on the other. Nobody will eat it. Our human society has been all along good in parts, bad in most of it–for one reason or another. Every society had in it something that was good and much that was bad. This is true of all countries, of all societies, all over the world through the history of humanity.

Now, here is a person who has undertaken the fantastic task–I would say almost impossible task–it is fantastic when looking at the task, it seems impossible when looking at us–but a great and glorious task looking at his achievements. We have seen what he **can** and what he **has** achieved. So his is a great and glorious task, a fantastic task and an almost impossible task all in one. It can be a success only if we offer our hearts to him in humble co-operation.

Now, it has been a disappointing feature of Sahaj Marg that in most places in the West, the Sahaj Marg society, whether it is a small one of ten abhyasis or a large one of two hundred abhyasis, is becoming converted into some sort of a social club where people meet to gossip. They meet not for the higher purposes of spiritual growth but for the lower ones of gossiping, of exchanging friendships, of exchanging so many other things which I would not like to talk about. It has become a market place. The commandment which says that we should not steal what belongs to another is broken in human relationships themselves.

Any institution can be created for the highest purpose, but in it the students can go for drugs and things like that and thus debase themselves, corrupt themselves, and possibly destroy themselves as well! It is not the fault of the school. It is the fault of the students. You can have a government where the highest ideals are laid down, but people lower them or totally trample them under their feet. A society can be free and noble, cherishing the highest values of human existence, or it can be corrupted and destroyed by the members of the society themselves.

The Sahaj Marg society is no different. The teachings of the Master are there before us. The values he wishes us to bring into our lives are there. The ideals are before us. And if we want to see what **can** be achieved, we have very fortunately still before us the Master himself to show us in his person, in his way of life, in his spiritual attainment of the Highest, what can be achieved. If we debase ourselves and convert this society into a house of gossip, where human beings are traded one for the other, and where the very roots of culture are being destroyed, and families are being broken up–it is a very unfortunate thing indeed.

We are playing with people. We are playing with other people's hearts as if they were billiard balls. Billiard balls are made of hard ivory or plastic. They can stand all the knocking about and the shocks that they are subjected to. The human heart is not like that. And in this process, we forget that we are playing with the biggest and softest heart in all creation, the heart of the Master. We do not realise or understand how every single action of ours contributes to his health, or destroys it. I am not speculating when I say this. You can see this for yourself. There are places where even if you throw him down, he will bounce back like a rubber ball. There are other places where he is sick from the moment he enters it. And what is it that contributes to his health or his sickness? It is nothing but the atmosphere we create around ourselves. I do not think any one of us is deliberately doing this. We all love the Master too much not to want him to be peaceful and healthy, and what we wish for most of all is to have him with us for as long as we possibly can. But what are we to do if we fail in the smallest things he requires of us?

The moulding of our behaviour, of our activities, the proper way of living a family life–these are the least things, things at the lowest level of our existence. These are the least things he can ask of us. These are things that we ourselves teach to our children. Every one of you is a father or a mother. You all know this. But what are we to do when adults themselves break down and seek to destroy that which they expect their own children to build? When adults themselves break down because in their utter selfishness they forget that the family life is what is important–not their own selfish desires and hungers of the body which we are seeing all around us– what are we to do? Such adults not only destroy themselves but also destroy the future about which Master has been emphasizing in his Delhi message, and again in Munich.

Master has repeated, again and again, the statement, "My teachings are difficult to understand today, not because I have made them difficult but because they have been designed and recorded for posterity." Yesterday he gave us an example to explain this. He pointed out that at the time the Vedas were written, only a few must have understood them. Today, after thousands of years have passed since they were written, there are scholars who know and understand them thoroughly, and many ordinary persons also understand them. So Master's teachings are for the future. Our presence in the present, and our good fortune in receiving the teaching direct from him, in having his guidance at every step of our sadhana, in being able to talk about and discuss his teachings and practice with him, this is an immense good fortune which we seem not to appreciate.

Those who possess valuable things rarely cherish them. We are forgetting the wonderful things we have, even discarding them thoughtlessly, and casting our covetous and lustful eyes on what is not ours. This is true whether it be objects or persons. We never value what we have, and foolishly seek what others have. This is most disappointing, not merely for us but for the Master. It is very important to realise this. If the Master becomes really disappointed, and he becomes really distressed, it will be a big tragedy for us. Forget yourselves. Think of your children! I think we all love our children too much to see their future destroyed. Who would like to see his children parentless, miserable, becoming a drug addict himself and thus adding to his already unbearable miseries–forgetting family, forgetting society, indeed forgetting humanity itself–all because the parents gave him nothing but a broken home full of misery, full of insecurity and without a foundation of love and security on which alone a child builds up its own existence? I don't think any of us really wish for such things to happen. Many of you perhaps suffered all these things too vividly in your own younger years to want this miserable fate to descend upon your children.

If we want to see ourselves in a safe and sane society living in a moral society full of spiritual values, contributing to human growth and development in peace and harmony with all around us, without one seeking to steal from the other; without one seeking to rob from the other or kill the other; then we have to create such a society for ourselves in our own lifetime. If we are unable to create such a society, then what will be the society that our children will inherit from us? We all have our failings. Our children are watching us all the time. Our children are much wiser than us. They seem to know intuitively what is going on. If this is the tradition, if these are the sets of values we are going to pass on to our children, what is going to happen to the future? Even in such a short span as thirty years or fifty years, what is the future going to be like? So this is not a plaything. Our lives are not playthings, and Sahaj Marg is not a joke, a plaything for us to play with.

If we are to follow Master's teachings, the minimum we have to do is to ensure that at least our own Sahaj Marg society is not corrupted. In a good brotherhood, we should not rob each other.

But unfortunately this is what seems to be happening. The very growth of Sahaj Marg seems to be a menace for its own existence. The growth in numbers seems to offer us more choice. When there are just two or three of us, there is very little that we can do. But when there are five hundred of us, well, the scope for internal dissension and mutual misbehaviour on all levels, including the moral level, is increased. And this seems to be unfortunately the case in some places. It is a shame that we, in our own society, where each one of us is supposed to be trying to achieve the highest ideal of spiritual growth and development, we ourselves contribute to the debasement of our own society. Is it not something that we should weep over? We should weep for shame.

We all say we love the Master. We try to help him, we try to serve him in as many ways as we can. But what is the one thing he wants of us? It is our own growth. He does not want anything else from us. He does not want money. He does not want food. He wants none of these things. He says all that he wants is that we should grow into what he wants us to become. That is his satisfaction, and the fulfilment of his work. If in this we cannot support the Master and contribute to his happiness, then we are failures–total failures. I don't think any teacher or guru should ask less of us. We see them all around us. They seem to ask only for their own welfare, their own comfort and prosperity. They ask for our money, for our physical services and so on, all for their own benefit, not for ours.

Here our Master is only saying, "Please accept my services so that you can become what I have become." I don't think there can be a cheaper transaction than this, in which the very universe is offered to us in exchange for the pittance of a human heart. I deliberately say "pittance" because by our behaviour we have shown what little there is of the **heart** in our hearts. People who can trade hearts at the drop of a handkerchief–I don't believe they have hearts. They have only something else pretending to be a heart. Such persons have yet to develop that which we call a heart.

These are the few thoughts that I wished to place before you in clear and unambiguous terms before Master leaves for India. I am only telling you what the Master wishes to say but is unwilling to speak about. So on his behalf I have tried to explain to you the contents of his two messages given at Delhi and Munich. Our abhyasis have found it so difficult to understand them. Master speaks in veiled and allegorical terms. I once asked him why he doesn't tell people in direct terms what they should and should not do. He answered, "If I give them such direct instructions and they don't obey them, then they are adding one more sin–the sin of disobedience of the Master. Then they really commit two sins–the first one about which I have to instruct them, and the second one the disobedience of the Master's instructions. I do not like to impose this upon them. So I don't give direct instructions to abhyasis."

So, this is the great charity of the Master, that he does not give us orders and instructions because he does not want to burden us with the sin of disobedience of the Master. So please don't expect direct advice. Master never advises directly. Don't expect personalized advice. He never says, "Mr. X, you don't do this." He only says things in a general way, and we should be alert and take up what applies to us. This is his way. He does not want to hurt our feelings by referring to our weaknesses and failings in a direct manner. Also advice given in a general way benefits every one of us.

So we must understand the Master's ways and his methods. We must understand how he behaves with us. Perhaps he is not a gentleman in the sense in which the English language understands it. But if ever there was a true gentleman he is it, precisely because he demands nothing while offering everything. He conveys his message and his thoughts and ideas on bits of paper upon which he scrawls these things for us. He is a gentleman precisely because he does not want anything of us–he asks for no money, he asks for no physical services; he does not ask for our obedience as we have just seen, and he does not want from us even our good wishes! He makes no demands of individuals, of society, not even of God Himself! This is my observation. Why? Precisely because he has risen to that level where such demands are unnecessary for his existence.

He does not need anything. But a man who needs nothing whatever, and who is willing to give us everything–if we have the good fortune to have such a person in our midst, and having him in our midst we waste our time in flippant activities, attending merely to the base and petty needs of the body, indulging in cheap romances and things like that–I again repeat that it is the greatest tragedy of the individual and, by contribution, the greatest tragedy of our society and our people.

I entreat you all to think over these things deeply. We make no demands. These are things which had to be said, which have to be understood, and most important, which have to be acted upon. The Master is there to give us the strength for all this. He gives us the teachings; he gives us the wisdom to understand them; and he also gives us the will power to act upon his teachings. He gives us all this so that we may develop to what he holds up before us as the highest ideal of human development. Thank you!

The Principles of Sahaj Marg

Volume 2

Sahaj Marg and the Problems of Personality

It is rather difficult to attempt a precise and brief definition of the word 'personality', except to say that it is the sum total of a man's behaviour pattern as apparent to an observer. The word personality itself is derived from, I believe, the Greek word *persona*, meaning mask, and when so derived, personality would mean the 'mask' or 'face' that an individual puts out to the world, or which he exposes to view. There are several modern shades of meaning ascribed to the word personality, including appearance, grooming, smartness, mood and so on, and perhaps some definitions also include mental states. However, broadly speaking, personality can be considered to be the something that is reflected in a person's appearance-cum-behaviour, and may be said to be the result of the interplay of two main factors, namely heredity and environment.

Psychology tells us that a man's exterior is conditioned by his interior, not in a physical sense of course, though that also can be true in certain cases, but in terms of a mental approach. That is, the man's mind makes of him what he is, or what he appears to be to the external world. It would be true to say that a man's personality is like an iceberg which reveals but a fraction of its totality for outside exhibition, and hides the largest part of its bulk from public gaze under the surface of the ocean. That this is true can be easily seen in everyone's personal experience of his relatives, friends and of such other humans with whom one is thrown into association in his life, however brief and superficial that association may be.

We are invariably made to wonder at how different a person appears to be on close association with him, as compared to what he appeared to be when first met or on casual acquaintance. It is perhaps right to point out at this stage that it is hardly ever one's

Reprinted from *Sahaj Marg and Personality Problems & Yoga Psychology and Modern Physiological Theories.*

own fault, because the person observed, or one who is being cultivated, rarely reveals the truth about himself until the casual acquaintance has ripened into something more solid and lasting to form the basis of personal confidence and uninhibitedness of behaviour.

This is as far as the personality of others in one's own experience is concerned. To bring the problem of personality to one's own door, as it were, it is a fair statement to say that probably no individual exists who has not, at one time or another, been surprised by his own thoughts or actions. In fact, in the ordinary run of humanity such a state of affairs is perhaps all too common, and perhaps forms the basis of self-hate and self-condemnation which, in the final analysis, is the cause of man hating brother man and condemning his brother. It is a fact of psychology that at the root of all man's troubles with brother man, and with his own environment, lies this suspicion and hatred of himself.

Man, it is said, is nothing but a cultured animal, and that culture is nothing but a thin and inadequate veneer superimposed on him by a demanding civilization, and through which the leashed animal is ever waiting and straining to break out into its uninhibited freedom permitted by the jungle law out of which it has evolved, but not yet outgrown.

It is, therefore, amply apparent that not only are personality problems ever present in one's relation to the external world, but such problems are perhaps more numerous and immediate, and demanding of solution in one's relation to oneself. It is here that the crux of the matter lies, and here is the psychological breeding ground of all the hate, tensions, frustration, jealousies and rivalries that today plague human existence at all levels of society, and within mutually excluding barriers of race, religion, tongue, culture, etc. It is with this latter aspect of problems of personality, that is of man's problems in relation to himself, that we here in this Mission are mainly concerned.

Man's problems are multifarious and enormous. There is firstly the problem of survival, of keeping body and soul together in an essentially hostile world. Secondly, there is the problem of existence, that is, once survival is made possible, to live in comfort and security. There is, thirdly, the ever-present problem of mutual coexistence with the members of one's own family, of one's own community, society and, in fact, this problem has attained intercommunal and international or global significance and importance in the last few decades.

Today's world is a world of maladjustment at every level of human intercourse, and of social and communal intercourse. It is a world composed of a conglomerate and seething mass of humanity split up into states or nations on a basis of geography, race, culture, religion, language or some such artificiality. What is of significance is that whatever be the reason, people are divided into camps and clans and they are tense against each other, and mutually warring. At the same time a veneer of so-called civilization makes it necessary for the individual to hide or mask his basic attitudes of aggression and tension under an externally assumed attitude of friendliness, cheerfulness and trust. This only serves to aggravate the internal tension further, because of the further strain imposed by such an attitude on an already over-strained existence. The remedy is worse indeed than the disease!

When we analyze the reasons for the existence of tensions we find that they are due basically to emotions of hate and fear, and to frustration. The so-called primitives also have these basic emotions, but with them fear is a legitimate fear of things one had to be afraid of, if one were to continue to exist. They hated with a pure hatred which left no burden on the conscience, and the need for which was again conditioned by the need to survive. They were, therefore, happily free of all the psychosis and neurosis which bedevil modern human existence. This is a picture of human existence as it is even today.

Man has, at least until very recently, customarily and naturally tended to turn to God for the easing of his conscience, and therefore of his tensions. Religion was thought to be the force which could relieve man of all, or at least most, of his sufferings, and religions perhaps did effectively cater to this important need of the human individual to some extent.

That modern living gives the lie to this belief or assumption is perhaps an uncharitable way of looking at the part that religions have played hitherto. But it is nevertheless true that religions, as they exist today, no longer appear capable of functioning as the principal organization, capable of relieving man of his miseries and tensions. This is largely because religions have tended to play upon man's emotions in keeping their hold upon him. They have invariably used two effective tools in maintaining their stranglehold upon the individual and society. These have been fear and temptation. Religions have alternately played upon these two notes holding out the temptation of a glorious heaven to be attained, or a terrible fear of eternal damnation in a hell full of brimstone and pitch. This attitude of the religions has, if anything, increased man's problems to almost insoluble levels since, apart from being made a hypocrite to all and to himself, he has been given the necessity of approaching even the Creator Himself in a hypocritical manner. There is no love for God in his heart, but only a horrible and ever-present fear of Him. Religions whose prime role is that of connecting man to God, have actually turned him away from Him, and can therefore be taken to have dismally failed in the fulfilment of the only function for which they exist. I do not think that anybody will dispute the fact that religious worship, or worship by external symbols and rituals of an externalized God, is kept alive by nothing except fear of a God whom we do not know, and a feeble hope of attaining a heaven which we do not understand.

Sahaj Marg, the modified system of raja yoga rediscovered by Samarth Guru Shri Ram Chandraji Maharaj of Fatehgarh, and now being offered to the whole world by our divine and beloved Master Shri Ram Chandraji Maharaj of Shahjahanpur, seeks to solve this problem in a unique manner by adopting the technique of *pranahuti* of yogic transmission, whereby the thought power of the Supreme Master is transmitted into the heart of the abhyasi. The immediate result, almost at the very first sitting with the Master or a preceptor of the Mission, is a feeling of peace and lightness. This has been confirmed again and again by innumerable abhyasis from their own personal experience of this method of sadhana.

It is a matter of fact that a de-tensioning is effected by loosening the knots of tension in the psychic area which immediately bestows upon the abhyasi a peace such as he has never known before. This is a total effect upon the personality, and not piecemeal efforts aimed at one or the other phases of it. Worry born of frustration and indecision are perhaps the first to go. Fear follows soon after, or if it is deep-rooted, it nevertheless leaves some time later– of this there is no doubt. I have heard Dr. Varadachari quoting, time and again, that famous sloka *Abhayam sarvabhutebhyo dadami, etat vratam mama*. I was never able to appreciate the deep significance of this utterance, and the great need for the fearlessness which the Lord promises here, until fear became the one obsessive emotion in my own life. That I am in the main rid of this is the greatest testimony that I can personally offer for the efficacy of this unique system of Sahaj Marg. The greatness and remarkable nature of the transformation is multiply enhanced when it is pointed out that change has gone almost un-noticed. I remember Dr. Varadachari once saying that all of God's activities are carried out in anonymity, and this I regard as the greatest testimony to His humility and that of my Master, that man can be helped without any humiliation for the gift received being imposed upon him.

We see, therefore, that under this system, attitudes of fear, indecision, worry, frustration all give place to changes of deep import and permanent nature, effected by the divine force and power of the pranahuti, giving in a relatively short time a person who now possesses courage, faith, and a sublime peace that pervades not merely the period set apart for meditation but his whole sleeping and waking existence; an individual who is adjusted to himself, to his immediate circle of family and friends, and to his environment. Such a person is an asset, for, by the change in his personality and attitudes to life, he is now capable of depth of thought, skill in action, courage in deeds, and all this so naturally and effortlessly, because they are not volitional but spontaneous. That is, his transformed human make-up is geared to these things and so it is natural to him.

It is important to note that these vital personality changes are effected without the abhyasi's knowledge, or effort on his part. There is no giving up of this or that, no heart-wrenching renunciation, no unnatural and ineffective anonymity imposed by name changes or adoption of specific garbs. Here in Sahaj Marg the force of the Supreme Master's transmission achieves all these permanent changes, changes of an irreversible nature, by seeking from the abhyasi nothing except co-operation in letting the force work upon him. Indeed, all that is necessary is **not** to impede or hamper the working of the force. Peace and harmony are easily established within the individual without any strain or tension. The entire spectrum of human personality is transformed by normalizing all the contributory or structural facets of that personality, and such a normalization restores the individual to his original nature which is one of repose in God with love, faith and surrender.

Superstition and Spirituality

Superstition is something very difficult to understand, both in its working upon the individual human mind–and through him of society–and the conceptual and emotional foundations upon which it rests and which subserve its working. That perhaps every single human being inhabiting the globe is superstitious in some way or other–some quirk of thought, some often surreptitious behaviour pattern and generally some religious or social observance–cannot possibly be open to denial. The only differences capable of arising out of a consideration of this supposition give an answer to the questions: What really constitutes superstition? What is really this superstition which is so little understood and yet almost universally prevalent and which, where it exists, makes the volitional and functional aspects of the human mind so slavishly subservient to its powerful and often ineradicable influence–an influence almost subterranean and primordial both in respect of its location in the human system and in its depth of functioning? It would be right to consider it almost a part of man's mental *terra incognita*–that part which Jung calls the collective unconscious. To understand superstition these questions must be answered as fully as possible and in a manner which must seek to define the areas of penetration, influence and function.

Superstition is commonly thought to consist of that area of human beliefs (and consequent actions) which are founded not on proven facts or on established cause-effect relationships of phenomena, but which relate to feelings of "excessive reverence or fear based on ignorance" (Chambers' Dictionary) and particularly relating to an individual's religious beliefs and rituals, and to some extent his social customs arising out of, or even entirely divorced from, such religious beliefs. Such beliefs are, therefore, widely held to be irrational and consequently form the subject of scorn and scathing criticism from the more educated and sophisticated minds, particularly the Western or European intellect. Such criticism is certainly valid and necessary, too, to clear the human mind of its cobwebs of a primitive and naturistic part but a wider examination will show that superstitions are not exclusively ancient beliefs. We have modern ones, too, and to this class the Western mind would appear to be susceptible, as these beliefs have a veneer of truth or apparent truth on them. That science does away with the need for God is one such; that better and better standards of material life can give more and more happiness is another; that love before marriage can ensure its blissful continuity after marriage or to put it in another way, that there can be no love after marriage if one does not love before marriage, is a third one; that education also cultures the educated individual is a fourth; that eating with metallic implements is cleaner and more hygienic than using one's fingers is yet another. Such examples can be many but what is commonly not appreciated is that these are as much superstitious beliefs as any that we suffer from in the Orient because there is no rationality behind them.

Superstition seems to change from time to time, i.e., once held beliefs are dropped and new ideas taken up. Also certain superstitions have subsequently become scientific facts (the earth revolving around the sun). So, where to draw the line is the question. Whatever it be, its hold is based either on fear of retribution arising out of non-performance of certain acts or rituals or on the hope of beneficial results arising out of the performance of such acts. The former preys on fear while the latter exploits man's incorrigible tendency to hope.

I have had my personal quota of such unreasoning fears and unrealised hopes, though perhaps the ordinary social and religious ones did not affect me as much as they affected others. Mine have broadly been confined to:

·The normal negative ones of fear of retribution arising out of non-performance of religious rituals: this I got rid of very easily as these superstitions were not deeply ingrained in my mind.

·What I may call 'futuristic' fears, arising out of a basic and fundamental fear of the future–a feeling of hopelessness resulting from awful imagination of losing one's job, etc.: I had a definite fear of the *dakshinayana* (the six months of the year of the sun's southern transit)

·A very deep and totally inexplicable fear of death and, strangely enough, not of my own death but of that of other loved ones. I would like to explain here that even though I am swayed by fear as an abstract emotion, I have never been afraid of my own death at any stage of my life. I have, however, been terrified, mostly during sleepless nights, of some near and dear one dying on my hands as it were.

I must relate here an incident which occurred a few years ago. I was staying in a double room in a hotel sharing the room with a colleague of mine. I woke up at five-thirty in the morning after a good night's sleep and found my colleague lying on his bed in what appeared to me to be an unnatural and death-like posture. The thought appeared in my mind that he was dead and this so terrified me that I started shivering physically and rushed towards the window to throw myself out–it was a room on the fifth floor. As I touched the window sill some sane instinct urged me to touch him and see if he were really dead. I struggled back to his bed and, with great fear, just touched him when he immediately woke up. Instantaneously I was normal and to this day my friend does not know that he saved me from suicide. I would like to reiterate that this is not just fear but a superstitious feeling that someone will die when I am there and this fear is less when more people are with me and is exaggerated when I am alone with just one other person. Until recently this fear was so obsessive that I frequently woke up at night to verify whether the person was dead or alive by observing whether the chest moved or not in breathing.

After I came to the feet of my Master in March, 1964, the first thing I confided to him were these abnormal and obsessive fears which threatened to ruin my life. He promised to help me. The first few months of sadhana eradicated all my religious and social superstitions and I am no longer bound to these. The second ones relating to the future also have disappeared. I am now confident that the future holds no evil or destructive potency and that it can hold nothing but good. The third did not disappear so easily, nor has it gone even now.

However, the Master's grace has worked wonders. Late in 1967 when he visited Madras, he casually asked me, "How are your fear problems now? I hope you do not suffer as you used to." I replied that though there was improvement, most of it yet remained. He said, "I have removed most of it but perhaps some shadow of it remains. Please sit in meditation." He transmitted to me for about twenty-five minutes. I got deeply absorbed and just before the end, I felt a dark face, a replica of my own, detaching itself from me and moving off sideways. I told Master the experience and he said, "I have removed everything, but still something may remain–the memory of fear itself and that you must avoid."

Since then I am a changed man. I no longer look about me for corpses to be terrified of. I sleep calmly. Occasionally, fear does come but it is not fear as such but a fear that I may be afraid, if such and such a thing should happen–that is, it is a fear that I may be afraid. When this happens I put my mind on Master's words and it immediately goes. The grosser fears have gone, but I expect complete freedom from such superstitious fears will come only when the cleaning process under Sahaj Marg has gone to the deepest sources of human samskaras–but come it must! The Sahaj Marg method with its 'triple-effect' transmission (to quote Dr. Varadachari, it is like Singer Oil, three-in-one) has cleaned me of all impurities, though within the scope of this symposium superstition is the subject. Under the guidance of Master and by His supreme grace, freedom of a total nature, impossible to even conceive a few years ago, seems now within sight.

Worship

The word worship has several meanings and among these the important ones are: to adore as Divine; regarding with adoration; reverent homage or service paid to God; and to be full of adoration. The act of worship therefore implies the recognition or consciousness of One to whom such worship is offered. A worship which does not have an object to worship is therefore a futile act.

The forms to which worship has tended, have kept pace with the development of human consciousness, and can be traced from the dim beginnings in animism, through worship of nature, spiritism, totemism, and on through ancestor worship, culminating in the present-day forms of worship in most religions where some form of personal deity is the object of worship. It therefore seems to be a law of nature that the way or method of worship should conform to the development of man, and where it does not conform, then a necessary conclusion would appear to be that man is a slave to the past, and has not risen to his full stature, whatever that may be.

Prayer, on the contrary, is generally thought to mean some form of formula used in praying, that is, a solemn request to God for something that one desires or seeks. In Sahaj Marg terminology prayer is equated with begging. Our Master has often said that "Prayer is begging whereas meditation is receiving." It is therefore clear that prayer and worship are not synonymous and do not imply the same relationship to the object of worship. Unfortunately, in the modern connotation, this has come to be so, at least in the generality of human understanding.

It is significant that at the summit of all world religions there is an exclusion or abandonment of ritualistic forms and modes of worship, and an effort is made to raise up the level of one's rela-

Reprinted from *Sahaj Marg* magazine of March 1971.

tionship with the Creator to a purely mental level, and thereafter, to the higher levels of spiritual understanding, being and identification. This form of approach to one's Creator is what is understood in the commonly used term 'mysticism', which therefore separates it from religion by eschewing the traditional forms of ritualistic and externalized worship of the deity. Mysticism transcends religion by seeking to establish a contact with the Immanent Divinity and since the Immanent is in the heart of all created things, the outer forms fall off by themselves. In the practice of meditation under the Sahaj Marg system this is what is attempted and achieved by most of the aspirants under our Master.

I have been frequently asked why there should be an eschewal of traditional disciplines and modes, and why the two, viz., meditation and traditional worship, cannot go on side by side. One stock answer, of course, is that when a higher and more enlightened form of association with the Ultimate is available, it would not only be superfluous but unwise to stick to lower forms which can drag one down from the higher level. But the real answer to this question came during a discussion some three years ago with Dr. K. C. Varadachari at Tirupathi, when some strong adherents of temple worship were present and put this question to the Doctor. Dr. Varadachari then explained that in the ancient days when temples were established, these were expected or designed to take the place of a guru to that large mass of humanity to which a personal living guru was not available, or to whom they had no access because of their level of spiritual development. It was customary to take one's child at a stipulated age to the temple and have its head shaved, signifying an act of surrender to the Divine, and at that stage the child was thought to be initiated by the Presence in the temple. The deity in the temple thereafter became the Ishta-Devata for the child, and as the child grew up, it was expected of him that he would meditate upon his Ishta-Devata, who in essence symbolized the presence of the guru, and thereby achieve the mystic path of worship leading to Realisation.

Temples, or rather the idols in the temples, were said to have been charged by great masters, and it was this charge or power which made possible this initiation. There was, therefore, no need to make repeated visits to temples after this solemn act of initiation had been achieved by surrender. A further point made was that in those days temples, or at least the more important ones, were in such out of the way places and accessible with such great difficulty, that a second visit was often completely precluded.

A second question arose as to why certain temples prosper and attract millions of devotees, whereas there are hundreds of other temples where one today finds only bats, owls and snakes. Dr. Varadachari gave a very illuminating and scientific reply and drew an analogy with the half-life period of radioactive material. He said that temples were initially charged by the masters who did the charging in such a way that the temples had power and authority over a definite extent geographically and temporally. When the power ceased to operate, the temples fell into disuse and became mere archaeological relics.

It is now amply clear that without a great master to charge temples, the temples by themselves have no meaning whatsoever, and that when a Master capable of charging anyone or anything by transmission is available to personally charge not only the material objects like idols but even the human heart itself, it would be the height of folly to desert the Master for the temple. It is well known in traditional religion that objects of worship in temples have to be sanctified by what is known as the *prana prathishta*, and unless this has been done there is no sense in worshipping any material object.

It is also important, at least in the case of newly erected temples, to know whether such prana prathishta is really done, which in effect means seeking to know whether the person who did the prana prathishta had the power of transmission. Without a great Master capable of transmitting the Divine essence, the prana prathishta cannot happen irrespective of the ceremonial or ritualistic forms associated with this act.

It is therefore necessary to understand what precisely our Master is doing, and how it is nothing but this very same prana prathishta now being done to human individuals, thereby converting such individuals into temples of God. In essence, therefore, what is done during transmission is to put Divinity back into the heart of the individual where it really belongs, and thus remove man's dependence from external objects and put it back within himself.

In meditation, the adoration is therefore directed to one's own heart, to the Divinity present therein, and by this act of transcendental worship the divinisation of the human being, in whom such a seed has been sown, is made possible, progressively and rapidly, to culminate in the ultimate achievement of total divinisation of the person.

Sadhana

I have been having some thoughts on what sadhana really means, particularly during the last one year, which I would like to place before you.

All human endeavour may be considered as consisting of two factors: first, the aim or the goal of the endeavour and second, the way of achieving that aim, i.e., the *lakshya* and the *upaya*. Either of these alone will be useless because any goal without knowledge of the means or the way to achieve it remains unachievable, and also knowledge of the way without knowing what goal we are aiming for is useless. It is, therefore, necessary that we have very clearly fixed in our minds the goal which we are aiming for, and strictly follow the path or the method which alone can lead to the goal.

Unfortunately, particularly in established religious systems, we find that very often the goal is lost sight of, and the practice or the formal ritual itself becomes the aim. This sort of practice may at the most give satisfaction that some sort of duty has been done, but nothing more. A more dangerous development is that such satisfaction in the fulfilment of religious rites invariably develops ego in the individual, which precludes the possibility of any development thereafter. It is no wonder therefore that religions have fallen into decadence and have become solidified to mere ritualistic practices, having lost sight of the goal at which the practices were originally aimed.

In our own sadhana, meditation on the heart is prescribed as the means to achieving our lakshya or goal. Here too we often find that meditation is done in a very mechanical manner and, as Master himself has apologetically pointed out by using a vulgar example, most people meditate as if they are going to the latrine, i.e., when the urge is there, the function is carried out and then forgotten till the need arises again. Sadhana in this sense therefore becomes meaningless and valueless. This means that meditation alone cannot be thought of as sadhana. People who meditate like this have the barest satisfaction of having gone through the process, and become complacent. As Master has pointed out in his *Voice Real*, it is like a man who has got a bit of turmeric and begins to think he is a grocer.

The method of meditation as prescribed in Sahaj Marg is meditation on the heart for half an hour in the morning and half an hour in the evening, and again for a few minutes at bedtime. I am sure that very few people can really say that even this minimum requirement of meditation is being performed by them. Even then the correct way of meditation is to get into the condition which our Divine Master grants us by the power of his transmission, and try to prolong this condition and, by thus slowly prolonging it, to ensure that the condition is maintained throughout the twenty-four hours. This is the first stage in our sadhana. At this stage constant remembrance may be said to begin. But even this does not constitute real sadhana.

The next stage is after we are able to achieve this established state of the condition, we begin to slowly perceive that we are making progress towards the goal established for us. We are able to appreciate what is being given to us by the Master, and we begin to sense that what we receive is infinite. We begin to understand that under no circumstances can there be any question of repayment to the Master for what we have received. At this stage gratitude begins to be awakened in our heart for the divine gift of grace that the Master is bestowing on us. In my humble opinion, even now our sadhana is incomplete because as we continue to progress, if we are true to ourselves, we now begin to understand all the complexities and faults of behaviour, etc., that exist in us, and from this stage onwards the need for co-operation with the Master in working towards the removal of all complexities from our own system begins to assume great importance. This co-operation must take the active form of analyzing ourselves to see what are the defects in us–mental, moral and spiritual, and try to overcome them with the Master's co-operation. Master is always there to help us in every possible way in all the fields of our activity, but unless we co-operate with him, whatever the stage of spirituality may be to which the Master may carry us, such spiritual attainment is unable to reflect itself in our outward behaviour and in our life generally. There has been quite some criticism in respect of highly evolved people who, by their behaviour and general living, have attracted public criticism that they are living in a manner not consistent with their spiritual attainment. The abhyasis of our Mission must take the greatest care and ensure that by ardent co-operation with the Master they are totally transformed inside and out.

If we are able to co-operate with the Master and try to eradicate from ourselves all our shortcomings, our progress definitely becomes faster, and the Master's work easier. With full co-operation from our side, we become pliable, *mulayam* as Master would say, and Master can then mould us at his will to what he wants us to become. Master has told me several times that the heart region is the gutter of humanity, and it is when an abhyasi is in the heart region, or *pinda pradesh* as it is called, that the Master has to descend into the gutter and do a herculean job of cleaning our system and prepare us for higher spiritual approaches. If we have any regard for the Master, it is incumbent on us that we try to reduce the burden of his task by co-operating to the fullest by crossing this region as quickly as we can. Our daily life must be conducted in such fashion that we are perpetually sunk in the condition granted to us by the Master, and working while in that condition, so that further *samskaras* [impressions] are not formed.

In my humble opinion, even this does not really constitute what should be the real meaning of sadhana. As our gratitude to the Master continues to increase, and as we are able to perceive the ever-increasing grace that is flowing from the Master, love for the Master begins to dawn in our hearts. I sincerely believe that only when such personal love and devotion for the Master begins, our real spiritual journey also begins. Up to now it has all been the mere play of Master's power arising out of his transmission and, in a sense, it can merely be called a *tamasha*. The real progress comes only when there is love because, as Master has repeatedly said, he himself is a mirror and only reflects what he sees before him. Therefore, when we love the Master, the Master begins to love us and thereafter our spiritual progress no longer depends on us but on him. It is like the child being carried by its mother and very literally from then it becomes the Master's responsibility to take the lover as His own and to take him wherever He wishes to. In this part of India, God is represented as love. In Tamil they say, *anbe sivam*, meaning God is love, but I believe God only loves those who love Him, and perhaps the second half of the phrase has been left out, deliberately or by mistake.

In my opinion, no yoga, whatever be its name, can have a successful culmination in the abhyasi's spiritual adventure unless the yoga culminates in *bhakti yoga*. Bhakti yoga here does not mean what it normally means in religious circles, i.e., *bhajan, sankirtan*, emotional dances and whatnot, but the real love in the heart of the abhyasi which very often is not apparent to anyone else except the Master himself. This love for the Divine Master is something which has no outward emotional content in it, which does not have to be expressed in tears of anguish on separation or tears of joy on reunion, but wherever the Master be, it continues to quietly simmer in the heart of the abhyasi who is now the lover longing for union with the Beloved. I remember Master once explaining to me what this devotion really means. He told me of an abhyasi of Samarth Guru Shri Ram Chandraji Maharaj, known among us as Lalaji Saheb. This abhyasi was so devoted to the Grand Master that often he used to prepare coffee in his home and take it to the Court and Lalaji Saheb would tell him that he had been longing for coffee at that time. This abhyasi also used to wake up by himself in the night and be ready with a bath towel and water anticipating Lalaji's visit to the bathroom. This is the degree of devotion that we should try to create in ourselves. There can be no question of real progress in spirituality unless we love our Master so much and so deeply that we evoke in him a divine love for us. This then is the culmination of sadhana where, having done all we can by giving our total love to the Master, he is in a sense compelled to take us up from there to complete our journey to the goal. I pray to the Master to grant all of us this capacity to love Him.

Sahaj Marg and Formal Worship

The Sahaj Marg system of meditation is based on the principles and practices of raja yoga modified and perfected by Samarth Guru Shri Ram Chandraji Maharaj of Fatehgarh who rediscovered the unique feature of transmission called in Sanskrit *pranahuti*. This has been further perfected and made easily available to abhyasis all over the world by our present Master Shri Ram Chandraji Maharaj of Shahjahanpur.

A lot of questions have been asked about this system of raja yoga and its relationship to formal forms of worship such as temple worship, idol worship, and so on.

To really answer this question one has to differentiate between religion and spirituality, because it is here that the difference really lies in an individual's approach to the Almighty. We know that there are many ways of approaching God, both practically and emotionally. In the practical way there can be the ritualistic approach involving primarily the hands, and sonal chants of mantras, and sometimes music and body movements, too. This is one approach. Another approach is by the silent recitation of prayer, where no sound is produced nor any bodily movements made, except lip movements alone. A third approach is restricted to thinking of the mantra or reciting the mantra purely in the mind without even lip movements accompanying such recitation. This the Shastras speak of as the highest approach with a mantra in mind. Thereafter we come to the meditative or contemplative paths where sometimes mantras are involved but very often no form of chanting is necessary. This goes by the name of meditation. But even in meditation under traditional raja yoga systems very often a form is taken up on which to meditate. The Sahaj Marg system teaches that God being an infinite and illimitable entity without graces, attributes

Reprinted from *Sahaj Marg* magazine of September, 1972.

and so on, we should really meditate on the abstract principle of divinity and if this is impossible in the beginning, Master recommends commencement of meditation on light, light being, according to him, the nearest to the abstract.

Even in religions, we are all familiar with certain forms or manifestations of the deities such as the *jyotir linga*, the *vayu linga* and so on. In certain forms like *spatika linga* the idol itself is invisible until milk or some such material of *abhishekam* is poured on top of it to define form. We also have the Sri Vaishnava cult propagating the worship of *saligram* which is a smooth round or ovoid stone, which the Vaishnavites say is the representation of the Abstract since it has no specifically human endowed form as representing the deity. We see that even in religion where a concrete object of worship is used, there is a trend towards making the concrete image as abstract as possible. All that Sahaj Marg does is to make this abstraction as complete as possible by transferring the abstraction to the mind itself and worshipping the Divine inwardly rather than externally.

I see no contradiction between the Sahaj Marg teaching and the teaching of religion when looked at in this way, that even religions teach a step-by-step approach to the Ultimate, starting with the lowest forms of worship such as worship of thunder, rain, water, the earth, trees and so on which existed in primitive times. As human beings evolved, they evolved for themselves more rational forms of worship by transforming the external forms of worship into anthropomorphic forms representing Divinity. Such human forms were necessarily endowed with multiple arms, each one holding a different weapon or appendage in its hands, to show that the Divine wields more power and more authority than a mere human being. This again became refined into abstract/concrete forms such as the saligram to which I have referred earlier.

The next logical step is automatically arrived at by the transference of external worship to an internal entity seated in our heart to whom the worship is offered. This is what yoga teaches. Where Sahaj Marg refinement comes in is in the form attributed to such deity seated in our hearts which is now made abstract to the highest possible extent.

A question is frequently asked, "What about the various forms of the Divine such as Vishnu, Siva, Muruga and so on?" I believe that Hindu scriptures describe these deities as descents of the Ultimate Divinity into human or super-human forms for specific purposes, such a descent being generally called an *avatar*. According to Master, avatar means a cosmic personality which descends, already endowed with certain powers which the avatar has to use for definite cosmic purposes in unfolding cosmic plans of human evolution. Master has clarified this in relation to what a special personality is. Master defines a special personality as a person who has taken normal human birth without powers descending with him, but upon whom powers are showered from above later on when he is chosen for the work. The difference is therefore clear in that avatars descend with specific powers, whereas the special personality is endowed with such powers after he is born, and such endowment of powers has no limit, whereas in the case of avatar there is a limit to the powers, the limit being the power with which he descends.

I believe that the *pancharatra agama* teaches that there are five principal forms of Divine manifestation. The first is the *Para* or the Ultimate which is formless, nameless, attributeless, and which is the source of everything in creation. This Para resides in itself as the creator of everything and also resides in the heart of everything that is created. Therefore, the Para is always defined in Vedic and religious literature as "smaller than the smallest and bigger than the biggest," and which is "all pervading, omnipotent, omnipresent," etc. The second manifestation is the *Vyuha* where there are four forms, viz., *Vasudeva, Sankarshana, Pradyumna* and *Aniruddha*. These are supposed to be the 'source forms' of the cosmic triumvirate of Creator, Preserver and Destroyer. The third manifestation *Vibhava*, which includes avatars who descend in the physical plane like the *Dasavatharas* including Rama, Krishna, etc. The fourth form of manifestation is what is called *Harda*, or the *Antaryamin*, being the spark of divinity residing in the heart of every created being. The fifth form is what is known as the *Archa* and this is the form in which God is externalized by the genius of man's thinking, and given forms such as we find in temples which we worship externally.

While, no doubt, human beings start with this *bahya-upachara* or external adoration of the Divine, it must be remembered that in all rituals of Hindu worship such external forms have to be endowed with divine power by a process known as *prana prathishta* which is done by a human priest or saint who is supposed to have the power of transmitting from within himself the divine energy to the idols or the other representational forms of God. It is only after prana prathishta is done that such idols, etc. become worthy of being worshipped. I believe that in the Sri Vaishnava cult there is a definite prohibition against worshipping man-created objects which have not been so sanctified.

It therefore follows that idols are preliminarily endowed with divinity beyond what any object in the universe automatically possesses as a creature of divine creation, and thereafter only can they be worshipped. The question also arises at this stage as to whether today there are people really capable of transmitting the divine charge, or whether all that exists is mere ritual connected originally with such transmission.

It is believed that a human being must necessarily start with external worship, but this is not the end of one's way of communing with God. We are expected to indulge in ritual or formal worship only for so long as we find benefit in it. After that we must necessarily seek a better approach to God, and at this stage comes the idea of meditation, when we do away with the need for an objectified form of worship by creating in ourselves the necessary instrument of worship.

Sahaj Marg has nowhere said that temple worship is wrong, nor does Master expressly forbid idol worship. Master has clarified that there is a correct way of worshipping an idol and this is to worship the idol as a representation of the Divine, i.e., we are expected to worship the Divine through this representation and not stop with worshipping the representation itself. If a person is capable of this, then there is nothing wrong in idol worship. Master

Sahaj Marg and Formal Worship 165

continues to say that when we are able to transfer our worship to the Ultimate, then where is the need to depend on a representation? I believe this is also the message of the Gita where Shri Krishna asks Arjuna to come direct to Him, instead of going through the devious ways of worship as enjoined in the scriptures. At the ultimate stage when surrender is possible, Shri Krishna again says, "divest yourself of, or renounce, all these forms of *dharma* and come to me. I will protect you and guide you. Do not doubt this." It is a pity that even Shri Krishna has to ask His closest friend and disciple not to doubt Him.

One common misunderstanding in most people's minds is that they must become very old before they can qualify for yoga. What is really necessary is that the mind must mature and if the mind can mature when one is a boy, there is no reason why such a boy cannot take up meditation. We are familiar with examples such as Dhruva, Prahalada, who were all young boys, but who were nevertheless able to approach the Divine in a direct way and achieve salvation. In fact, under the Sahaj Marg system no preparation whatsoever is needed for a person to begin meditation because, as Master has emphasized again and again, meditation is an instrument for the purification of the mind and its preparation for communion with the Ultimate. That is, meditation is a means to an end and not an end in itself. This being so, anybody who is willing to try it or practise it is qualified by that very willingness, and needs no further preparation or qualification.

When we become established in meditation and inner awakening commences, what we find inside has more attraction than what is outside and so, slowly, the mind is weaned away from the external world. Thereafter, meditation becomes deeper and deeper as our being becomes established at deeper and deeper levels. Then a gratitude begins to grow in our heart for what we are receiving as divine grace, and this being impossible to repay in normal terms, love for the Master commences to grow until it culminates in *bhakti*– a true bhakti–which is nothing but a loving adoration of the All-giver. Thus, this Sahaj Marg way makes it possible for us to approach the Almighty first practically and finally emotionally, and so ensures a complete inner and outer development of man, balanced in every way.

The Goal of Spiritual Endeavour

All spiritual endeavour is the pursuit of an inner way to achieve the definitely predetermined goal of inner development of the self to its perfect state, which various systems call the Godly state, the divine state, the perfect human state, the state of cosmic or supercosmic or universal consciousness and so on. The emphasis, be it noted, is on **inner** development and neither the way nor the goal have much to do with the externals of human existence.

In this endeavour most human beings know nothing–indeed, **can** know nothing–about either the way or the goal, though one's own inner longing and aspiration towards an unknown and unrecognized goal do often act as pointers to the fact that there is a state of existence open to us, of which we may know nothing, but nevertheless the very existence of our own intuitive craving for it acts as a pre-proof of its existence. It is like the appearance of the first star after sunset, indicating that more do exist if we would but have the patience to await their appearance. But of the way, the inner way, the same thing cannot be said, except to concede logically to oneself that where a goal exists, a way must necessarily exist to lead one to it. At this stage, given a serious seeker, the search to discover the way commences.

This seriousness in the seeker is the first prerequisite for success in the spiritual adventure. As Master has said, there are numerous worshippers of God, but few **seek** Him! There seems to be a mysterious force or law working in the universe, which ordains that where a sincere seeker exists, Nature so modifies the condition of his personal existence as to make him a sort of magnet, which inevitably attracts to him persons and events which will play a significant and active role in the furtherance of his search. As his personal search deepens, the law works, and more and more in his favour, strengthening the forces of attraction towards himself, finally, at a certain stage, bringing to his very door a guide who can then take charge of him and assume responsibility for his further progress on the inward path. The truth of this is vindicated not only by Master's own statement that "the cry of a true aspirant will bring the Master or Guru to his door," but also by the innumerable testaments to this very remarkable occurrence given by aspirants in whose case precisely this miracle of the Master seeking them out has occurred. Given the capacity to hand oneself over to the Master completely, to surrender in fact, the goal can then be said to be in sight!

But, alas, it is at this stage that difficulties seem invariably to arise, coming from the tussle between faith and reason to establish overlordship over the poor precariously perched individual. What faith says "yes" to, reason often says "no" to–and the tragedy, particularly in modern times, is that we are educated out of our native innocence to a state where reason alone predominates, and where the dictates of reason are required to testify to the rightness of every thought, word, or deed that we indulge in. And in this predicament, doubt comes in as our most formidable enemy. To add to our confusion and ineptness in handling the situation to our advantage, doubt is generally misunderstood as representing scientific curiosity–which it is not. In scientific curiosity we seek that of whose existence we have an inkling or glimmer–but in doubt we question the truth of that which we see, feel and know to be right. And the moment doubt appears on the scene, the will is divided against itself, reason is bemused, and the danger of losing the path becomes very great. It is at this stage that great courage becomes necessary in putting aside the behests of the voice of reason, and so to strengthen faith. The successful performance of this will soon open our eyes to the fact that reason had somehow misled us, and as faith advances, there comes a stage of total dependence on the Master, which can be fittingly called a state of surrender. Surrender is not a ritual act to be piously and ritually gone through, but is a state of existence which comes into being when one's dependence on the Master has become complete.

The Goal of Spiritual Endeavour

Here we meet the second problem: all our life we have been taught to be independent, to stand on our own legs, to manage our affairs ourselves and so on. How, then, are we to negate a lifelong and deeply inculcated teaching and accept the opposite state? A proper understanding of the real meaning of this state becomes necessary. Surrender does **not** mean an external dependence for material fruits of one's actions. Surrender does **not** mean the impotent dependence on external powers to support or bolster our weaknesses. Surrender does **not** mean outside help in crises of existence. All such connotations are wrong, and are largely responsible for the criticism of the doctrine of dependence on the Master. The right meaning is that we recognize the all-pervading, omnipotent and omnipresent nature of the Master's spiritual essence, and this being so, our endeavour, action, becomes something arising out of His will, not ours, and therefore they must have a definite plan and goal and this being so, He works, not we; He achieves, not we; and we become instruments of the Divine will of Master. A sure belief in the Cosmic Person carrying out His plans rids us of belief in, or dependence on, ourselves, because our judgement of causes, effects, events, is no longer useful or even necessary. And so the earlier dependence we had on our own selves becomes naturally transferred to a total dependence on Him.

What happens when we come to this state of surrender? Hesse's beautiful imagery comes to my mind where the seeker at just such a desperate moment comes face to face with a model of a human figure that really consisted of two persons, back to back, first one being himself. This side was blurred, while the other one, of his Master, was strong, well developed. As he watched, the figures became crystal clear, and he could see inside. Then he saw something was flowing from his own figure into his Master's, and he thought or felt that his figure would completely flow into his Master's so that only the Master would remain, while he disappeared entirely.

In Sahaj Marg we have this, and in addition we find that as the abhyasi becomes 'empty' in the real sense of the word, his Master flows into him, so that what was nothing more than a mere mortal to start with, with all the weaknesses, frailties and limitations of humanity, becomes divinised until he becomes Master in spirit and essence. This, to my mind, is enriching the individual to the divine state. I would like to complete Hesse's beautiful imagery by adding that there is this reciprocal flow, from us into Him, and from Him into us–and only this latter flow of Him into us can really complete what Master calls the *laya avastha*, the state of complete mergence of one in the other. The individual is **not** destroyed by being taken into the Master; all that Master does is to empty us of all that is merely human, and then pours Himself into that vacuum to recreate us to His own state of Being. This then is the culmination of our search, of our endeavour, that we become He by He becoming us!

Dvandvas or the Pairs of Opposites

Human life may be said to be nothing but a confrontation with what Hindu *dharma* calls *dvandvas*, translated as the pairs of opposites–life and death; pleasure and pain; happiness and sorrow; riches and poverty; good and bad; virtue and vice; light and darkness; health and sickness and so on *ad infinitum*. Even a merely superficial examination of the problem of existence reveals that all human effort is aimed at removing one of the opposites, the negative one, and establishing the opposite one in its place, permanently if possible. Much of human effort is squandered in trying to establish the positive component of the physical pairs of opposites, namely health, riches, comfort and so on. When these are achieved we tend to seek the same positive existence at the mental level too, such as virtue, wisdom and happiness. The struggle, alas, never seems to end because just as we think these have become facts of our life, the negative aspect of the same pair tends to come into the picture somehow, we know not how.

Philosophies teach us that where things go in pairs, both must exist together–that is, where health exists, sickness must coexist with it; where there is wealth, poverty is indeed an unseen component of that wealth itself, and must inevitably follow, sooner or later. The ancient Chinese recognized the ephemerality of worldly phenomena, and the duality inherent therein, and very pithily stated this truth by saying that every stick has two ends!

In the words of the Gita, we are taught to **rise above** the pairs of opposites. What does the Gita teaching really imply? It says, "Don't seek happiness because sorrow must follow it; don't seek wealth since poverty must follow it," and so on. What we are asked to do is to negate both, and this teaching has been responsible for the life of renunciation adopted by many all over the world, culminating in strict asceticism. The crux or essence of this teaching is 'give up all you have before you can take up the real life.'

In the Sahaj Marg system of raja yoga, our Master has evolved a simple and natural method of yogic practice where such total renunciation and asceticism become unnecessary, at least as these are traditionally understood and practised. Our Master teaches that to give up something we have requires enormous will power, and such renunciation entails great mental strain on the renouncer. Very often those who have renounced family and home suffer from such monstrous tensions that any higher development becomes impossible, for the mind continues to be attached to all that has been left behind and, in a very real sense, true renunciation does not exist. In true renunciation the mind must have achieved liberation from all that it was attached to, if progress is to follow.

Master further holds that once a person has accepted certain responsibilities like wife, children, etc., he is duty-bound to discharge these responsibilities, and Master indeed teaches that to run away from home and family is a sign often of cowardice and selfishness. So under the Sahaj Marg system there is no place for this traditional interpretation of renunciation.

What then does Master teach? He says we must cultivate an attitude of 'non-attachment attachment', that is, we perform our duties, discharge our obligations in all spheres of our existence, while remaining unattached to all these. The raja rishis like Janaka are stated to be examples of this ideal of human living.

Master's most important teaching is that to 'give up' creates strain and enormous tensions. So we are not required to give up but to create an attachment to higher values and purposes, when **automatically and naturally** the unnecessary things of life drop off. That is, detachment has to be created by developing attachment in a different direction. When we attach ourselves to the Divine, the world falls off. We are no longer part of it, though of it. We are in it, living in it, participating in its activities, but are apart from it all. This may be the condition of 'the living dead' that Master refers to. We are alive while we are really dead to this existence!

In examining this problem of the pairs of opposites, we discover that, in reality, there are no pairs of opposites at all! It is because of our fragmented perception and limited understanding of what should be 'total' that this phenomenon occurs. We are all familiar with the phenomenon of light. Physics, the branch of it which deals with light, teaches us that light is nothing but radiation, a part of which we perceive as light, visible light. In Figure 1 below, the area between A and B is visible to human eyes. This region is called visible light–while the ultraviolet and beyond, and similarly the infra-red and beyond, are invisible to us.

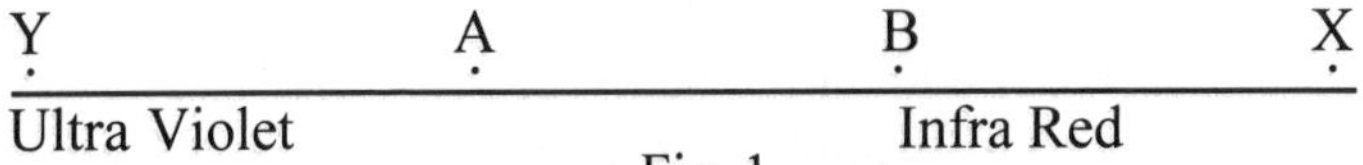

```
Y              A                    B              X
·              ·                    ·              ·
Ultra Violet                   Infra Red
                    Fig. 1
```

We know that there are forms of life which perceive precisely these ranges of light, or parts of it. That is, there are life forms capable of, say, 'seeing' light, in the region BX and others capable of seeing light in the region YA, both of which are beyond human vision! What does this imply? It implies that there is no set region or area of light which can be called visible, since the visibility depends on the life form referred to it. So visibility is purely subjective.

Analyzing the phenomenon of sound, we find the same thing happening. Human ears hear only certain wavelengths of sound with definite limits, whereas there are life forms whose ears or hearing instruments 'hear' beyond this range. Physics further teaches us that all these vibrations, light, heat, electricity are but one, namely electro-magnetic radiation. Some parts of it we, humans, perceive as light, some as heat and so on.

Happiness and sorrow are amenable to similar analysis.

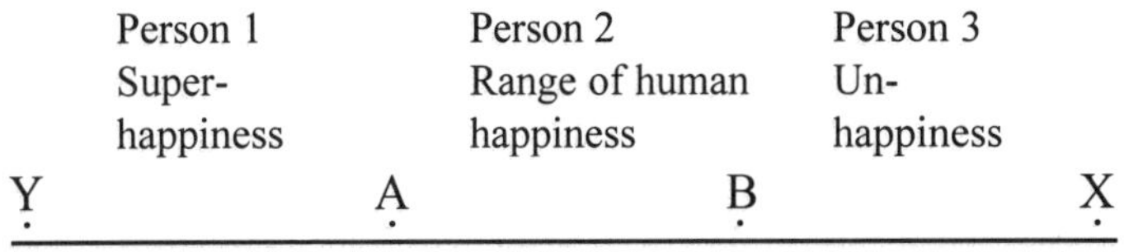

```
        Person 1          Person 2            Person 3
        Super-            Range of human      Un-
        happiness         happiness           happiness
Y                    A                   B                X
·                    ·                   ·                ·
                         Fig. 2
```

In Figure 2 let us assume AB represents the normal range of human happiness with B as the border between happiness and unhappiness. It is a matter of everyday observation that some find happiness (or seem to exist happily) on, let us say, the BX range, while others exist at the YA range. To person three, BX is the normal range while all to the left of B is something superior, superhuman happiness, let us say. To person two, BX is unhappiness, AB is the normal range from the happy/unhappy state of B to happy/super happy state at A. To person one, AB represents as does BX, unhappiness in increasing degrees, while YA is the normal range for him, and superhuman levels of happiness must lie beyond (to the left of) Y. Even a single individual, as he grows in maturity, finds that his ideas of happiness keep changing.

This explains why some people suffer when they see the unhappiness or misery of others. For person one, whose normal happiness range is YA, those living in the range BX must appear to be miserable. I have seen Westerners suffering intensely when they see poverty conditions of India. The concerned people may not be 'really' suffering, but appear to suffer, because the Westerners are putting themselves in the Indian's place and feel what they would have felt had they themselves been in the Indian situation. The same goes for the suffering of animals, etc. In all these cases we tend to 'see' or 'feel' from our own emotional standpoint. This is why when an individual improves his standard of living, it is almost impossible to go back to the earlier standard. What was once an acceptable and comfortable way of living can now no longer even be thought of! To each individual his own range appears to be normal, **until** he is made to grow (emotionally, mentally, etc.), when he sees beyond his range and understands that there are no fixed limits to happiness and sorrow (A and B) as he thought; but the stick (to use the Chinese example) is indeed an infinite one, without ends, and like all infinite things, assumes the form of a circle girdling the universe. Therefore, we must re-draw our figure of the range of happiness and show it as a circle, when the whole theory of the existence of dvandvas or the pairs of opposites collapses. Dvandvas just do not exist.

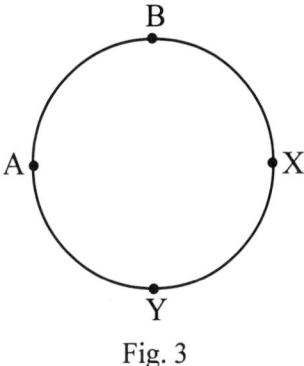

Fig. 3

The Taitriya Upanishad classifies happiness or *ananda* as human happiness, the happiness of the deva, the happiness of Brahma and so on, level by level up to *paramananda* or ultimate bliss. We can now see that the rishis have classified happiness in this order purely from the human standpoint, but when seen from the Divine point this classification also will collapse because at the Divine level or Ultimate level the pairs of opposites have ceased to exist since the Divine is at the 'Centre'.

This also offers an explanation for the paradox that even as humans develop spiritually stage by stage, they yet continue to be faced with happiness and unhappiness, health and sickness, vice and virtue and so on, which the developing aspirant is unable to understand. This analysis, I believe, clarifies this apparent paradox because it reveals the fact that at all levels whether of an avatar or of Brahma or of devas or rishis, the person at these levels continues to be faced with such situations exhibiting these dvandvas. It is only when one reaches the Ultimate level that the dualities drop off and one is faced with an unchanging vista of existence in eternity.

From the centre of the circle, we then see the whole panorama of Divine existence around us, appearing to limited and segmented visions as happiness or sorrow or whatever, but to the enlightened *gnani*, it is nothing but the manifestation of Divine energy, affecting persons as they themselves allow it to affect them. In the ultimate analysis this is true of life and death. In fact to say 'life and death' is, I believe, incorrect. The correct statement would be 'birth and death' because these are the phenomena that appear to us as interrupting the flow of eternal life. What is born certainly dies but it happens only to the body which the 'life', or to state it in another way the 'spirit' or 'soul', adopts for its manifestation. Therefore, birth and death are only phenomena which the soul adopts, whereas life is eternal and free of these dvandvas. To human vision these exist, but to a divinised vision life is ever present, or eternally present, without beginning or end.

Therefore, renunciation is meaningless. What we need is a Master who, by taking us to the level of liberation, puts us in the Centre and so liberates us from the dvandvas and makes our life one of constancy, steadiness, in a state of being akin to His!

The Disciple

Much has been written and said about the Master's role in the development of a disciple in spiritual sadhana. And much of what has been written on this subject is the outcome more of wishful thinking, imagination and preconceived notions rather than of knowledge of what is called a Master. One of the spiritual truths is that a Master cannot really be 'known' unless he who seeks to know him has the requisite spiritual stature to know. It is a truism that we know progressively more as we develop, whatever be the field of knowledge. It is in this context that the term 'understanding' is often used to replace the word 'knowing'.

Another aspect of spiritual life is that spiritual growth reflects itself in increased understanding and not vice versa. As a disciple grows, his understanding increases. In intellectual life we rather tend to reverse this equation and to put the cart before the horse. This arises out of a misunderstanding whereby facts are taken to be knowledge! The Bhagavad Gita reveals this clearly in tracing the development of Arjuna under the guidance of his Master, Krishna. Arjuna assumes Krishna to be a mere human being, and treats him as such–as a friend, playmate, and even finally as his own charioteer! But he had a love for Krishna that was unsurpassed, and this compelled Krishna to befriend him and to reveal himself to Arjuna in a stupendously grand vision. The moral of this is that the Divine, or Divinity, manifests and reveals itself only as its wish, and can be 'known' only when a revelation takes place. The revelation comes not as a result of yogic or other practices, but as a result of the Master's will to reveal Himself–and it is a very very important fact that **love** alone can compel (yes, **compel**) the Master to do this.

But does this mean that spiritual practices are useless? No. It is the practice or sadhana that prepares the human mind to accept

Reprinted from *Sahaj Marg* magazine, March, 1974.

understanding when it comes. It does this by the process of 'cleaning' by which all past impressions are wiped off, transforming the mind into a pure instrument to accept what comes to it in meditation. A normal human mind rarely views any fact or phenomenon as an isolated bit of information input. All judgements (even legal ones) are on the basis of past precedents–what we normally accept as 'experience'. It takes a lot of understanding to realise that this so-called experience most often acts against us by preconditioning us to think and feel in intellectual and emotional ruts, and robs us of the facility of 'pure' action, where each act is a pure act of creation, guided by the parameters of the moment alone, and totally untrammelled by the past. This is what spiritual practice helps us to achieve, thereby endowing us with the ability and willingness to accept revelation when it comes. Sadhana is thus merely a means to an end.

One rather intriguing fact is explained here. We are familiar with the inexplicable fact that there are often abhyasis who appear to be very devoted and carry out the prescribed spiritual discipline with enviable thoroughness. But these very persons appear to stagnate. Why? An answer would be that they have confused the means with the end. To them the sadhana has itself become the goal, and they have verily missed the wood for the trees! This points to the fact that meditation can become mechanical, and therefore static–a danger to be carefully avoided. Under the Sahaj Marg system of meditation, the abhyasis are taught to avoid this pitfall. In our meditation we are required to keep the goal constantly before us. The firm idea that we are moving towards the goal is a very necessary one. It is this that makes our sadhana a dynamic process.

This brings awakening in the disciple himself because we have seen that the mental attitude of the disciple in undergoing the prescribed sadhana is more important than the sadhana itself. In fact, according to our Master, a stage is reached when sadhana falls off, and, that which can fall off is only a thrashed material. What should be the attributes or qualities of a perfect disciple? I am raising this question because Master, in one of his books, has stated that we should find a perfect Master for our development and has also posed the question "where to find a perfect disciple?" Master has often said in conversation that to find a perfect disciple is more difficult than to find a perfect Master. There are the normally expected characteristics of obedience, service, devotion, sustained practice, etc. All are familiar with these conceptual requirements. The emphasis is usually on sustained practice of the method. Traditional yogic teachers have often emphasized the practice as being the most important, much to the detriment, I fear, of the disciples. It is in the Sahaj Marg system alone that top priority or top importance is given to the mental aspect of an abhyasi's life rather than to the physical practices to be followed.

It is of course necessary that a disciple obeys the Master implicitly. The great Indian mystic Kabir is stated to have said that while a disciple should not take alcoholic drinks, nevertheless, if the Master orders a disciple to drink, the disciple should not merely drink but should drown himself in a vat of wine so that the liquor should pour into him through every pore of the body. This emphasizes the degree of obedience that is called for. By obedience and by following the Master's guidance, not only in spiritual sadhana but in all aspects of one's life, one comes to realise that the Master is not just a Master of one's spiritual life but is an all-pervasive Master with franchise over the sum total of one's human functions. The development of this attitude strengthens one's attachment to the Master and begins to develop in the disciple a feeling of total dependence on the Master.

There is a beautiful story highlighting the need for such total dependence, which goes thus. A mystic was wandering in the desert, and was almost dying of thirst. He stopped thinking of God in his search for water. Suddenly, he met a traveller and begged him to give him some water. The traveller turned to his camel to get some, and when he turned round with a glass in his hand, he found the mystic lying on the sand, his body in the process of rapid putrefaction, dying. The traveller was amazed at this miracle and asked the mystic to explain it. The mystic answered that when he asked the traveller for water, he had swerved from dependence on his Master, and this was the punishment!

All extant systems of yogic practice teach that after a certain state of spiritual elevation has been reached, there is no longer the need for a Master. The Sahaj Marg system is unique in reversing this trend of thought by teaching that, as a disciple develops, his need for the Master increases and, at very highest levels of spiritual attainments of elevation, a Divine Master alone can take him on to further achievements. Therefore, instead of dependence on the Master falling off, the dependence on Him for everything we need–physical, material, mental or spiritual–progressively increases. At this stage a disciple may be said to become a pure instrument of the Master's will, and ego falls off. Instead of the disciple acting for himself, by himself, he becomes an instrument in the Master's hands used at the Master's will for unfolding the Master's plans. No unused instrument can remain sharp and rust-free. It is only a used chisel which remains bright and sharp but it must be recognized that the chisel does not act by itself but allows itself to be used according to the artisan's will. The disciple must similarly be able to perfect himself under the Master's will and guidance and later, to surrender himself as a mere instrument into His hands for His use to achieve His purpose. This may be said to be the state of surrender.

At this level, the instrument offers no resistance or impediment to its use; and, to use an analogy, that pane of glass is perfect which allows the total quantum of light coming from one side to pass through to the other side. A disciple who can achieve this stage of utter transparency where he does not exist for himself, such a disciple alone can allow the Master's will to pass through him to act for itself. Therefore, we must try to become 'non-existent' to the rest of the world or universe, very much like a pure plate of glass which is often unperceived.

I remember one amusing incident when a new airline's office was opened. A full office front of plate glass was kept so impeccably clean and transparent that a prospective passenger who had just purchased his ticket walked out right through the glass front, not perceiving that there was a pane of glass in front of him. The perfect disciple should be similarly 'transparent' or non-existent, because ego manifestation from within himself would have ceased, and the Master alone perceives him as an instrument working at His pleasure. Such a one would fit the definition of a perfect disciple.

What Is Mine?

Our life is dominated by two ideas, the idea of self expressed by the word 'I' and the idea of possession expressed by the word 'my'. The idea of 'self' is the idea expressed by the term 'ego' in general usage. An average person's life is obsessed by the need to assert himself at each and every opportunity, and thus to establish the supremacy of his own ego above others. The word 'I', therefore, is the single most used word, particularly in conversation!

To consolidate this ego-supremacy, and to make that supremacy visible to all, the person feverishly accumulates material possessions, thus consolidating the 'my' aspect of his existence. To a great extent, perhaps to an overwhelming extent, possessions are merely props to reinforce one's own ego, and therefore show the inner weakness of the ego. Not having self-supporting, self-endorsing inner qualities, the ego has to seek such support in objects of external value only. Such persons who seek riches and affluence have to parade their wealth and the grandeur of their possessions precisely for this much-needed reinforcement of the ego. The already bloated ego continues to swell and bloat further day by day and, to keep pace with it, the accumulation of material possessions goes on feverishly accelerating side by side. The entire life purpose of such a person is nothing other than a mad dedication to increasing accumulation of possessions.

This also explains why such ego-centred persons have not merely to possess things, but to possess the **best** of everything. It is not enough that they have much, but what they have must also be the best. This means that their need for purchasing power is far higher than it need be for comfortable living because, to them, the best means the most expensive! It is a laughable but tragic matter that generally such persons have little or no judgement of quality.

Reprinted from Shri Ramchandraji Maharaj's 75th Birthday Souvenir, Hyderabad, 1974.

What is Mine?

They go more by outward appearance than by inner worth. So they seek glamour, ostentatious presentation, dressed-up appearance and so on. The majority end their lives with a vast accumulation of useless, glittering trash of very little real value to anyone–least of all to themselves. Such a moment of disillusionment may turn a few fortunate ones in the right direction and give them a new orientation of a more purposeful nature, but by and large, they become frustrated cynics and end their lives in despair.

What is it that they have done wrong? Where is it that they have wandered off the path? The answer is a simple one. They made the fundamental mistake of linking their happiness, satisfaction and the idea of success to material possessions which, by nature, are perishable. If they had been able to de-link the desire for possessions from the ego, then, lacking food to feed it, the ego itself would have had a chance to collapse to normal dimensions.

Master's fundamental teaching relates to this aspect of man's existence. He asks us not to identify ourselves with our possessions. The whole difficulty of life, and the tragedy of existence, begins with such a false identification. When we learn to perceive that I am what I am, whether I have possessions or not, then the first light of *viveka* or discrimination dawns upon us. We are what we are by the fact of our existence, **not** because of what we possess or what we have studied and so on. A man may be very wealthy, but even if he should lose all of it, he is still what he was yesterday. This great fact of being we must learn to appreciate. Being, true being, needs nothing to condition or garnish its existence. It is! A materialistic attitude to life has therefore to be abandoned before one can set foot on the path to right living. It is the attitude which is important, not the fact of possession or non-possession. Given the wrong attitude, poverty can be as damaging as riches.

Does the 'my' aspect of existence then have to be thrown away? No! There are spiritual values which we must cherish, nurture, and make our own in as possessive a way as we can. They must become so much a part of our lives that they are our lives. This is to be pursued as a goal in itself. What are these things or values which Master allows us to be possessive about, in fact exhorts us to possess? There are only three of them and they are: the Master, the Mission and the method.

The Master is an object of possession of which a true abhyasi can never be dispossessed. The physical frame of Master has been adopted by him to prove to us that he exists. It is a creation of his to make known to us His presence, and to invite us to go to him for help and guidance. The real Master is something other than the physical Master we perceive. This real Being is indestructible and eternal. Once we possess Him we can never lose Him. It is up to us to tie Him to ourselves so closely that we can never be parted from Him unto all eternity.

What about his Mission? Is it not material, and therefore subject to laws of materiality, and thus perishable? Yes, but only if we look on buildings, structures and such like objects, as the Mission. The real mission is his Mission, looked upon as a mission in life. Every man has a mission in life. What is his Mission? It is that of creating a new world of a spiritual order where all creation can live a spiritual life in peace and tranquillity under his blessing, and in his benign presence. Such is his Mission. So when we take his Mission and make it ours, we participate in his work and by doing so we become, in degrees, more and more like him. Perfection in the work done can alone make this possible. Making the Master mine is not enough. The Master's Mission has also to be accepted as mine. Why? Because without a mission, the Master would not be here with us! Such a personality does not grace this world of ours without a purpose. Therefore the Master is not separate from his Mission. In a sense he is his Mission! Hence in accepting him, we have to accept his work, too, as ours. This is seen to be inevitable!

Having achieved this, the third possession comes easily, naturally and understandably. It is the method. How does Master carry out his Mission? The answer is that he has a body of teaching and a system of practice, together called 'method'. This is his own method for doing his work. Having taken his work, the method too has become mine, and so we complete the prescription given by Master. We thus see that the only three things which are really and truly mine, and mine not merely for the duration of this life but for all eternity, are Master, Mission and method.

In reality these three are but one. They form a triad. Master without his Mission doesn't exist. It is his Mission for which He has descended here among us. To fulfil it, he has infinite powers and a definite technique, the combination of the two being 'method'. Therefore, it is fallacious to think of these three things as separate. It is a greater fallacy to think we can have one of them without the others. We either take three-in-one, or one-appearing-as-three, or none at all!

Even in ordinary life we, most of us, make this mistake. We accept a job, we then take the salary it offers, and demand the rights we think we acquire with it, but refuse to support the employer's aim and to accept responsibilities that go with the job. So here too, at a mundane level, we seek to divide what is really one, and suffer by consequence. Duryodhana made this tragic mistake of separating the Lord from his army, taking only the latter, and suffered defeat at the hands of the wiser Arjuna who took the Lord Himself, knowing that where the Lord went, everything went with Him. In the spiritual existence the need to perceive Master, his Mission and his method as a divine totality is paramount.

Brothers and sisters, we therefore see the futility of accepting merely the Master and stopping there. True! He can give us something. He may even liberate us if He wills it, but all this is child's play in which we should not indulge. Our goal should be to become like him in every way, and this means to work like him, to teach like him, accept responsibility like him and, finally, achieve the mastery that he has achieved, and so culminate our spiritual endeavour by being like him. For this, our identification has to be so totally complete as to embrace the person, his work and his teaching. Such an identification alone can be called *layavastha*.

I pray that Master bestow upon us his grace, his love and courage to make this great spiritual effort possible to all of us.

Father and Son

In his Presidential address, Shri Kumaraswamy referred to our beloved Master as the father and to all of us as his children. But I do not think that any of us realises what this association of father and son really means. I would like to say a few words on this subject before I formally release the Souvenir. I do not wish to think of myself as a *chela* or a disciple or an associate of the Master. I have always felt myself to be his son, in every sense of the word.

A baby is born into a happy family. It is tiny, and requires devoted and loving care to bring it up. The parents lavish such care on it, care of an extraordinary kind. Nature has endowed the baby with a father and mother so that they look after it in every possible way. The baby is not conscious of itself. It does not know what it wants. But nature, in the shape of the parents, looks after it. It is cleaned when necessary, fed when necessary, and so exists under the loving care of its parent until the age of three or four when the first glimmerings of self-consciousness begin to develop in the child. At this age it begins to know itself as a person, with a form and a name, and also begins to understand its own bodily needs. It now begins to ask for what it wants.

The parents' vigilance for the child's physical needs now relaxes a little as the child itself begins to look after itself, increasingly relieving them of their attention in this field. Their duty now goes to the higher level of preparing the child's mind and intellect; and in developing its character and shaping it.

A time soon comes when the child becomes a boy. He now starts taking interest in his father's work, and wants to actively participate in it. Perhaps the father is a painter. The child watches the father at work and, having watched for some time, wishes to emulate him. The father's heart is puffed up with joy and gladness.

Reprinted from *Sahaj Marg* magazine, November, 1974.

Here is his own creation, wanting to join him and help him in his work! The father buys a small brush for his son, and puts it into his tiny hand. Then holding the hand that is holding the small brush, he lovingly guides it in its first effort at work. A few strokes are painted. The child pauses to shout for its mother to come and admire its work. The mother rushes to see it, and hugs the child to her bosom, making much of its first effort and praising it while the father stands aside proudly, with secret gladness and joy in his heart.

The boy slowly gains increasing proficiency and confidence in his work. By the time he has become a mature youth he has mastered his father's craft sufficiently to stand shoulder to shoulder with him in the joint execution of their work. The father and son are now joint participants. This signals the beginning of a lifelong partnership between the father and the son. As the son develops in strength, maturity and proficiency, he takes on more and more of his father's work, while the father watches his son growing and developing under his own loving care and guidance.

A day at last comes when the father, having grown old and tired, tells his son, "My son! You have learnt all that I could teach you. You have become as proficient in the work as I have. I am grown old and weary, and the time has come for me to transfer the responsibility to you. God bless you in your work!" Now the son takes over not merely the work but the responsibility for it also. He is now the craftsman himself. But the father's role is not over. He cannot be dispensed with, ever. Why? Because the son, however old and however proficient he may be, faces moments of frustration and doubt. He may be one hundred years old, and his father many more years older. Yet the son sometimes goes to his father as a child of yore, and seeks comfort and advice. The father lovingly fondles this old man who is yet nothing more than the child of his love. He fondles him and talks comfortingly to him, and gives him fresh confidence and strength with his wise words. The son goes out, once again erect, with his shoulders held back, a grown man again.

Whatever the father may have achieved in his work is but the foundation upon which his son will build. The hut a father built will become a house, a palace, and in turn the succeeding generations will continue to build upon it, enlarging it into a kingdom, a nation, and so on until the work embraces the whole world in its embrace.

The father but laid the foundation! But without that foundation a super-structure could not be built. The father's foundation is everlasting because he laid it with his vision on the distant future. Therefore, the father's work is all important, indispensable. But so too is the son's. Because if he does not build upon his father's foundation it remains a mere foundation, to be hidden under the sands of time. What makes the son take up his father's work? It is his overflowing love for the father that leads him to it. This love for the father in the child's heart made it take the first faltering steps towards its father's work. The same love helped the boy to gain proficiency in it, and the man to gain mastery over it, until one day the son, now a fully grown man, not merely exercises mastery but becomes in his turn the master craftsman. It is love and love alone that can bring this about, where the son is transformed into the father.

Brothers and sisters, in our spiritual life, too, this same pattern of growth is visible if we look for it. When we take human birth, nature looks after us. Spiritual growth is made available to us by tradition and heritage. By these practices we attain a stage similar to the four year old child, that is, we attain self-consciousness and now should know what we want and where to look and seek for it. At this stage our conscious association with our Master begins. He now consciously and openly takes up the work of guiding us to our goal. A day must come when we long to share a tiny part of Master's work out of the immense love for him flooding our hearts. Master smiles angelically and entrusts a little to us. We proudly feel we are doing it and helping him, but ours is the tiny fist of the five year old child clutching a brush in its hand, both lovingly held in the Master's own hands. Thus begins our real association with our Master, our spiritual father. And if we are true to him and really love him, we must, each and every one of us, yearn to work more for him, so as to relieve him and permit him to rest. Any arrogance or pride is a terrible mistake because it is the Master who works, and helps us to work. His creation is supreme for it is the spiritual foundation on which the universe of the future will be built. Whatever his sons build is only on this grand foundation. Without this foundation the son cannot build anything. Even when the last generation has built and completed the magnificent and Godly edifice of the new universe planned by the Master, it is but the culmination of His vision, His work.

Every father's heart longs for such children who will build his creation for him. It is the duty of every one of us to become such devoted children dedicated to the furtherance of his work. Let us not merely talk of being his children and parade in empty fashion. The love for him in our hearts alone can enable us to become true spiritual children of his.

If we worship him without this love in our hearts, we are merely going back to the formal religious worship, empty of spiritual content.

If we garland him without this love in our hearts, we demean him and convert him into an idol of flesh and blood.

If we give him a donation without this love in our heart, we are merely indulging in bribery and corruption. All these become shameful things if there is no love in our hearts for him. But love transforms them into acts of noble prayer and sacrifice, which alone is true. This is my short message to you on this glorious occasion when we are assembled to celebrate our Master's 75th birthday and to adore him and pay homage to him.

I now come to the pleasant duty of releasing our Souvenir. It is but a book, but it represents the culmination of much thought, effort and organization. It is the crystallization of such loving work undertaken by many, and as such I have pleasure in releasing it as a small and humble token of that invisible love of ours which goes with it.

Karma Yoga or Work and Its Reward

Those who work expect to be rewarded for it. In simple human terms this is a universal expectation, and much work goes into computing the reward, or remuneration as it is nowadays called, both by those awarding it and by those receiving it. Most current disputes centre around this problem, and the definition of what is fair compensation for a specified input of labour.

There is a beautiful parable attributed to Jesus Christ. A farmer, or husbandman, as he is called, is recruiting labourers to work in his fields. From the morning people come to him for employment, and he fixes their wage for the day at one talent. He goes on recruiting workers, almost up to the closing time, fixing the same wage for all, which fact, however, the workers do not know. At the end of the day, when they are paid off, they are shocked and upset to find that those who were employed early in the morning are paid exactly the same as those who joined the workforce just before close of work. Naturally they protest to the landlord that this is grossly unfair and against all concept of rewarding work. He merely replies that he had fixed the wage for each worker when he was employed, and the worker had agreed to it. That was all, as far as he was concerned. It may be concluded that if he chose to pay the same rate irrespective of how long a person worked, that was his own affair.

In this parable we see one concept of reward. The generosity of the husbandman is to be emphasized. He rewards a person for **agreeing to work**, without being bothered about the **quantity** of work put in. In other words, the employer is rewarding the workers' **willingness** rather than the ability or quantum of service rendered to him. This may be considered to illustrate the problem of work and reward at one level.

Reprinted from *Sahaj Marg* magazine, November, 1975.

Karma Yoga or Work and its Reward

In the Bhagavad Gita, Lord Krishna teaches that man has the right to work, but has no right over the fruits of such work. He teaches the correct approach as being one of renunciation of the fruits of labour and calls this karma yoga. It is of course a very difficult idea to accept. It is not merely an idea, it is an ideal. But if we think deeply over this, what is the conclusion that we can draw? Surely Shri Krishna does not deny us the right to exist, which is what his teaching would imply if man were to **receive no reward** for his work. It is implicit in one's existence that the means for such existence will be provided but one has to leave this to the Provider, and not waste time on calculating the reward that one should receive. The Provider knows what to give, and if man applies himself to the calculation of what he should get he is, by implication, questioning the knowledge, and more so the generosity, of the giver. So the proper attitude for human beings is to work without thinking of the reward they will or should receive. This puts the question of work and reward at a higher level of human endeavour, by making man work in the confidence that his needs will be met fully and completely. The mercenary attitude is done away with, and if this teaching is universally adopted, it will at one stroke do away with all meanness and corruption attendant on this problem.

Master, while discussing the benefits accruing out of Sahaj Marg sadhana, once told some abhyasis that there was indeed a minimum benefit in that no one practising this sadhana would ever suffer for lack of food or clothing!

But what is it that work really gives us? Is it merely a reward to be received slavishly from another person? Or is it something higher than this? To my mind, if Shri Krishna's teaching is correctly interpreted, what it really means is that one thinks in terms of reward only so long as one thinks that he is working for another person, and therefore the other should pay or reward the work done. Karma yoga teaching, properly understood, should mean that one should not think he is working for another but for one's own self! If this idea comes, then who is to reward the worker? From where is the reward, if any, to come? Surely the Self is the one to reward its self!

When we study the results of work, divorced from any concept of reward, an illuminating knowledge dawns upon us. We find that what work really confers on us is the ability and power to undertake bigger, higher work. Whether it be in the physical or mental/intellectual fields of human aspiration and endeavour, this fact is absolutely true. Every piece of work, undertaken and successfully completed, endows us with the ability and power to go up to the next higher level of work. Is this not a reward? Why then are we universally blind to this? It is because we have conditioned ourselves to thinking that reward must come from outside ourselves.

Let us examine this a little further. What happens to a physical worker who neglects his work? He loses the capacity to do his work efficiently and correctly. His muscles become flaccid, and continued idleness makes them ultimately atrophy. So a stage comes when **the work has to be withheld from him**. This is the ultimate punishment, that work has to be denied to him. Who has punished him? The logical answer can only be that by non-performance of the duty entrusted to him, **he has punished himself**. The same conclusion attends non-performance of duty at other levels too. In all cases the worker loses his ability and power to work, and work is withheld.

If, however, the worker works correctly and efficiently, increased capacities and power develop within him, the consequent reward being that **he is given higher and progressively higher work** and so is enabled to develop himself to the limit of possible growth. The conclusion is that as we develop ourselves more and more by active and efficient conduct of the duty entrusted to us, our employer, or Master, gives us higher and yet higher work to do, thus affording us the opportunity of developing ourselves to higher and higher levels of human attainment until we finally arrive at a stage of perfection in work, approaching the divine capacity for work.

Master has, for the first time in the annals of human thought, introduced the concept of power grossness which results from power given **not being used**. This idea of power grossness is powerfully illustrated in Shri Krishna's statement that even He, the Ultimate Being, the Purshottama Himself, cannot remain idle for one moment. The explanation he offers is that such idleness on his part, even for one moment, would lead to the destruction and collapse of the manifested universe. Looking at this from the Sahaj Marg point of view of power grossness taught to us by my Master, we see why the Divine Himself cannot remain idle without work. As Master jokingly explained creation to me, God **had** to create the universe and keep it going, so as to utilize his powers, as otherwise He himself would lose his powers! Thus we see that work is inevitable for growth. It is only by work that a person can grow. The reward of work is higher work. The reward of correct performance of higher work is the highest work. And what Master does to help us grow is to give us the first work he bestows upon us. Here begins, to my humble thinking, the real sadhana. How we perform the very first duty allotted to us by Master governs our future development. If we do it well, conscientiously and with dedication, higher work is given to us, having within itself the possibility of further growth that is put before us. If we fail, we punish ourselves. The reward, to my thinking, that Master can give us is thus tied up in the work that he gives us. And this reward we earn by proper performance and nothing more. The punishment can only be denial of future work, thus closing upon us the door of self-development.

A great truth of the spiritual dimension is that power is given simultaneously when work is given. In support of this statement I relate the case of a newly created preceptor, upon whom Master bestowed some work. The preceptor did the work. His senior preceptor, who was in charge of the centre to which he was attached, wrote to Master, praising the work done and recommending that the person should be rewarded. Master's reply was illuminating. He wrote that on the day the new preceptor commenced the work entrusted to him, at the very moment he commenced it, he was put in a particular region of spiritual existence!

This analysis reveals that work alone can be the reward of work well done. By doing our work well, all that we can aspire to is for more, higher work and nothing more. But 'nothing more' is misleading, for, as I have shown here, work alone makes growth possible and therefore when work is given to us, it is not merely work that is given to us, but the possibility of infinite growth that is opened up to us.

The Bhagavad Gita once again gives us a clue to this important and universal truth, when yoga is defined as 'skill in action' or in other words, skilful performance of one's work. The true yoga, or sadhana as I have called it earlier, is therefore nothing but the right performance of work bestowed upon us. This is true yoga, or yogic sadhana at the highest level. This implies that there can be no yoga where such 'skill in action' is not developed. Master once told me that all who participate in His work are really performing the work of Nature, that is, they are participating in Divine work.

Here it is important to bear in mind that physical rewards, in material form, are things of which we can be deprived by men or circumstances. Power and abilities developed by us by right performance of our work are 'within' us, are non-material, and therefore remain ours forever. We can never be deprived of them **as long as we continue with the right performance of our duties**. Such are the indestructible, undiminishable fruits of work properly done.

In closing this analysis of karma yoga, I conclude by quoting the words of an anonymous poet:

Work Is Man's Great Function

He is nothing, he can do nothing,
he can achieve nothing, fulfil nothing
without working.

If you are poor–work.
If you are rich–continue working.
If you are burdened with seemingly unfair
responsibilities – work.

If you are happy–keep right on working.
Idleness gives room for doubt and fears.
If disappointments come – work.
If your health is threatened–work.
When faith falters – work.
When dreams are shattered and hope seems dead – work.

Work as if your life were in peril. It really is.
No matter what ails you – work.
Work faithfully–work with faith.
Work is the greatest remedy available for mental and physical afflictions.

May my Divine Master make it possible for each and every one of us to work for Him, and thus enable us to grow to the ultimate limit of growth offered us by the Sahaj Marg system of yogic sadhana.

The River of Love

Every mighty river is born in some mountain range as a tiny humble rivulet, containing but a small quantity of water. This water is derived from atmospheric precipitation in conformity with the laws of nature. And the same laws of nature force precipitated water to flow down in many such small rivulets, giving them the power to overcome all obstacles on the way. The tiny rivulet cuts its way down through the soil, flows around mighty boulders blocking its path, leaps across chasms and springs down great heights as a waterfall, all in obedience to the same laws of nature!

As they flow down, each small rivulet flows into another, each adding to the power of the other, and thus on and on until a small river emerges, turbulent in its onward flow towards its destination–a destination which it neither perceives nor knows anything about. All that guides it on and on is its obedience to laws of nature. As it flows on, more tributaries swell its flow. Each of them is now a river in its own right, and now it is rivers that merge and flow on. It becomes a big river, ever more powerful and turbulent, gathering strength and might as it flows on. One day it reaches the plains as a majestic and mighty flow of an immense volume of water. Turbulence is a thing of the past. All the noise and visible force of its mountain existence is now no more. It is placid, seemingly gentle, but mighty with a mightiness few can perceive in its onward sweep. Its very volume propels it on to its destination.

On and on it flows, gaining more volume, gaining more tranquillity and calm, ever fed by more and more rivers of increasing grandeur and size, and thus ever gathering unto itself more of invincible might and power, but withal seemingly gentle and placid, until at last it arrives at the predestined goal and, in majestic triumph, it merges with the ocean!

Reprinted from *Sahaj Marg* magazine, November, 1976.

The ocean is thus swelled by many mighty rivers flowing into it in obedience to the laws of nature. The water of the ocean, in turn, is taken up by the laws of nature and re-precipitated all over the surface of the earth. In this process the waters of a river, which could at best serve but a small part of a country, now offers itself in the service of enormous areas of the world. Thus the ocean can be viewed as a mighty reservoir of power, created by small contributions from many, to be used ultimately in the service of all! In a sense each river is surrendering itself, its identity, to Nature so that it can be used in the service of Nature itself. In this process it, too, is regenerated by the return that it gets when nature pours itself unreservedly to the ocean. A river not only serves a universal function but finds, to its wonder and delighted amazement, that it is itself regenerated again and again, thus, in a sense, gaining an external existence so long as the cycle set up by Nature is not interrupted by selfishness anywhere. The river thus becomes eternal, giving itself completely to the ocean only to find itself getting back what it has given, manifold, giving that too to the ocean, once again receiving the life-giving waters–and so on until eternity.

Our Sahaj Marg sadhana reaches a culminating point in the surrender of the self into the Universal Self of the Master. It is a culmination in sadhana but only a beginning in spirituality! All abhyasis ask how this surrender is to be achieved, or how a state of surrender is to be arrived at. Master has taught many things about it. The first step is meditation, to be followed by constant remembrance. After this a stage comes when we must have got rid of the idea that we are 'doers'. It is Master who is the real doer, the real *karta*. When this attitude becomes established the fruits of action, the *karma-phala*, also belong to him. All ideas of reward, of punishment, etc., evaporate away here, to leave a vacuum into which He can flow in increasing measure. But do we find fulfilment even now? Alas! No! Why is this so? I think it is because we still enjoy what is done, or enjoy the results of action in a subtle manner.

Master once said, "Everyone gives me his sufferings, his pains, his disappointments, but few give me their happiness and their enjoyment and health." If we meditate on this idea, we can commence giving or surrendering to him even our pleasures, successes, happiness, etc.; but still fulfilment seems to evade us. What is the reason? I feel that the reason is that we are unable to give up what gives us most happiness, most pleasure, most satisfaction–in one word that which gives us bliss. It is love! It is the love of others that we receive in our lives that gives us everything we seek in life. We are able to surrender to him everything else, but we are unable to give up the love that we receive all through our lives. Here lies the real problem of surrender!

It is love that begot us; love nurtured us through the initial years of our life; love strengthened and fortified us as we grew into adulthood; love makes life possible thereafter, and brings into our life a flowering and fragrance that warms our heart and cherishes us and fortifies us to face life to its very end. Every one of us participates in this divine play of love. In a sense each one of us is a tiny rivulet given birth by love. Each of us is a rivulet capable of, and with the potential for, becoming the mightiest of rivers. As each rivulet merges into another, and as a stream thus formed of many rivulets merges into a river, and as that river too merges in its turn into a mighty river, which ultimately flows placidly into the ocean, we too in our lives must merge in a total manner into something greater, mightier than ourselves. We are attempting to do this. The love that we receive fortifies and strengthens us. But then what is it that holds back fulfilment? We are all too willing to let other loves merge into us, into our self, and swell it, but we are unwilling to allow this accumulated love to flow into the ocean of Master's universal love. In effect we are not rivers of love, even small ones, but merely small ponds which tiny streams flow into– and stop there! Stagnant water in time stinks and becomes unfit for any use. So we too become stagnant. The love that we receive stagnates in us, and putrefies in us. And thus we too become unfit for anything, even useless to ourselves, unless we allow the accumulated love in our lives to flow into Him, and thus bring life giving flow and power into our lives.

By surrendering the love that we receive, we keep uninterrupted the cyclical flow of love. When we surrender this to Master, the mighty ocean of His love is swelled, ever more and more, until it too merges into the universal repository of divine love. From there the universal power of the Master showers it abundantly back on all humanity of which we too are a part, and we thus derive our love-sustenance from it! Thus a cycle of love is established by which we derive increasingly more and more of the love that we surrender to him–provided we do not selfishly treasure the love that we receive and lock it up for ourselves in our little hearts in miserly fashion. If, unfortunately, we do this, then the love that we receive stagnates and finally corrupts us and thus does a disservice to those who had given us generously of their love.

The acme of surrender is therefore the surrender of the love we receive, and it is this which brings about a state of spiritual surrender in us. It is not merely a duty to surrender all the love that we receive to the Master. It is the real way of surrender itself! This is true surrender!

Yoga Through Love

We of the Mission and our sisters and brothers of this great city of Madurai–which as my learned predecessor pointed out, has been steeped in culture, in learning, in religion–are all fortunate in having in our midst our Revered Guru Shri Ram Chandraji Maharaj of Shahjahanpur. I would like to point out certain important aspects of a guru's or a great personality's visit to any place. It is said that great personalities do not go anywhere, or say anything, without a purpose. So when our Master comes here to Madurai, there are several very important reasons why he comes to us. Of course the first and most important reason, at least to us, is that he is amongst us physically. And we who have come to love him, adore him, and cherish him beyond anything in this world, for us it is a great occasion when we can be together with him, speak with him, laugh with him, and partake of all the physical sensory methods of relationship between human beings. This, to us, however highly spiritually evolved we may be, is yet a very important thing, that we should be able to be personally with him wherever we are.

But there are more important reasons than this for his presence amongst us. Of course, he glorifies as much in our presence as we glorify in his presence. He also enjoys himself when he is with us. He jokes with us. But as Master says again and again, even his jokes are pregnant with meaning, and those who understand them, they alone know that he does not joke. His jokes convey the greatest wisdom, the greatest teachings. So, that is one very subtle way in which he teaches us by his physical presence. Whatever we may read in literature, that becomes something very impersonal, but when we talk to him, when he jokes with us, laughs with us, we learn a lesson which Arjuna probably learnt when he consorted similarly with Krishna. To my mind, the greatest teaching of the

Reprinted from *Blossoms In The East.*

Bhagavad Gita is that a human being can start with God who is present on this earth merely as a human being–play with him, eat with him, sleep with him–and yet, by the Lord's grace, when his eyes are opened to that infinite vision which alone can make us see God, realise that same friend of his, that the same *sakha* of his, is also the Almighty. We always try to see God in some abstruse, abstract way, not realising that most often, or perhaps always, God presents himself to us only in a form in which we can recognize Him. That is the human form. So when masters come to us, it is the Almighty himself who comes to us. It is in a form which we can recognize, in a form which we can learn to love, from which we can receive our teachings. So, that is another great function of masters when they come to us in their physical form.

Another aspect is that he does his spiritual work from wherever he may be. In Sahaj Marg, at least, this great innovation, spiritual innovation of transmission makes barriers of space, barriers of time non-existent. But yet when he comes in the immediate presence of his own disciples, he is able to look into us with a much more detailed vision, and thereby diagnose our spiritual condition in a much closer, much more evocative fashion, and deal with us adequately. He can do everything from wherever he is, but when he is with us he can do it with greater precision. It is like a doctor: in an emergency we can always telephone him and tell him the symptoms and get something prescribed. But no patient or the patient's attenders or friends are ever happy unless the doctor comes and pays a personal call, because then the evaluation is very personal, very specific. So, the Master is able to do these things when he is with us, very personally. That is another reason for his presence among us.

Then there are various cosmic factors. As Master says, great saints are like vacuum cleaners. They do not draw just the dirt or the uncleanliness or the grossness from individuals. They draw it from the very atmosphere itself. Therefore it is said that if the world has one saint of calibre it is more than enough, because he sucks into himself all the rubbish that we are throwing out from our lives.

So, these are some very important reasons why the guru–the Master–comes amongst us.

And last but not least is the very ordinary one of having his *darshan*. I have known people flocking to him in hundreds and thousands just to have his darshan. They come and just file past to have a look at him, and go back with, I think, a somewhat childish impression that the darshan is enough to absolve them of all that they have done, or not done, and to lift them up to the highest. Now, it is not so easy to have darshan. Darshan, in its true meaning, means 'to see'. Master told me several years ago that many people come to see him, but few people really see him. Now, what is this real seeing which constitutes true darshan? Our Master is able to look inside us, to analyze us spiritually, find out our shortcomings, find out our strength, find out what we lack and fulfil those lapses, and thus develop us spiritually into something approximating to his own stature. We, on our part, should be able to look into him, going beyond the physical form which is a very big limitation for most of us. We just look at this form and think we have seen him. We evaluate him by what we see with our physical eyes.

There may be some remnant of longing in the heart, something which makes us long for higher things; but yet this vision of the eye, this superficial eye, makes us very foolishly depart, thinking that we have got something which we have not got at all, because of this wrong idea of darshan. So, a true darshan is one where a disciple is able to see the Master for what he is in himself, not what he appears to be; because this appearance of his is a very deceptive thing. This is true not only of this Master but of anybody. Even the great avatar Krishna was subject to this limitation. Rather, those who were with him were subject to this limitation and they thought he was only a magician, a trickster. It is recorded that he showed himself in his *vishvaroopa darshan* so many times, but those around him, the Kauravas particularly, just laughed at him, and at what they called his tricks, his magic.

Now, it is necessary that we do not similarly fool ourselves by thinking that our Master is playing tricks on us, because he looks very simple. He is very simple. As Master says again and again, in nature everything is simple. There is no complexity in nature. We find that everything in nature is utmost simplicity itself. It is only when man steps into the picture and starts producing man-made things that we find complexities coming out in machinery, in our environment, in our behaviour patterns, in life itself. Now, the only way to go back to that simplicity is to see what simplicity really means. When we see it in our Master we should try to emulate it. Don't just copy it but try to emulate it. Make the way of his life the way of your life. Try to become Him.

Master says the ultimate stage of spiritual advancement is what he always calls *layavastha*–the state of merger. Normally in literature this means merger with the Infinite; but we do not know the Infinite, we do not know how to merge, in fact we do not know what merger really means. Because, we are only knowing from our physical experiences, the coming together of two physical things, whether they are trains, cars in collision, whatever they may be. They just come together and we call this a merger. But a merger is something where the two become one in essence, in practice, in form, in everything. So, to achieve this laya, there are certain prescribed methods which we call yoga. We need not go into all that here, because subsequent speakers who will be speaking after me will explain to you in detail what all this means. But it is this laya to which yoga refers. Yoga is, of course, traditionally translated to mean 'union', but my Master goes several steps beyond that. He says it is not mere union, not mere coupling of two things, but it is an actual merging of one with the other so that there are no longer two things; there is only one thing where there were two before. This is the true meaning of laya. This is the true meaning, or should be the true meaning, of yoga.

Now, one of the great obstacles to the yogic pursuit has been the traditionally accepted belief that yoga, or yoga abhyas, is a very difficult thing which is beyond the reach of common people; that it cannot be practised while leading a family life; that we require to put into it not merely our heart and soul but all the twenty-four hours that we have at our disposal. My Master says this is not correct, because though it may have been correct in an epoch when it was possible for these things to be done, Nature never denies itself to any seeker at any time during the world's persistence in time. And Nature here is something synonymous with God. Master says there is no difference between God and Nature. Nature with a capital 'N' is synonymous with God; nature with a small 'n' is what we usually refer to by nature, *prakriti*, our inner nature and things like that. So, the first obstacle that we have to overcome when we start practising yoga is this idea that it is difficult. There is nothing difficult about it. As Master said once in Denmark, very humorously, "The difficult thing about this is that there is no difficulty. That is the difficulty." So when we remove this idea of difficulty from our minds, we overcome perhaps the biggest obstacle that we set ourselves, or set before us. That is the feeling that it is difficult.

Now, practice alone can prove to us whether something is simple or not. We may all talk from stages and say, "Well this is a very simple thing. The name Sahaj Marg itself means it is simple. It is another meaning; the other meaning is that it is natural." Then you may say, "Okay, you say it is simple, but I have been always told, my grandfathers were told, my great-grandfathers were told that yoga is a very difficult thing. You have got to be a celibate; you have to renounce your life; you have to go into the jungle and things like that."

But when you read the Gita, to which my learned predecessor, our Judge Mr. Somasundaram referred, it is somewhat confusing to find that Arjuna was nothing approaching a yogi. Of course, he was a great and very valorous warrior. But if you read the Gita or the Mahabharata in detail, you will find there was Dharmaputra who was a giant among men, who was *dharma* personified, who was the son of Dharma, and he was not able to achieve what Arjuna achieved. Then there was Bheema, who was an elephant among men, and he was not able to achieve what Arjuna achieved. Then, wherein lies this greatness of Arjuna that he was able to see the Lord Almighty in the *vishvaroopa darshan* which Krishna himself says even Gods, even *devas*, even the greatest of Rishis are pining for, but He has not shown it to them? But here is this very human warrior, a wielder of a bow and an arrow and he got this vision. What was it that led to this? If we go into the Gita or the Mahabharatha a little analytically we will find that he got Krishna's full grace, full vision, all his support, not by any yogic practice or any such thing, but by the mere fact that he loved Krishna above all else. He had nothing in his mind above his love for Krishna.

So, we find the great truth which is there glaring, staring at us from the pages of the ancient literature, which everyone of us has missed, that by love alone Arjuna conquered Krishna. There was nothing else, there was no yoga abhyas, there was no *ashtanga yoga*, no *pranayama*, nothing of this sort. The only craft which Arjuna knew which he could practise with some authority, aiming at perfection, was his archery. There were numerous archers in those times. Why, Drona was himself the greatest of archers and Drona did not have the vision. Drona was their teacher! And here is a disciple getting a vision that the teacher himself did not get. Here is a disciple who got the grace of the Almighty which was denied to the teacher himself. What about Bhishma? All that he got was a bed of arrows in the end. When we read our ancient books, scriptures, they are very valuable, but the secret is hidden. It is like the seed, which if you cut open, you find only nothing in it, as is referred to in the great *Brihadaranyaka Upanishad* by Yagnavalkya and his disciples. "What is there when the seed is cut?" he asks. The disciple says, "nothing," and Yagnavalkya says, "From that nothing, this whole tree has come." So, when we read the Gita our mind goes towards complexities, towards glamorous passages, towards erudition, and we lose the substance of that great ancient teaching. It has not been said in so many words that Arjuna got it out of love, so we forget it and we try to do everything that other people have done and we miss the boat.

So, the starting point is that yoga begins with love, with nothing else. And where there is love, fear cannot exist, doubt cannot exist. Now, when we approach yoga merely from the point of knowledge–acquisition of knowledge, acquisition of physical valour, physical strength, of siddhis–then of course we are faced with limitations, very practical limitations, sometimes insuperable limitations. But when we approach the yoga with only love in our hearts–not that we want to become perfect in physical form, not that we want to become perfect in our jobs and earn more money, or that we should be erudite and that everybody should applaud us as wise people; but this love says I want to become what he is–then yoga is the matter of just a moment. It is nothing more than that. Because where love exists, all barriers are broken, all barriers are transcended, and the guru's grace flows because love knows no barriers of any kind. God Almighty himself cannot deny to us what our love demands. This is the teaching of my Master.

If people have read one of the books that have been published in this Mission, there are two important aspects there. One of his own brother disciples of our great Grand Master Lalaji Saheb used to wake up at night before Lalaji woke up, intuitively knowing when he would get up, intuitively knowing what he would need. He was ready with a pot of water, with a towel, whatever was the need of the hour. Lalaji Saheb, our Grand Master, was working in the Courts and when Lalaji wanted coffee in the court, this abhyasi knew what he wanted and he would go with coffee to him. There was no telephone. It was something which you may call the telepathy of love. It is not mere telepathy, it is love responding from one heart to the other heart. But yet there was this fact that it was my Master who is present before us today who became Lalaji's chosen representative, successor, and therefore the recipient of his complete love. I asked Master, "What is the secret?" Master said, "When two are present physically it is easy to love each other. Only the true lover can also love when the physical form is absent." In his own poetic fashion, he put it that 'any moth can immolate itself in a living flame, but the moth that can immolate itself in a dead flame alone gets what it requires, what it wants, what it seeks'.

So love which depends on physical form, physical presence, physical aspects of existence, is a transitory love. It is not love at all. You can call it by so many other names–affection, attachment, passion–all these names or terms are applicable. But true love exists beyond eternity because the presence is unnecessary for it. When the physical form is necessary, the presence is necessary, there is a limitation of time, there is a limitation of space. But when we have transcended the physical form and then the physical form perhaps disappears from our vision one day, and that love continues to grow beyond all possibilities of growth, then you know that here is a true lover of the Ultimate. Such a person has transcended eternity itself because all the physical factors have been obviated from his vision, have been erased from his vision. He is now Master not merely of his Master, but of eternity itself. So the Master becomes, don't think I am being disrespectful when I say this, but the Master becomes the slave of such a lover. He becomes the servant of such a lover and therein lies the service that Divinity offers to humanity. It descends to the level of being a servant so that it can raise its devotee to its own level and allow it to be its Master. As Master has said again and again in his literature, a Master is the servant of the whole universe. He is a Master because we call him a Master. But for himself he thinks that he is the servant of the universe. He is there to do service; but as he once reminded me, I think very very necessarily, here is service without servility. We are not servile when we offer this service. The Master is not servile. He is a servant without servility. His service is there without servility. That is, he is teaching us how a Master can be a Master and yet be a servant; or to put it the other way, how we, while being servants, can yet become Masters. That is the great teaching of the Gita again, "*Oordhva moolam adhassakam asvattam prahuravyayam.*"

One of our great preceptors Dr. K. C. Varadachari used to say that this *sloka* gives a hint that you should start reading the Gita from the eighteenth chapter backwards and not from the first chapter forwards. You start with surrender–"*Sarvadharman parithyajya mamekam sharanam vraja.*"–you start from that and then everything comes automatically. Yoga becomes established, *gnana* becomes established, abhyas becomes established. And he used to claim this '*oordhva moolam*' idea was introduced only to give a hint to the true seeker that we should not begin at the beginning, we should begin at the end. And what is the end? It is the *lakshya*, the goal. Do not start with yoga abhyas; do not start with difficulties that are facing us. Don't talk of what we are going to lose or what we are going to gain, that is all in this mundane existence. Start **there**. If that is our goal, we are sure to achieve it because nothing can stop us. We have lost sight of everything else and therefore they have lost sight of us. This is a technique which he has offered to us in his own teaching, that even when intruding thoughts come, you just ignore them. Thoughts have power only because we attend to them. Where we have no attention, there is no power reciprocally from the other object. So, when we have in our vision only the ultimate lakshya, the goal, everything else falls off by itself. What to talk of thoughts? The world itself falls off, the very universe itself falls off. And then, by his immense grace, by his immense mercy, which alone has brought him to us, we are able to reach that goal in the shortest possible time. As Master said, we just turn our face from this existence and there is the other existence waiting for us.

Judge Mr. Somasundaram reminded you that great personalities remind us of something. Now what is it that they remind us of? In Sahaj Marg, my Master says they remind us not of this world of which we are only too aware. They remind us of our real home from which we have come here. Once he explained this to me with a very beautiful simile. He said it is like a girl who gets married and goes away to her husband's home from which she has come. But as she has children, her family affiliations grow stronger and stronger. In the course of ten or fifteen years, she has forgotten the home from which she came. So like that we have come down to this world as if we have been married and given away, and we have forgotten our original home. The only thing that the process of meditation is really meant to teach us, is to remind us that there is something above from which we have come here, and it is our business to get back where we belong. This is not our home; that is our home. In meditation we experience certain states of existence which make us slowly forget this world. It is not as if we relinquish our hold on this world or we renounce something. In true renunciation we do not renounce anything. The objects which have been enslaving us, they renounce us. It is not we who are attending, it is the whole grasp of our attention which is making us slaves, and when our attention goes to something higher, automatically this attraction falls off. Then there is no power in external objects of the world to attract us, to enslave us, to hold us in bondage.

When we start meditation, this memory of our original home is strengthened in us little by little. And as it grows, we find what Master very beautifully calls a state of non-attached attachment. That is, we are not detached; but we are attached in a very non-attached way because attachment to our duties, to our families in this non-attached fashion is a very necessary thing. One of the primary teachings of Sahaj Marg is, we have a duty to perform and we cannot throw away that duty in the selfish interest of our personal self. Any man who is married owes a duty to his family, to his wife, to his children. He has to protect them and see that they are brought up in the right way. Master gives a hint. He says, "Don't think your family is your family. They are God's children entrusted to you. They are in your trust. Look upon them as you would any other trust." Suppose I give a million dollars to somebody and say, "Create a trust and administer it." You administer it. That is all. But when we become attached then the trust becomes something else. Distrust perhaps comes into it. Mutual differences come into it and very often we go to the extremes of separation and things like that. But if we can discharge our duties by treating them merely as trusts which the Divine has put upon us, everything becomes easy. This is another great lesson of the Gita where Krishna says, "Even I cannot be without work for a moment. If I stop working for a second, the universe would collapse." When that is true of him, it is much more true of us, because he is without bondage. He is not enslaved by anything. He is the creator of work itself and if for him there is not a second of rest, it means that for us there is no rest at all.

"*Asanthasya Kutha Sukham?*" they ask. Where can you find peace in this world of non-peace? It is not our business to look for *shanti*; nor is it our business to look for health, fame, riches, etc. Of course yogic literature promises us so many things, but we forget all that. As I said earlier, it is not that they are valueless or that we are trying to belittle them. As Mark Antony said, "It is not that I love Caesar less, but that I love Rome more." Here, it is not that we love the world less or its objects less, or the teaching of the great rishis less; but it is that we love our Master more than anything else. So this alone can lead us to the goal that we are aspiring for. And once we have this idea of the goal, and the love for the Master develops, there is no question of our not reaching our goal in the quickest time. All these things, Master says, he can commit provided we take upon ourselves this small duty of learning to trust him, to love him and ultimately, what true love means, surrender to him.

The Beauty of Sahaj Marg

Nature is beautiful. Great artists, great scientists, great thinkers and philosophers have all expressed in words of moving rhapsody and inner ecstasy the beauty of nature as they have perceived it. The common individual has also felt and experienced this utterly fascinating beauty in the various aspects of nature, though he may not have been able to express it as the great personalities have been able to. This is not for lack of desire to express the felt beauty and the resultant ecstasy, but merely because of inability to translate experience into language. Every individual has had such moments of revelation when the inner ecstasy could be expressed by nothing more than tears of joy, of happiness.

Further, where the inner person has developed in himself the ability to perceive this grand panoramic beauty of nature, he finds, often to his amazement, that the beauty which he perceives in the benign manifestation of nature is also present in the more awesome, frightening, destructive and violent manifestations of nature. When he begins to perceive this, understanding begins to develop in him that nature's functions are at least in three directions, namely the creative, the protective, and destructive aspects. When this perception of nature's beauty becomes total, then there is neither love of beautiful nor fear of the terrible. At an advanced stage of perception, even that force of nature, the ultimate destruction which we call death, begins to lose its hold of awesome terror, and he begins to perceive the beautiful aspects of death. As he grows in his faculties of perception and understanding, death begins to have for him the fascination that any other aspect of nature has. Death becomes merely another phenomenon of nature, one of so many in its ever changing aspects, all beautiful and all necessary. Indeed, at one stage he begins to perceive that in nature, whatever is necessary is necessarily beautiful, too.

Reprinted from *Sahaj Marg* magazine, November, 1977.

In comparison with a vast, sky-embracing panorama of a magnificent sunset, a tiny flower in a meadow does not attract one's attention. But one who has learnt to perceive beauty develops the vision necessary to perceive beauty not merely in the grand, the vast, but also in the tiny, the invisible, too. He then begins to understand that beauty is not dependent on the scale of manifestation. Beauty is independent of the dimensionality associated with space. So, scales of magnitude become meaningless. The tiny, the microscopic are as beautiful as the grand, the panoramic exhibitions of nature's beauty.

Then he finds that this beauty is to be seen, can be seen again and again, day after day. He begins to understand that what was beautiful in its beginning yesterday is still beautiful today in its full bloom. He also sees that what has withered after living out its lifespan also continues to be beautiful. So he perceives that the time dimension, too, has no hold on beauty. Anything beautiful continues to be beautiful, notwithstanding the factor of time, and the changes in its form and appearance. Then dawns the realisation that beauty is a permanent and everlasting aspect of nature, and one who can see it, sees it.

Nature is orderly. There is nothing unnecessary in nature. Each manifestation of nature occurs precisely when it must. Hence we perceive the system behind it, the system which governs the appearance and the disappearance of the various manifestations. And the existence of a definite system reveals to us the law of the operation of that system. This, in turn, leads to the inescapable conclusion that the laws must have a lawgiver, one who made the laws and set them in force. Such a lawgiver we call God, the Almighty, etc.

No system can be considered perfect where the results of its application result in imperfection. Nor can a perfect system be developed by one who is himself imperfect. So, by observing the perfect results of the operation of any system, we are able to understand the perfection of the system operating behind the results, and then to perceive the perfection of the person who has designed the system which he sees in operation. So, a perfect person alone can produce a perfect system which will give perfect results.

The person comes first, the system next, and the results last. Therefore, enlightened people worship God, not nature. The primitive worshipped the fruits of nature, because they saw the results only. Partial enlightenment, advancement, saw the emergence of worship of the forces of nature, a step higher up in the ladder of evolution. Subsequent advancement in the spiritual essence of a person took him beyond the powers of nature to the wielders of those powers, the sun god, the moon god, the god of rain and so on. Yet further growth and maturity of a spiritual nature brings in the idea of one behind the many. And so, God, as distinct from the pantheistic vision, comes into the picture.

When we study the system of Sahaj Marg, we immediately appreciate its simplicity, its naturalness; and our experience has already taught us that true beauty, indestructible beauty, lies only in nature, in the natural. All that is natural is beautiful. So the first beauty of Sahaj Marg is its naturalness. It goes with nature. Every element of its teaching and practice are in tune with nature. Even the ultimate renunciation comes about naturally, without effort, without tension, without misery. We see that in nature, nothing seems to take effort as we understand it. Everything is spontaneous, natural. Whether it be the emergence of a tiny flower, or the birth of a microscopic life form, or the grand and awesome serenade of thunder and lightning, all seem to operate without application of effort. They emerge naturally when necessary, when appropriate. So the primary beauty of Sahaj Marg lies in its utter naturalness.

We also see the utter simplicity with which nature operates. There are no complex machines in nature. Scientists may sometimes call them complex, but that is because they are yet to understand the way a particular aspect works or operates. Everything in nature is essentially simple. In Sahaj Marg we see the same simplicity, both in its precepts and in the practice that it offers. This simplicity is the second beauty that we perceive in this system.

As we practise the system we find unfolding within ourselves far-reaching changes, changing the very basic foundations of our existence. They happen without any effort on our part, beyond the simple practice of a simple system. These changes open up for us vistas of development unknown in the past. The present practice not merely does away with the grievous burdens we have brought within us, but by doing so opens up a glorious future of a perfect existence which comes within our field of perception, and into which we naturally grow. We see the perfection which it offers and as we understand and bring it into the centre of our being, we realise that the perfection we see in nature is becoming ours, too. The perfection of the results which the practice of the system brings into being is utterly beautiful. It testifies not merely to the beauty of the results of Sahaj Marg practice, which is the third aspect of its beauty, but reinforces in us a total faith, a total perception of the beauty of the system itself, its perfection.

As we go along the path of this sadhana, we see the Master, really 'see' him for what he is, what he has been all along, but which our limited vision made us blind to. We see in him the perfection which alone could have made it possible for him to develop the system which we have found in our own experience to be beautiful and perfect, because the results of its practice have been seen by us to be beautiful and perfect. So Master stands revealed as the perfect, and the beautiful.

Herein lies the beauty of Sahaj Marg. It is beautiful because the creator of the system, the system itself, and the resultant product of the operation of the system are all perfect, and hence beautiful. This is the beauty of Sahaj Marg.

Surrender and Freedom

Preceptors are often asked how an abhyasi can progress speedily to the goal. We find this question cropping up again and again. There would appear to be many answers to this question, such as obedience, discipline, regular sadhana, regular cleaning, following the ten maxims, etc. All these are, of course, necessary. However, surrender seems to me to be the thing that is most necessary; and once a state of surrender is achieved, all the rest become automatically established.

This idea of total surrender to the Master seems to pose certain difficulties, the most insistent fear in the minds of abhyasis being the idea that surrender implies total loss of freedom, loss of personal identity, etc. Our sisters and brothers of the West seem to face this problem in greater measure. One preceptor of the West actually asked Master this question. He asked, "Master, you are always talking of freedom, yet you ask abhyasis to surrender. Does surrender not imply loss of freedom? How to reconcile these two things?" Master answered, "The only freedom is the freedom to do the right!" I would add that since surrender is right, and necessary for spiritual growth, it is an act of freedom to surrender oneself to the Master. In fact I consider surrender to be the highest expression of one's freedom. It is the perfect expression of freedom itself.

I often wondered how to bring about this state of surrender. I found a hint in Master's writings, where he says that to achieve this state one should create a feeling of dependency on the Master. This idea of dependency creates its own problems in the minds of abhyasis. It seems to imply that the abhyasi is a helpless being, bereft of freedom of choice, of freedom of action, etc. I, too, felt in this same way until one day, during meditation session with abhyasis of the Madurai centre, some ideas came to me. I understood that

Reprinted from *Sahaj Marg* magazine, January, 1978.

we are all utterly dependent on so many things for our very existence. We are dependent on air more than anything else for our life, for without air to breathe, we would die in a minute or so. We are dependent on water to a very great extent. I remember the experience of Master in this connection. Several years ago he was caught in a cyclone while travelling between Vijayawada and Madras by train. He was stranded halfway for nearly three days at one point, surrounded by flood waters on all sides. The train could go neither forward nor backwards until the water had subsided enough for the railway officials to certify the track as being safe for train movement. When he later came to Madras after this harrowing ordeal, he told me, "It is easy for a person to go without food even for twenty or thirty days, but it is impossible to go without water for more than a day or two. Even that is too much, I feel! This is the mystery of His creation!" We must remember that this was during a time of severe flood, when Master's train was surrounded on all sides for miles around by torrential water almost up to the floor level of his carriage.

It is not enough that there is water all around us. It must be fit for drinking. As a poet has said, "Water water everywhere, but not a drop to drink!" So we are greatly dependent upon this second element of nature for our survival. Then we are dependent upon food for our living. Here we see a law which seems to operate in nature. Air is vital for our very existence, water for our living. As the element becomes grosser, our dependence seems to decrease accordingly, but nevertheless the dependence is there.

A baby is dependent totally upon its mother. Without the mother it could not survive. But the child does not feel it is a slave of its mother. Then, as human beings, we are dependent upon one another for love, for help and so many other aspects of our social existence. We are dependent upon energy sources, whether animate like animals, or whether inanimate like the sun, coal, oil, etc. So we find that when we analyze this subject adequately, it reveals total dependence on so many things; but are we thereby made slaves to these things? I think not. Our human condition is a state of exist-

SURRENDER AND FREEDOM

ence in dependence, while being free to live as we choose within the parameters of that dependence.

The next idea that came to me was that of slavery. From time immemorial strong men have made slaves of the weak. In slavery, too, we find slaves are totally dependent upon their owners. The same dependence is there, but now it is associated with total loss of freedom. Further, the owner/slave relationship is one where the strong exploits the weak mercilessly. In slavery we have the phenomenon of total dependence coupled with total loss of freedom. When any trouble comes, the slaves bear the trouble first. If it is war, they face the bullets first and are the first to perish; if it is famine in the land, they are destroyed out of hand. Even minor misdemeanours are punished by death.

In the relationship of a Master and his disciples, what is it that is different? First and most important, it is a relationship where the Master protects, cherishes and nourishes his disciples within the widest meanings of those words. Protection is total. The disciple is protected even from awesome death itself. That is what liberation means. The disciple is cherished beyond even the Master's own relatives, sons, daughters, etc. As Lalaji told our Master, "To me the spiritual relationship is more important than blood relationship," and the nourishment, the spiritual sustenance through transmission is permanent, everlasting. In our experience we find, again and again, the Master sacrificing his health so that we may grow. He spends from his meagre resources so that we may be looked after. He works ceaselessly and tirelessly so that we may be at rest while progressing on our spiritual journey. And have we lost our freedom in any way? I cannot see any loss of freedom, not even an iota. We are free to live our lives within our own cultural and social environments. We are free to pursue our careers and lead a family life. We are free to come and go as we choose. All that is required of us is the practice of the three or four elements of Sahaj Marg sadhana, namely meditation, evening cleaning, night meditation on prayer and observance of the ten maxims. So any loss of freedom is illusory. It is a mere figment of the imagination.

Master gives us the beautiful illustration of a mother and child. If a child should be attacked by a tiger, the child runs to its mother.

The mother does not hesitate to protect the child even if she should be killed in the process. Nor does the child wonder whether its mother can protect it. It runs to the mother naturally, and the mother protects the child in a similar natural manner. This gives us a clue to the state of dependence. It is a natural state created by Nature in its boundless wisdom and mercy so that by interdependence all may grow on the evolutionary way. Dependence, therefore, is a help. What we could not do for ourselves, natural dependence makes available to us. No human being would like to face a situation where he had to manufacture the very air that he breathes! Is such a thing possible? Nature gives it to us free of cost, without putting us to any effort for it.

I feel surrender is more a realisation of this dependence. The dependence is already there, whether we like it or not. Our realising it only ensures that we co-operate fully. In the modern world of today we find a great deal of work on avoiding pollution. Why is this? When we realise that without breathable air we would perish, we think in terms of keeping the atmosphere clean and unpolluted. When we realise that without potable water we cannot live very long, we take steps to keep our water resources sweet and clean. So realisation of dependence makes us aware of the need to preserve these elements of nature essential for our life and well-being.

Earlier in this analysis, we have seen how the subtler the element, the more vital it is for our life. The grosser elements are less vital. Now, transmission is the subtlest energy that exists. It is that from which everything else is born. When we realise this, then we see the need to preserve the source of transmission, our beloved Master, in a healthy and happy condition. We begin to see how he is the most vital necessity to us. Then we begin to become disciplined. We begin to cherish him, to love him, to seek to protect him in our puny but loving way. So discipline itself arises out of surrender, which is but a total awareness of our dependence upon Him.

I hope these few thoughts may make it possible for abhyasis to realise that surrender is not what we have apprehended it to be. It is a most desirable state, one in which we are not merely promised all, but in which we receive all.

Work and Play

The other day, during meditation, I suddenly recalled something I had learnt at school perhaps forty years ago, and had forgotten completely since then. Before satsangh I had been asked some questions about constant remembrance, the right attitude to meditation, and about one or two other allied subjects. There had been a short discussion following the answers I gave. Now, during meditation, my mind seemed to throw up a single sentence at me, and at first I was at a loss to understand its implication. The sentence was something all school-going children have learnt before they are ten years old. It was, "Work while you work, and play while you play." While being involved in the transmission session, my mind seemed to enlarge this sentence to amplify its meaning, as it were, in an effort to find its relevance to the moment then passing.

On first thought, the meaning of the sentence seems to be self-evident, and if someone claimed that it had deeper implications than its superficial meaning, people would tend to laugh at him. Don't we all work when we are working, and don't we play when we are playing? This would be the question that any one of us would automatically ask; if we were to deny it, they would be annoyed. It is the very simplicity of this old saw that hides its deeper meaning, so vital for its true understanding. Simplicity seems to be the greatest deceiver of all. We meet it again and again whenever subjects other than merely superficial ones are being studied and the subjects appear simple. Simplicity is the veil that hides deeper values and meanings. Our Master has said, "It is my simplicity that deceives people." In this school-taught sentence, too, its simplicity hides a profound meaning.

A little self-examination shows that we are often not working when we are at work. We are merely at our place of work. The

Reprinted from *Sahaj Marg* magazine, March, 1978.

work lies before us, waiting to be done. But alas! Our minds are elsewhere. The mind may be far away on a projected holiday. It may be on a distant play field following an unseen match with the mind's eye of imagination. It may be at home worrying about a sick person. Or it may merely be indulging in gorgeous flights of unfettered fantasy. But at work it certainly is not. So what happens to "work while you work"? It is a difficult thing to accept, but it is too general to avoid attracting attention. I dare say that no individual exists who has not, at one time or another, caught himself in this activity of not working while at work.

The play situation is not much different. Perhaps more people really play when they are playing, but here too we find persons have their minds and attention elsewhere than upon the activity at hand. So, play ceases to be the recreation and relaxation that it should be and was designed to be. We find, therefore, that neither our work hours nor our play hours are fully productive of the gains and values that they should produce for us if properly participated in.

How is this relevant to spirituality? Every abhyasi has undoubtedly found in his own experience that while he is supposed to be meditating, his mind is wandering where it likes. When he becomes aware of this, the mind is brought back to meditation. This is true of a majority of abhyasis. But there are abhyasis who let their minds wander because it is such a pleasant thing to do. Such persons only **think** they are meditating. Actually, the mind has been let loose to wander at will. Is it any surprise that such abhyasis progress slowly, and some even don't progress at all? If they really meditated when they are supposed to be meditating, results must follow "as the night the day," as the saying goes. Not satisfied with thus ruining their meditation hour, they destroy their working hours by worrying about lack of progress on the spiritual path. I have found this with quite a large number of abhyasis, who speak of everything other than Sahaj Marg when they come for sittings, and speak of nothing but spirituality when they should be at work; a queer but often tragic inversion.

Work and Play

When Master is in Madras, I have often been tempted to go late to my office. But he would invariably chase me out of the house at 9 A.M. saying, "You must now go to your office. Work is more important than wasting your time here with me. If I want you I shall ask someone to call you." In the beginning of my association with him, I used to try to stay on, but he would never allow it. He was quite definite that during work hours, the abhyasi should be at work. Is this not exactly what the school lesson says? And it is precisely what Master teaches us, both by precept and practice. I have often wondered at the concentration with which he works. It is total. One can see the same attention given to eating. When he eats he thinks only of the activity of the moment. Dinner time is no time for idle talk or laughter or even for serious discussion. Dinner time is for eating. An important lesson I have learnt from my Master is that anything that is worth doing must be done with one hundred per cent attention. Nothing less will suffice. This is true dedication.

We all take up abhyas as a sort of game. And so we don't benefit to the extent that we should. If we take it up as work, work upon ourselves, and set to it with one hundred per cent attention, it must yield one hundred per cent results. Then we will see that a brief hour or two of work upon ourselves converts long and dreary hours of daily work to play. Advanced abhyasis of Sahaj Marg have invariably wondered at the sudden and immense capacities that seem to flow into them which makes it possible for their regular work to be done more and more efficiently in less and less time. A stage comes when an abhyasi can say truthfully, and with confidence, that his work is but child's play. When is this possible? Only when we really work when we are expected to work, and really meditate when we are supposed to be meditating.

We listen a great deal to what Master says but we don't hear him. We observe him hour after hour, day after day, but as Master himself says, rather sadly, "Everyone comes to see me but nobody really sees me." Why? Precisely because when we are listening to him speaking, the mind is elsewhere, thinking of something else.

And when we are looking at him, only the eyes are focussed on him; the mind, the true seeker, is elsewhere.

So by lack of attention to what we are doing, whatever it may be, we lose all the benefit we should get from that activity, whether it be work or play. This is only too true of Sahaj Marg. As Master says again and again, we are not incapable of attention. On the contrary, we all have considerable capacity for it. All that happens is that attention is where it should **not** be! It is in the office when we are meditating. It is at the playground when we are in the office. It is upon unwanted thoughts during meditation. And so on and on. All that is necessary for success on the path is to bring attention back to where it belongs. As Master says so simply and beautifully, "Just divert the mind, and It is there!"

Idol Worship

There is a widespread and general belief that worship of forms or images representing a chosen deity, made of metal, stone, wood or some other material, is idol worship. This is no doubt true. This is indeed the general meaning and the way in which it is generally understood. To verify whether some additional ideas I had about idol worship were appropriate or not, I looked up the word 'idol' in the Chambers' Dictionary. This is how the word is defined: "A figure: an image of some object of worship. A person or thing too much loved or honoured. Any phantom of the brain, or any false appearance by which men are led into error or prejudice which prevents impartial observation, a fallacy." This definition appeared to vindicate certain ideas which I had been brooding over for several years, and which seem to me to follow from a correct understanding of Sahaj Marg teaching. The second part of the definition is the significant one, in this context.

Our Master has repeatedly stressed the need to preserve one single channel of thought so that the total powers of the individual can flow and act in one chosen direction. This is the aim of our sadhana. A division in this, by having two objects, means that only part of the power of the mind is available in each direction. The more channels, the less the power in each. The emphasis that Master lays on the need to preserve but one channel is so immense that when talking of God and the guru, he makes bold to say that two cannot find place in one heart! In *Voice Real* Master writes, "They say that one must love his guru as much as he loves God. In my view that is quite impracticable for there can never be two parallel objects of love. The human heart is not a caravanserai..." He then goes on to say, "It is also an answer to the question regarding the relative position of guru and God." That means we have to ignore

---

Reprinted from Shri Ram Chandraji Maharaj's 79th Birth Anniversary Celebration Souvenir, Bangalore, 1978.

either of the two. For this Swami Vivekananda reminds us saying, "Know thy guru as Brahm." This is a challenging idea, and apparently quite a revolutionary one, too. But those who have studied the Hindu Shastras know the importance given to the guru. The guru is spoken of, and worshipped, as God incarnate. He is all and everything. There is no difference between God and guru. It is but a distinction without a difference. It follows that when we seek to separate or divide the idea of God from that of guru, we sin in that we create a division where none exists–and so slip from a natural unity into an artificial diversity. In other words, when we think of two where there should be only one, then idolatry, the worship of idols, comes into being. When this is true at the sublime spiritual level of deity itself, how much more true must it be at lower levels!

The paramount importance of maintaining one, and one alone, in our remembrance cannot be exaggerated. But what do we find in actual practice? We find that even those who express wholehearted abhorrence of idol worship still continue to indulge in it. I am not referring to the traditional form of idol worship where man-made images are used. This form of worship has been abandoned. Yet they are idol worshippers in another sense, perhaps a subtler sense. The idol of stone or metal representing deity has been replaced by flesh and blood idols used to represent Master. Such idols are many. To some abhyasis the father has become such an idol. Master is no doubt maintained in the background, but it is the father-idol that is in the forefront, and which receives the abhyasi's love, veneration and prayers. The father has been idolized! To other abhyasis the preceptor has become such an idol. I believe that any abhyasi who says "my preceptor" when talking about the preceptor who is serving him has fallen into this form of idol worship. Here it is the preceptor who has been transformed into an idol, or idolized. Here again, the Master may be in the background, but is that Master's rightful place?

If I say that many preceptors have lapsed into such idol worship, I may be pardoned for it. It is, however, true. There are preceptors for whom the father, and even the father-in-law, have become objects of veneration. There are preceptors who venerate the

Idol Worship

preceptor who has guided them and served them. In a few cases there are several such master-figures in the mind. When Master says that very gods are functionaries of Nature, and are there to serve and not to be served, can we deify preceptors and relatives in this way?

This preceptor worship is often carried to extreme lengths, apparently absurd but really tragic in the extreme. Master himself told me of an incident which occurred several years ago. He had arrived to a particular centre by train. As soon as he got down from the train he was mobbed by a large gathering of abhyasis, some wanting to garland him, some wanting to carry his luggage, and all wanting to touch his feet. Master requested them to leave him alone and allow him to proceed. Master told me, "Look here! I asked them to stand quietly and to let me proceed. I was quite tired and could not stand still while all of them touched my feet. They know I do not approve of this. I requested them two or three times but they did not listen to me. Then Mr. X, the preceptor-in-charge of that centre, came up to me and found that I was being put to some difficulty. He said a few words to the abhyasis and all became quiet. Look, what wonderful discipline he has maintained!" I pointed out rather sadly that this was not real discipline. A group of abhyasis who would not obey the Master could not be said to be disciplined. It was no doubt a good thing that they at least obeyed the preceptor. But what would one think of an army where the soldiers would not obey the commands of the supreme commander, but would obey orders given only by their captain? Can such an army be called a disciplined army? Certainly not. But our society has degenerated to such an extent that we choose to worship only idols, but not the Reality.

On another occasion I was shocked to hear of a particular preceptor being referred to as the *bhagiratha* who had brought down the Ganga of Sahaj Marg to his area. I may be pardoned if I say that to me this was blasphemy. That it was another highly respected preceptor who made this reference only made my sorrow keener. Can any preceptor claim even the smallest share of credit for the work? Is he the real doer? I must say that preceptors generally do not fall into this error. But abhyasis idolize them to the extent of ascribing to them the credit which should go to the Master. Where our credit is given, there goes our gratitude and this is followed by our love. So, wrongly ascribed credit can be disastrous in leading to the creation of an idol for us. We have heard Master saying, "I have prepared him for the work. He will do good work." It is this masterly preparation which enables the preceptor to work. This is true of every attribute of power that a preceptor may possess. All is given by the Master, according to the work allotted. So to whom is the credit due? In *Voice Real* Master writes, "Whom should I therefore be indebted to, to God or to my Master? To me the answer is quite clear, and I owe everything to my Master alone." Master's message is quite clear. All credit goes only to our Master. When we give credit where it is not due, that too is a form of idol worship. We should beware of falling into such errors.

There is a growing propensity for abhyasis to have their own favourite preceptors. This phenomenon has grown rather alarmingly in the last six or seven years. We are all familiar with the concept of *kula-daiva* or family god. There are temples which seem to attract pilgrims on a national scale, while some temples seem to be destined to be nothing more than village shrines. We seem to be importing these ideas into Sahaj Marg practice and thus corrupting it. Many years ago I had myself fallen into this error by becoming overly attached to a particular preceptor. That he was a lion-hearted giant among men, an intellectual and moral giant, a greatly adorable person, all this did not make my spiritual error one whit less. One day Master was with us in Madras, surrounded by abhyasis in his bedroom. Sister Kasturi was also present. They were all inside in Master's bedroom while I had been sitting out in the garden with my favourite preceptor. After I had been outside for a couple of hours sister Kasturi called me to fetch Master a glass of water to drink. I brought it to him, and after he had finished drinking it, I turned to go away. Sister Kasturi then told me, "Brother! Master is here in your house. Why don't you sit here with him for some time and talk to him?" Master gave a short laugh and said, "He is Mr. X's *chela* [disciple]!" The four words of this short sentence from Master profoundly shocked me into an awareness of my great folly.

Idol Worship

It was as if I was woken up out of a long sleep of ignorance. I am grateful to Master that he thus shook me awake quite early in my spiritual sadhana under his feet. I understood then that there can be one, and only one, in our heart. There is no room for a second one, however great such a one may be. Master makes so bold as to say that for one who is totally devoted to his Master, there is no room even for God! God comes to us as the Master so that Master may reveal himself to us as God! This is the secret of spiritual sadhana, the culmination of such sadhana.

When we select preceptors to be our favourite preceptors, we fall into all sorts of errors of conduct. Master emphasizes the great need for etiquette in abhyasis. The first error, or breach of etiquette, is that we start inviting such preceptors to come to us. If they are treated as brothers and sisters, nothing is wrong in it. But this is generally not the case. They are invited in the place of Master, and then this becomes a sin. This tendency to invite chosen preceptors is growing, and the disease is prevalent to a greater extent in some areas than in others. Unfortunately, this tendency seems to have invaded the centres of the Mission in Europe and the USA, too.

What is it that happens when we invite a chosen preceptor? First of all, it is an act of the greatest disrespect to Master. Our business, as abhyasis, is with our Master. The preceptor is no doubt there to serve us, and if we need spiritual assistance and guidance we should refer our problems to the preceptor, who has been made responsible for our progress. If the preceptor himself needs clarification or guidance in serving us, then it is up to him to seek it from Master. It is the preceptor's job to seek help from the Master, and it is for Master to decide what should be done. If Master thinks some other preceptor should assist the local preceptor by visiting the concerned centre, that decision is solely Master's to take. It is entirely for Master to decide who should be sent, where and when. If abhyasis start inviting other preceptors to visit them it means that they are taking the matter into their own hands, and this, if looked at from the proper standpoint, is the beginning of indiscipline. In fact it would not be improper to label it an act of indiscipline. This is the second fault. It is also possible that abhyasis unwittingly do a disservice to such preceptors. Preceptors who are thus repeatedly invited are exposed to the danger of egoism. We should remember that all preceptors are servants of the one Master. They are given work according to their level of approach and their capacity and willingness. Master prepares people with definite ideas of work to be allotted to them. So, everything is done by them. Therefore, any idea of one preceptor being superior to another is wrong, and abhyasis should not allow such ideas to come into their minds. Nor is it our business to think in such terms. Even if a preceptor becomes like the Master in every aspect of his being, he still cannot be Master. He can be masterly in his approach and in his work, but he is not the Master. Master himself has said that there can be only one such Personality in the whole universe at one time.

We, as abhyasis of the Mission, should totally avoid having favourite preceptors. This is one aspect of idol worship. When we invite them to come to us, this deepens. In some cases this goes to grossly impertinent levels, too. I was once with Master in Chi. Umesh's house. It was early in the morning, and Master was seated in an easy chair, smoking his first hookah, with some five or six of us seated around him on the floor. Some abhyasis from another centre came, prostrated before him, and immediately requested Master's permission to go to my house. Master asked them why they wanted to go there. They said that they wanted to have a sitting from another preceptor who was then staying with us in my house. Master asked them, "When I am here, why do you want a sitting from that person?" They smiled, said nothing in reply, and went away. Then Master looked at me and asked, "Why do they want to go there when I am here? Are they not satisfied with my transmission?" What could I reply to this? I could only bewail the folly of the abhyasis concerned and pray that light may dawn upon them.

If this is not idol worship, I don't know what it is. What have we to do with anybody else when Master is with us? And is he not always with us, wherever he may be physically? We all mouth this belief without really believing it. This disbelief, or lack of faith, reflects itself in our behaviour. If there is real faith in us, our

Idol Worship

behaviour cannot fall into error. I remember an anecdote related to me soon after I had come to Master's feet. Sister Kasturi had accompanied Master on her first visit to Tirupathi. Knowing it to be her first visit, some well-meaning abhyasis offered to take her up to the Tirumala hills and to show her the famous temple there. Sister Kasturi is reported to have replied, "When I am with the Creator Himself, what have I to do with His creation!" When Master is with us, we need not go to any preceptor unless Master instructs us to do so, or Master has approved a general programme of individual sittings in which we may then safely participate.

I have sometimes felt that worship of stone or metal idols is less dangerous than the worship of flesh and blood idols. Inanimate idols cannot reciprocate our emotions of love, reverence and adoration. But when we make an idol of a living human being, such an idol can reciprocate our emotions, and herein lies the greatest danger; because such reciprocal feeling draws us deeper and deeper into the web of infidelity to the Master.

Our Daily Bread

Every human being has needs, definite needs, the basic needs of existence for water, for food, for clothing, and for shelter, all of which have to be satisfied if one is to exist. There are needs related to our physical existence. Then there are emotional needs, the fundamental need being the need for love. One also needs a sense of security, a sense of being wanted for one's own sake, and so on. I would say that the physical and emotional needs are fundamental and basic. These needs have to be fulfilled somehow. And all religious prayers rightly address the Creator Himself for their fulfilment, thus recognizing the source of all well-being, of all fulfilment.

In the Lord's Prayer of the Christian religion, one line of the prayer says, "Give us this day our daily bread." I have often wondered why the prayer was phrased in a way which appeared to limit the generosity of the giver to nothing more than one's daily portion. Why did the one who prayed not pray for more? Why not ask for our needs for our full span of physical existence to be guaranteed by one single act of prayer? Is it that the individual can think of nothing more than one day's needs, or is it that he doubts the capacity of the giver to give more? Or, even worse, does he doubt the generosity of the Almighty?

Many years of thought did not give me any answer to these questions. But recently, one morning during meditation, the answer came to me; I think this great Christian prayer has been verbally expressed out of an intuitive feeling that anything in excess of what one needs is bad for the person. On analyzing this further, much material comes to mind, providing food for further thought. What happens when a man is very rich? Having easily fulfilled his physical and material needs, the mind is diverted into how to uti-

Reprinted from *Sahaj Marg* magazine, November, 1978.

lize the excess available. The mind turns towards luxuries. Luxurious living becomes attractive just because the person can afford it.

When one raises one's standard of living, the mind pursues that line of thought; and more and more luxuries begin to be sought. A frantic drive for fulfilment eggs the individual on and on. There is no end to it. Originally, wealth made luxury possible. Now, the drive for luxury makes the person expend all his energies on the accumulation of more and more wealth to create increasingly more luxurious living conditions. So the mind is diverted from one's true goal to false and impermanent material goals. Wealth does us this disservice by diverting our minds away from the true goal of human life, the perfection of the human existence by achieving a balanced existence. Wealth can also do more positive harm, by attractions of negative sorts being made possible, of indulgence, thus degrading us physically and morally.

If a man is very strong physically, then he can become an oppressor of weaker persons. Instead of using his strength for the good of others, he begins to use it for self gratification and to enslave other beings to his debased will. One who should, by virtue of his strength, be a protector of the weak, becomes their oppressor and often their destroyer.

What about the craze for knowledge? How much knowledge does a person need? All that we need is sufficient knowledge to take us through life to our final destination. Here, too, excess is unnecessary, and any effort in acquiring knowledge beyond our needs is but a foolish waste of time and energy. Excessive knowledge can create intellectual arrogance in its possessor. Such a person is no longer a servant of society. A truly knowledgeable person serves society and is known by his attitudes of love, humility and charity. If knowledge is sought for its own sake, it too becomes a mighty weapon to destroy its possessor. Arrogance and pride come in as negative character traits. Such a person seeks self-glorification. He seeks the limelight. Service is no longer his purpose. Rather, he seeks to be served by those less endowed than he is. His goal is no longer that of self perfection, but has been debased to that of self-glorification to pander to his vanity and pride. So, the pursuit of knowledge, too, is seen to be a dangerous one.

Thus we find that all that a person needs, whether of the means of physical sustenance or of physical strength or even of knowledge, is but the bare minimum necessary to carry one through the stormy ocean of life to the other shore of personal spiritual liberation. That is all that a person needs. This is beautifully and simply stated in the Lord's Prayer I have referred to earlier.

Anything in excess is bad for the individual. An ancient Tamil proverb says, "Beyond measure, even nectar becomes poison." This is true of all things without exception. It is unfortunate that physical well-being and luxurious standards of living have been equated with civilization. True civilization is not dependent on these things. As Dostoyevsky has said, civilization does nothing more than develop the capacity to feel more and more sensations. That is, civilization, as it is understood, deals only with the sensory world. True civilization is, however, something which goes far, far beyond such mundane concepts. True civilization is the creation of a society where all individuals strive for personal perfection by aiming at the proper goal. This can only be achieved by bringing balance into our existence. Nothing should be sought for in excess of what we need. Everything in excess is poison. This is what our Master has so beautifully taught us, the idea of flying like a bird on two wings, the spiritual and material wings, with the two in perfect balance. Such a balanced person is the truly wise person. He may not be rich. He may not be strong. He may not even be intelligent. But nevertheless, he is wise because his mind is focussed on the true goal, and all his energies are harnessed to the effort of realising that goal.

Craving, Reality and Adoration

I have been asked to say a few words before this session comes to an end. But I think we are all talking only in terms of 'time philosophy', which alone comes to an end. Just now we have celebrated our Beloved Master's birthday. I personally do not look upon it as coming to an end of one year. It is eternal, without a beginning and without an end. We all live in time-oriented, space-oriented, movement-oriented phenomena and we are bound by them. Now for a Being like our Master, I do not think any of these things exist. It is an Existence in existence, it is a Being in being, and Life in life.

One of the grandest concepts of Sahaj Marg is that we fly on two wings of materialism and spiritualism, and therefore, our efforts must be in both the directions. We should not try just for spirituality alone. We will have to strive for material perfection also. This applies equally for our Mission as well. Today, we are almost two and a half thousand people assembled here, the largest number, larger than the Basant Panchami function. We are very happy, very satisfied. Even though I am internally very happy, yet I would shudder to think what it is going to be in ten years' time. If the Mission grows at this rate, by 1990 we will be several lakhs. That means we will have to organize not with individuals, not with groups, but with humanity in masses, in nations. Every abhyasi should ponder over it and try to perfect himself for such an eventuality.

We all have the services of our volunteers. They have done a good job. In the beginning of our sadhana, we feel we are serving our brothers and sisters. As we evolve, we feel that we are serving our Master. But further on, we don't know we are serving. Everyone has to develop that attitude where service is an expression of

Reprinted from *Sahaj Marg* magazine, July, 1978.

one's being. I think this is what our Master does. He does not know whom he is serving or why he is serving. He does not even say he is serving his Master. The very idea of service does not occur to him. He is not conscious of it. This is the highest service.

Now, service implies simplicity and discipline. Service essentially means discipline. When there is service of the magnitude of Divinity itself, the service has to be highly disciplined. Equally important, the person who receives such a service should be disciplined. Many of us are disappointed that Master does not come here and meet us; he does not give us *darshan*. Most of us are disappointed that we don't get individual sittings from Master. I heard some of our elder brothers saying that they don't have personal communication with Master as they used to have earlier. I was telling them, "Wait a few years more and we will need a telescope or a binocular to see him." So, when the Mission grows, we should also grow spiritually. The idea of separation in terms of space and time are to go away. Our human ideas of time and space alone prevent our union with Master.

I think much of our indiscipline is because of lack of appreciation of His grace. I think it was Shankara who said three things are there which are expressions of Divine grace. In no other way can we achieve them. The three are:

i) birth in the human form
ii) craving for Realisation
iii) and, most importantly, to be gifted to come to the feet of the guru of calibre.

Shankara says these are impossible without Divine grace. If these are there, that proves we are already recipients of grace. For every one of us, the first one is there. We all have the human frame. The third one also is there, the guru of calibre, our Master. If we are not progressing, it can be only in the middle situation where we lack craving for spiritual realisation, which is a must. So, whenever somebody complains of lack of progress, it is due to lack of craving in him. Anxiety we may be having, *lalach* [greed], but there is no craving. We run to Master, touch his feet, push him down, and do everything else, out of anxiety, greed; these are expressions of animal passion. We are only actuated by greed, to possess something (we don't know what it is, either) which others are getting. It is a very low human attitude, not craving. So, it is not enough to be born human beings; it is not enough to come to the feet of the Divine Master, if there is no craving. Master also says, again and again, that 'craving is necessary'. (When craving is absent, indiscipline manifests itself in our behaviour.)

Let me give a small example. We have put up a counter for *chappals*. When the evening programme ended there was a line formed by a few disciplined people. But within ten minutes it was like one of the *Anna-Dana sabhas*. Everyone was scrambling for their chappals and everything was in a mess. So in ten minutes all the organizational effort was destroyed; and it took three hours to find chappals. The protection that our chappals had was lost because we, in our ignorance, in our haste, in our greed, misbehaved and we lost our privilege. The same thing happens with every walk of life. We don't get a thing if we don't deserve it. By our misbehaviour we are damaging the reputation of our organization. People do not think. Our organization is judged by our behaviour and by our actions. What would an outsider have thought on seeing this scramble? So, discipline is a must. When there is craving, indiscipline goes away; if indiscipline goes, craving will automatically come. It is discipline alone which brings craving. A disciple should necessarily be disciplined. But here Master calls us his 'associates'. I hate to be called an associate of Master. I want to be his disciple. Can anybody be an associate of Master? Master is very intelligent. He flatters us by calling us associates. We are happy and satisfied with being patted on our back. We don't know the meaning behind it, which is that we are not fit to be his disciples.

And then, when we fall at Master's feet, we are not conscious of his service. Not only this, we are questioning Master's attitude. When there is enough food in the kitchen, we do not go and rush for it. If we rush for food that means we don't have faith in our father and mother that they can provide enough for the whole family. Every time you rush and push, you are only questioning the donor–Master. He is verily the embodiment of love. It was Narada who said about God, "He is the embodiment of unspeakable, indescribable love." Anything which is spoken about is limitation. Master loves. He does not know he is loving. The only expression of Master's existence is the absolute outflow of love from eternity, to such an extent where there can be neither beginning nor end. It is *anadi*. Then, why this foolish anxiety to drag out of him that which he is giving us, and which we don't know we are getting? All our indiscipline stems from this ignorance. By so doing we are not going towards Reality. We are going towards artificiality.

I think it was Vyasa who relates this story. Of course it is hurting to human ego, but it is instructive. It is about a man who had developed in himself the capacity to grunt realistically like a pig. He went to a village and started grunting like a pig in an exhibition, and made lots of money. Now, an advanced guru was going through that village and he saw there was an opportunity to teach a lesson to his disciples. So he took permission from the organizers and opened a second stall where he claimed the audience could hear a more realistic grunting of a pig; and he said it was free. He brought a pig and naturally the pig grunted more realistically. People came there but were disappointed because it was the actual pig which was grunting. Therefore, they went back to the human being who grunted like a pig. Thus, our human tendencies are moulded in such a way that we don't want the reality, because unreality is more glamorous, more charming, more attractive, and more enticing to the senses.

I was very happy to find in the first day's coverage of our function in the *Indian Express*, where Master has been described as a "Personality without Personality". People find it difficult to describe Master. Reality cannot be described. If it is described, it becomes this or that. Duality comes into the picture. If one is distinguished by his personality, the limitations set in; such a person cannot be called a Master. 'Personality without a personality" is a beautiful expression.

These are the things which I thought I should express. I believe in sharing of thoughts, not lectures or talk. It is somewhat sad when we find abhyasis taking sittings from preceptors rather than from Master. This is like that story of the pig. I often wondered why this happens. Preceptors are also human beings. Sometimes they make an effort and give a sitting from lower levels because of which you can be put into samadhi stage. It is significant that samadhi is described as *pashana tulya* condition [stone-like condition], whereas our samadhi is *sahaj samadhi*. We prefer the substitute to Reality rather than Reality as such! Whatever be his attainment or his progress, the preceptor is never a substitute for Master. He is acting for and on behalf of Master. I do not mean any disrespect to any preceptor brother. What I am trying to tell you is, when we are going to Reality we must be wedded to **Reality**. If we are seeking experiences we are still bound within the consciousness which is time bound. Here, we have to free ourselves from this stage into which we have got ourselves by past experience.

We should go to Master alone. It is our duty to adore Master. Love can be selfish. When love is associated with humility and devotion, it is adoration. What is the difference between love and adoration? Love is selfish. Adoration is totally selfless. There is humility in it. In effect, adoration becomes surrender. Adoration means we are perpetually in that in which we want to be. It is already a condition of *laya*.

Serving the Master

I have been very fortunate in accompanying Master on some of his travels. Wherever I have gone, I have noticed the eagerness which abhyasis have shown in serving Master. The eagerness is generally so overpowering that a scramble frequently ensues among the abhyasis, each one striving his best to be the one to serve the Master. It is a common sight to see one abhyasi trying to help Master get out of his chair, while another abhyasi anxiously looks for his slippers. A third one is ready with Master's walking stick, while a fourth may be holding out a towel or napkin. All are eager and anxious that Master should accept the personal service so proffered. And surrounding the few happy ones who have managed to grab something with which to serve him, are the disappointed many who could not take timely action. This I have seen repeated again and again, wherever I have gone with Master.

Is Master happy with the services of the abhyasis so eagerly and anxiously offered? Sometimes yes, but often no. I have no doubt that Master is happy to see the idea of service developing in the minds of the abhyasis. Nevertheless, one reason why he may not be happy is that few abhyasis, if any, take the trouble of finding out what exactly he wants. The wrong sort of service is offered. This generally comes about because we are anxious to serve the Master not for his own sake, but for the sake of the pleasure it affords us, or the reward that we expect such service to earn for us. In thus trying to serve him, we generally hinder him or obstruct him. So, the first thing that one wishing to serve him sincerely must do, is to try to ascertain his needs and wishes, and then act appropriately. It is the rare abhyasi who seems to be able to sense the need of the Master and to offer him a glass of water, or a pillow to rest upon without being asked for it. When this is accepted, all the others

Reprinted from *Sahaj Marg* magazine, January, 1979.

look on, unhappy that they did not think of doing so. What is the secret in such cases? The secret is not to **think** of what Master needs, but to intuitively feel it, and act to fulfil that need. Love for the Master–a totally absorbing love for him–alone seems to make this sort of intuition possible. Thus, only an abhyasi who loves the Master can really serve him. The others can only try to guess what he wants or needs, and generally end up by obstructing him, and causing annoyance and displeasure to all.

Now, what is it the Master really seeks of us? What is it by doing which we can really and truly serve the Master? After all, anyone can help him to put on his slippers. Why rush to do it? Similarly, not much service is involved in handing him his walking stick, or in opening the door of the car for him to get in. These are trivial things, and also things in which his need of our services is minimal. Then what should we do? Is there service of a higher order than merely physical action? Yes! One can serve him by assisting him with the work of the Mission. The work of the Mission is his life work, the purpose of his mortal existence. In assisting him in that work we certainly serve him in a more vital and necessary way. This does not mean that we should not help him find his slippers or his stick. We should certainly do it when necessary. But we should not stop with this level of service. We should strive to rise ever higher in the levels of service available. We can offer our service in writing about his teachings and his work. We can offer our assistance in maintaining books of accounts, or by running the printing press. Engineers can offer their service by helping with designing and construction of ashram facilities and so on.

Thinking about these things, I often wondered whether there was one way of serving him which one could call the highest way, or the noblest way, or perhaps even the most loving way of serving him. It came to me one day during group meditation with abhyasis at Mysore, that there is such a way of serving him in the highest, noblest and the most loving way. What is it that he wants from us? Is it physical service? He can get this from servants. Is it work of the ashram? He can pay staff to get this done. Is it giving a little money or donation? Certainly not, because one prayer from him can open the wealth of the universe and put it at his feet. Is it wisdom-filled advice? He is the very repository of all wisdom. Is it skill in action? He is the source of all skills. Love? Can it be love? Regretfully, almost with tears in my eyes, I got the answer. No! Many love him, but do all therefore or thereby serve him? No! No doubt it is a high and noble offering. But service? No! Then the answer came to me in a bliss-filled flash of light without luminosity. What is it he wants us to do? He wants us to **become** that which he wants us to become. And in doing this lies the greatest service to the Master. He serves the Master most nobly, most lovingly, who becomes what the Master wants him to become. A simple answer. An illuminating answer. A soul-searing answer. A tear-evoking answer. All these, yes, also an understandable answer.

Is this not, after all, the very thing that every father wants of his children? What can exceed the grief and despair a person feels when his progeny turn out to be nothing; all his dreams and aspirations shattered; all the loving work bestowed upon them brought to nought; a lifetime of dedicated work ruined just because the person on whom all this was lovingly showered refused to become what he was expected to become. There is no greater disservice a son can do to his father than by this non-becoming, nor can there be a greater service than in the becoming. If this is so with our worldly parents, how much more so of our spiritual father, who is our mother, too! Can his grief and misery be any less if we fail to come up to his expectations? And can his joy know any bounds if we become what he wants us to become? Master's work upon the abhyasis and his love for them is his service to us. In fully availing of his services and becoming what he wants us to become, lies the greatest service that we can, in turn, do to him. The greatest service we can do is, therefore, to utilize the loving service he offers to us in the most devoted and dedicated manner. In the total acceptance of his service to us lies the totality of the service that we, in turn, can offer him.

What is it that we have to do to become what he wants us to become? The animal man has to become humanized and then we have to proceed on to the destination. The way is before us–meditation, cleaning, prayer, and constant remembrance. We have already covered the journey from 'what we were' to 'what we are'. Now, 'that which we are' has to become 'That', 'that which we ought to be'. This is but another way of saying that our sadhana must be correct in every way. Then only can the goal be attained. Many meditate, but few meditate as Master asks us to do. Many only **think** that they are meditating. Many also use objects of meditation not specified in Sahaj Marg. During cleaning, cleaning is not done but thoughts are allowed to breed in indulgent fancy. Remembrance is rare, and if at all it is there, then it is about other things and not that which we should remember. And so it goes on, the sad chronicle of our imperfect sadhana. How can such abhyasis ever truly serve the Master? Our sadhana is purposeful, goal-oriented, and at the same time amazingly simple and undemanding. If, in its practice, abhyasis don't progress, then one can only conclude that the will to progress to the destination is lacking. The motive force is lacking. That is, even the desire to serve Master is lacking. If one accepts the idea that only the abhyasi who meticulously carries on his sadhana and proceeds unlingeringly towards his goal is really serving the Master, then all other aspects of service are seen to be merely lower orders of service, at best. There is the danger that such service can even degenerate into hypocritical attitudes of self-seeking. Every currency needs to be 'backed'. Similarly our service to the Master must be backed by love, devotion, and correct practice, as these alone help us to become what he wants us to become, and thus set the seal of true service upon our efforts.

Life and Liberation

All life is struggle. Wherever we look, we see life involved in this frantic struggle. The animals of the earth, the aquatic life in the rivers and oceans of this world, the birds of the air–all are undergoing this struggle, and man is no exception. Just take a fish out of water and see how frantically it struggles for life. Throw a land animal into water and see its frantic and untiring struggle **to get back into its own element for survival**. Thus each type of created life has its own native element in which alone it can live and function.

Man thinks he is in his element. And because he can fly and swim, he imagines he is in his element in all the elements. He imagines that just because he has discovered and perfected vehicles that can take him deep under water, and also high up into the atmosphere and into the near vacuums of space beyond, he has conquered the elements. Why then does he still struggle for existence? Why is he miserable? The poor think that once their poverty is eradicated they will be happy. But look at the rich and the affluent. They, too, are miserable. A stonecutter is able to sleep in a jolting lorry on a bed of crushed stones under the hot sun, but a rich man is unable to find sleep even on a comfortable cushioned bed, with his room air-conditioned for the very purpose of insuring restful sleep.

The rich imagine that power and position will give them satisfaction and a sense of well-being; but the higher they rise, the more enemies they create, and the effort merely to retain their position seems to need efforts far beyond their capacities. Stresses appear, leading to breakdown of the physical constitution, mental embitterment, emotional imbalance, etc. Sleep is the first thing they lose, then progressively, health, peace of mind, happiness–and if they do not check the all-round decline in time, life itself.

Reprinted from *Constant Remembrance* (Newsletter of the Mission in USA) Vol. 10, 1979.

Perhaps they abandon the quest for wealth and power, and seek solace in intellectual pursuits or artistic pursuits, instead! It does not take them long to recognize that here, too, the happiness and peace of mind that they are searching for, eludes them. We thus find unhappiness, misery, and struggle to pervade all of human existence, and none born into this physical existence is free from it.

The animals, birds, and fishes struggle only for physical existence. We humans struggle physically, mentally, and emotionally as well; having come to this conclusion, we rest, embittered and cynical misanthropes. Had we gone one more step ahead in that reasoning, we would have stumbled upon the real answer. 'Spiritual' is the term missing in the sequence, 'physical, mental, and emotional.' The true fact is that the land, air and water, which we consider to be our elements, and which we have conquered, are **not** our true elements. Hence, we are like fishes out of water.

There are certain varieties of fish that spend a fairly long time on land when they come out to spawn. Are they happy there just because they are able to live a little longer on land than other species of fish? No! They are constantly flipping and flopping about, anxious to get their job done and to get back into their true element. Whales live in the oceans, and dive to the farthest depths, but they have to surface once in a while to breathe, because they are mammals. So the ability to live in an alien element is at best a temporary ability. For permanent existence–and existence of wellbeing, of peace of mind, of harmony–one's own natural environment is essential.

And here we come to the crux of the matter. What is man's natural habitat? Where is it? The Master answers that our real home is **there** where we have come from; and all our struggles of this physical existence reflect our deep longing to get back there, where we truly belong. A fish out of water frantically struggles for very life. It does not know why it is doing this. It cannot know that it has to get back into water. But it struggles strenuously nevertheless. If it gets back, it swims away serenely, once again in harmony with its nature. Our struggles are like that. That is why all humans, without exception, struggle here in this life: the poor as much as the rich, the sick as well as the healthy, the powerless as well as the powerful, the ignorant as well as the learned; all struggle. It is a natural struggle to get back where we belong, and in this struggle we are as blind as the fish that knows not what it wants, but is pressed forward by its inner nature to struggle, and go on struggling, until it gets back to its element or dies in the process.

If we recognize the true nature of our struggles as the effort to get back to our original element–our real home as Babuji calls it, the spiritual abode of truth, bliss, and harmony–then our efforts begin to have a definite orientation. Our efforts, now geared to a definite goal, become purposeful. Forgotten are the merely human aspirations of health, wealth, power, and position. We recognize them as being temporary and ephemeral because our very existence here, being in an alien element, is temporary and ephemeral. That is, our efforts now take on the character of a guided approach to our goal of realising (finding and establishing ourselves in) our true, original home.

This is the reason why abhyasis feel at home in spiritual gatherings. Wherever such gatherings are held, abhyasis say how like Basant Panchami the atmosphere has been. During those few days all worries evaporate, all problems disappear, and amazingly, even thoughts of 'home' are gone. When abhyasis wonder at this last phenomenon–that even the home and family are forgotten–the answer is, "How can one remember a home when one is in it?"

This is the liberation–however temporary it may be–that Master allows us to experience, which gives us peace, harmony, and well-being. All that we have to do is make it permanent, and this is the spiritual pursuit in which we are all involved, and which, by Babuji's benevolent grace, all sincere practicants of Sahaj Marg will achieve.

The Friend Within

The happiest period of a person's life are the years of childhood lived in the bosom of the family. They are carefree years, full of the laughter and sunshine of life that makes it the glorious era of one's existence. As we grow older, the greater is the longing and the nostalgia associated with the memories of our childhood and youth. What is it about our early years that make them so universally happy ones? They are the years filled with growth, both physical and mental. Every event has the wonder of a discovery, an aura of newness, about it. There is no staleness. This freshness, this wonder, this uniqueness in everything that one sees, touches, perceives, envelops the early years of our existence. The childhood years are like the unrolling of a new carpet. It is untrodden, new, springy, and glorious in its pattern, colours and texture. The future will be nothing but treading on the same carpet again and again, wearing out its pile, slowly destroying its colours, dirtying it and wearing it down until it is nothing but a pitiful skeleton of its former gorgeous self. This is one aspect of the matter.

There is a second aspect, more important, I think, than the first. In childhood we are the cherished and loved members of the family. We are with our parents, brothers and sisters all the time, waking or sleeping. All their love is unstintingly showered upon us. We have little or no work, and virtually no responsibilities. Cares, we have none. Life is one long and joyful episode filled with love, happiness, tenderness and care. Our every joy is shared by those around us. Our little sorrows are comforted away by hugs and kisses of love. Our pains are smoothed away by loving hands. We are sung to sleep. When we do something of which we feel happy or proud, the parents are there to praise us and make much of us. Should we suffer a trifling hurt or injury, their sympathy and love

Reprinted from Shri Ram Chandraji Maharaj's 80th Birth Anniversary Celebration Souvenir, Ahmedabad, 1979.

is immediate. We have only to run to mother for it. In short, for everything that we want, we do, or feel, someone is there to praise us, cherish us, support us, love us.

This goes on till a child becomes a youth. The spontaneous turning to members of the family now ends. Aid is more selectively sought. The boy or girl still seeks guidance. They still need someone to make much of them. The need for a pat on the back when some success has crowned our efforts is still very much there. The ego needs constant bolstering. But the ebullience, the bubbling over of the earlier childhood phase have, alas, disappeared. The youth now seeks all these things, but only from one or two. The mother is always a part of this scene. Fathers seem to easily lose their appeal, to regain it only when they have become grandfathers, and then, too, only for their grandchildren. In short, when the child becomes a youth, it has weeded out its large family circle of admiring well-wishers to just one or two individuals. The circle of confidence has shrunk. The youth's dependence is on just one or two others. Therefore, he has to depend increasingly upon himself. I feel that as self-dependence is taught and instilled into children, and as they become more and more self-dependent, the joys and happiness of childhood vanish like mist when the sun rises.

A stage comes when the youth, having grown and matured into an adult, competent and educated to face life on his own, acquires a family of his own. There is enormous happiness, even bliss, in this stage of life. There is ecstasy of family existence, of parentage. There is joy and happiness in gaining increasing command over the domestic and official environments, reflecting one's growth and development on the social scale. Yet all this is accompanied by a sense of loss, of something that seems to have eluded us.

Till forty years one was invited to birthday parties, marriages and similar happy and joyful events. Now one seems to have more of hospital visits on his hand. There are more calls to the crematoria than to birthday parties. Sorrow seeps in through every available avenue. The flawless armour of our ego had begun to develop hairline cracks even as we were in college. Now the cracks have widened, and seem to allow all the sorrows and miseries of existence to seep in and rob us not merely of peace of mind but of sleep itself. More than anything else, we have no one to turn to. In our middle age, few have the good fortune of still having their grandparents alive. Even if they are alive, they need all the physical assistance and emotional succour that we can possibly offer them. There is little that they can offer us. If we are fortunate enough to have parents, they, too, are often unable to help us in any tangible form. More than anything else, we just cannot turn to them for solace as we used to do in the years of our childhood and youth. Our ego will not permit it. In short, as we grow older, we are increasingly thrown upon ourselves. We have to shoulder the burdens that the younger generation we have brought into being puts upon us. Their questions have to be answered, their cares removed, their needs satisfied, their joys shared and their sorrows removed by our love. Not only have we to bear our burdens, burdens which, in childhood, our parents bore for us, but we have the burdens of the elder and younger generation, too, to bear. At this stage in our lives, when we are in our middle age, we live the care-worn and tormented existence of one who has to bear the existential problems of three generations.

There is no wonder in the fact that it is generally in middle age that most persons seem to turn to religion for solace and guidance. In the average person, middle age seems to constitute the threshold separating the mundane years from the religious life. One turns to religion, to God, or to a guru, precisely because there is no one else to whom we can turn. As we grew up we became more and more 'self-dependents'. Side by side, as we grew older and approached middle age, loved ones began to leave us for the beyond. The family circle is depleted. Friends too, are lost. If we have the bad fortune to live a long life, a really long life, then miserable indeed is the existence of such a person. He has no one, literally no one, to turn to. The only recourse is to God. It is then that we realise that all our life we have been placing our dependence on non-eternal things, animate or inanimate. Being non-eternal, they vanish sooner or later, beaching us on the barren sands of an unknown shore where every footprint holds nothing but terror for us. It is then that we realise that had we placed our dependence on Him who is everywhere, and in our hearts too, this misery would not have fallen to our lot. We realise that God is not a subject to be thought about and cultivated in our old age, but should have been the most vital, most necessary *vyavasaya* of our early years. Religious traditions have recognized this need for one to be connected to God early in one's life, as evidenced by rituals associated with such an act still practised in all religions of the world. Unfortunately, they have remained mere rituals, the inner presence having been lost in the paraphernalia of the rituals themselves. The vital connection was therefore missed. The Divine connection remained unmade. The seat of the friend remains vacant.

The spiritual connection, the connection of the individual with God, is therefore not merely vital for our existence, but is a very early need, too. It should be effected as early as possible in our lives. Postponing it to the later years can have grave consequences. Yoga seeks to make this inner connection of the self with the Self and to create for us an eternal friend within ourselves. Such a friend is a permanent, eternal entity, ever available to us, not separated from us by time or space. It is significant that in Sufism the Master is called "Friend"! The guru or Master is indeed the sole friend that we have. All the others, worldly associates, are only acquaintances, persons with limited capacity, often with even less of willingness to help. It is not enough to have a Master. It is vitally necessary to internalize His presence within us, to seat Him upon the throne in our hearts from where He can guide the course of our existence to its destination. Only a Master who has 'filled' our heart can help us in all things, in all ways, and make of our existence that which it ought to be.

True Abhyasi, Right Aspiration and Real Goal

We are coming to the concluding part of a most auspicious, most spiritually significant, and what is most important, a most spiritually elevating and ennobling experience that has been the substance and the essence of these three days that we have been together here; where we have tried to offer our humble homage at the holy feet of our Divine Master by celebrating his birthday. Such occasions are extremely important; and when we come to such celebrations of unbelievable spiritual magnitude, importance and value, it is essential that we understand how we should comport ourselves, how we should behave generally; what should be the way of life that we should adopt not only during these three days but throughout the rest of the year so as to draw from Babuji Maharaj the very essence of existence itself, which Master calls 'Life in life'! So I personally consider these celebrations as something of a retreat into ourselves where we establish contact, through Babuji Maharaj, with the inner essence, with His own inner essence which he has implanted in us, and thereby seek, and receive, the spiritual revival, the grace, his wisdom-filled illuminating words which help us to carry on for the rest of the year, till we come again for the next *utsav*.

Now, these are called concluding lectures, but I am an optimist and I believe that what ends can only begin again. So I look upon the concluding address as the inaugural address for the next session, and in that spirit I would like to place before you certain points which my beloved Master has offered to us yesterday, and the publication of which he has approved. This will be printed and issued to all centres in due course, but since the message contains exhortation and since the advices contained here are extremely important for us, I think I should take this opportunity of your pres-

Reprinted from *Sahaj Marg* magazine, July, 1979.

ence here and reveal to you Master's thinking. Master says, "The abhyasis aspiring for the Highest alone can be said to be the true members of Shri Ram Chandra Mission." I repeat, "The abhyasis aspiring for the Highest alone can be said to be the true members of Shri Ram Chandra Mission." Here Babuji Maharaj has tried to emphasize that one does not become a member of the Mission by just walking into our centres, taking three meditation sittings, practising it in a rather haphazard fashion without devotion, without dedication, without interest, nor by wearing the badges that we are all wearing on our hearts. What is essential is that the teaching should be inside the heart. We should receive the transmission here, right inside the heart. I once heard a preceptor rather humorously remarking about a most unreceptive abhyasi to whom he had been giving a sitting. When the sitting was over the preceptor said, "My dear friend, I did not ask you to sit in meditation to whitewash your outside. It was your inside which I was seeking. But I could not penetrate into it. You are so unreceptive." So, a true member of the Mission, of this august, this glorious and what will prove to be an everlasting Mission, is one that should seek the Highest. No lesser aims can qualify us for membership. No lesser aspirations can qualify us for membership. He who seeks the Highest alone is a true member of the Mission.

The second point which Master has emphasized is, "If they continue this aspiration for some time, devoting themselves to the Almighty, then comes the grace to foment the real aspiration." Here is a great secret which Babuji has revealed. First he talks of the highest aspiration, the aspiration for the Highest, and now he says that if this aspiration for the Highest is continued for some time then the grace of the Almighty, our Babuji Maharaj, descends to foment in us the real aspiration. So the real aspiration is something else again. Now, how to know it? How to understand it? How to even find out what is this real aspiration? So the first aspiration for the Highest is but a step in the real aspiration which is opened up in us, which is fomented in our heart. Craving is created for it. We are all talking of craving and the need for craving every day. But yesterday Babuji Maharaj opened up this secret that the level of aspiration at the beginning, which we call the aspiration for the Highest, with a capital H, is yet a lower level of aspiration than that which should develop, provided one has the right aspiration in the beginning. Aspiration for the Highest is therefore not the highest aspiration. So the right aspiration confers upon us not merely the membership of the Mission, but draws or enables us to draw from the Almighty sitting here, the grace that is pouring down on us, which in turn will foment in us the real aspiration, i.e., instead of whitewashing the outside, the grace now starts getting inside and fomenting that which must be fomented.

The third point which Master gave us: "We want that fountain in us which may spring forth all the time doing worldly or Godly work." Now what does this fomenting create in us? What is the wellspring of creating, which springs into us? What is it expected to do? It is expected, first, to spring forth. Now it is a sort of a desert land, uncreative, unproductive. But by the fomenting power of the grace that descends into us, and that awakes the real aspiration in us, springs–which he calls the fountain–are opened up in us. It springs forth because there is a gushing out. There is power embedded in us which pushes the things out of us for creative work in the two fields of Divine and worldly work. Here Master emphasizes the fact that Sahaj Marg does not emphasize the Divine aspect of life or the worldly aspect of life. As he has said again and again, this path is that of the bird which flies on two wings, and there has to be perfect balance of both. So our business is to allow the first part of the real aspiration for the Highest, thereby acquire His grace which will foment in us the real aspiration, which in turn opens up the wellsprings lying dormant in our hearts, covered up with all the grossness of ages and ages of existence. When they are pushed aside by the innate strength of Divinity, by the innate power, latent seeds of Divinity fountain forth and enable us to perform in both the fields of Divinity and materiality. What does it do? Master says, "It removes the rust already settled on the instrument we have." Any tool which has not been used for some time will have a covering of rust on it. Now, if you wipe it off externally–it is possible to do it–and leave it unutilized, then within two days you will again find rust on it. So what is the true and only efficacious method of removing the rust which we have covered ourselves with? It is to allow the inner fountain to spring out, which by enabling us to work perfectly in the twin fields of materiality and spirituality automatically, from inside, throws out all the rust, and by its continued creative functioning in these fields, further covering of rust, further addition of grossness, as we usually say, is prevented altogether.

Next Master gives us what I consider to be a very, very important exhortation. It is not just advice, it is an exhortation! He says, "It does not look nice to have the idea of being a Guru before time." As Babuji Maharaj explains, even the merest tyro in spirituality seems to assume that he has got on to some sort of a pedestal in spirituality; and by that little, tiny, minute elevation which we get even from the first glance of the Master, one should not begin to think that one is superior to his fellow brothers and sisters. One is still very much part of humanity. This brotherhood, this idea of brotherhood, should not be lost. One should not try to think that he is becoming a guru in any sense.

Master once explained this to me, when we were flying back from abroad, from Beirut to Delhi, and we were talking of divinisation. Master said, "The higher you go, the lower your vision must descend." I could not understand it for a moment. But you know, I found myself looking out of the window of the plane and it suddenly struck me that when we are in the air, we only look at the ground, whereas when we are on the ground we are looking up into the sky all the time aspiring to reach the stars in heaven. So this is one aspect of invertendo, that we always look away from where we are; and the Highest has to look down to the lowest, and the lowest has to look up the Highest.

So, as one proceeds and by my beloved Master's grace and his immense mercy, as we ascend higher and higher, our vision has to come lower and lower, and it must reach a level where, as Master says, "A true Master is one who has submitted to the entire creation." It is not merely submission to humanity, not merely compassion for existence or compassion for the living things, or even, as I have observed in Master, compassion for vegetable life. Perhaps you all know that when our Shahjahanpur Ashram, the headquarters of our worldwide organization, was to be built, the project was delayed for six months because there was a standing crop of *arhar dhall* on part of the estate which Master refused to touch. He said, "Well, it is a growing thing. It is a living organization. It must come into fruition and for that we must allow the time. My building can wait. This cannot be destroyed for that."

This is the idea with which we have to face life. This is the idea with which we have to see what life is. Life does not mean human beings alone. Life is that which pervades the entire universe. And if our ancient seers are to be believed there is life even in stones. The only thing is that they have adopted, or got into their existence, such an immensity of grossness that there is no movement, there is no sensation, there is nothing in them. It is life at its most dormant, most static aspect. At the other end you have the spirit, not embodied, untramelled by desires, not bound down by grossness, freedom in the universality of the spirit. So this is the compassion we have to develop. It is not a compassion in the aspect of pity. I remember one great preceptor once told me that if we look at true saintly persons, you will find there is always a film of moisture upon their eyes. Now, it is a fact of observation that the more material a person is, the more metallic the eyes become; they glitter. There is a metallic glitter in their eyes; whereas the more elevated spiritually a person becomes, his eyes become softer and softer, and at one stage you find a film of moisture covering both the eyes. It is not tears, but there is a permanent film of moisture and the preceptor explained to me that it is the permanent wellspring of compassion flowing into their eyes, and it is reflected as a compassion which is universal in nature, not for you or me in a particularized sense but in a universal sense. So at this stage it does not look nice to have the idea of being a guru before time.

The sixth point is "If anybody has such an idea for the good of the Mission there are other ways which can help the growth of the Mission." That is, if a person truly wishes to serve the Mission and wants its good, wants it to grow, wants it to expand, not out of personal egoistic tendencies but out of that immense gratitude that what I have received, others too must receive, then there are other ways of serving the Mission. It should not stop with me. What Master has given to me is not for myself alone. It is like a river which flows from the Himalayas down to the sea. We are permitted to take that much of water that we need, but we cannot dam up the river at our doorstep in a selfish manner because the river must flow; and if you dam it up, the river starts stinking because it is now stagnant. Life must flow, rivers must flow. Here, too, the good of the Mission means service must flow out of the heart of every abhyasi. The right aspect of service, service without bias, service without preference, service without seeking rewards, is important. I emphasize this point particularly because very often we have abhyasis coming to us, coming to Master himself, saying, "Babuji, I wish to offer my services to the Mission." And while their offers are very sincere and very genuine, they are somewhat premature because the concept of service is not properly understood and there are yet differences in our minds of what types of service we shall offer, how that service should be accepted, and in what form that service should be remunerated. Only when all these three aspects, which are lying dormant in our minds (not really dormant but suppressed by us because we wish to appear sincere, we wish to appear spiritual, and therefore they are kept dormant, hidden from the Master, as they think, but only really hidden from themselves), are understood and sublimated, are we ready for real service.

Now it is only when this three-fold idea of qualities of service, etc., disappear from our minds that the *sadhaka* becomes a true *sevaka*. There is a difference between a sadhaka and a sevaka. A sadhaka does for himself, while a sevaka does for the Master. I must emphasize here something which I am telling our brothers and sisters wherever I go—that when we serve, when we offer our services to the Master, there is often this immense temptation offered to us by abhyasis. They come to us and say, "Sir, you have done so much for us. You have spent so much of your time on us. You have been getting up at four o'clock and going to bed at midnight giving sittings and we are very grateful to you." I say this is a temptation because preceptors are human beings and if they get into their heads the idea that they are serving humanity, the first crime in spirituality commences, because none of us are serving

True Abhyasi, Right Aspiration and Real Goal 255

anybody except the Master. We are only servants of the Master. It is my Master's desire that I should transmit to the abhyasis. So I do it. It is our Master's desire that we should congregate and feed the people here and house them properly. So we do it. That is why I emphasized three days back when I had a volunteers' meeting, that our brothers and sisters who are here, they are Master's guests and therefore should be treated as such by us. Even brotherliness is not enough. They are Master's beloved guests and if we have the idea of service, it should be something like what you offer to your *sambandhi*. When the bridal party with the *baraat* comes, how much fuss we make about them. How many sweets we offer to them. How much attention we give to their every least comfort. This should be the aspect of service because here Master is the supreme bridegroom and all of us are brides, in the ancient principle that there is one *purusha* only and all the others are only females, whatever be their sex. So this should be the aspect of service.

Next, Master gives us a point concerning transmitters, of preceptors, but that concerns only the preceptors. And so I come to the final point Master places before us which is, "Our aim should be to reach the highest point."

So he has created, as it were, a spiritual circle by starting with the aspiration for the Highest and ending with the aim which should be the Highest. Now, an aspiration and an aim–there is a distinction which our beloved Master draws here. An aspiration is really not an aim. When does an aspiration become an aim? When the aspiration is solidly backed by our will to achieve. And as Master emphasizes again and again, will can be created in us. Will can really become fruitful only when there is interest. Sadhana starts, or has started for most of us, when we heard of it from some friends or some abhyasis whom we know. They said, "You know, there is a Mission called Shri Ram Chandra Mission and I find it a very good thing because I have benefited by it." One man says, "My anger has disappeared," another says, "I found peace of mind," things like that. So we come, we enroll ourselves, we start sittings and then as we go on doing this meditation, we find that in our own experience we are able to confirm the experiences of others who introduced us to the system. This confirmation in our own experience of the values which we sought makes our interest deeper, and the deepening of interest makes us more and more disciplined in our sadhana; I would not say perfect because perfection comes only at the last. It makes us more and more sincere in our efforts, and our sadhana becomes deeper and deeper. So, when experiences–or shall we say, what we should call experiences, not the things which are brought out in cleaning, but the true spiritual values which are revealed to us as they deepen progressively, our interest is elevated to the level where it becomes a commitment to our sadhana; and when that reaches its culmination, you find the tendency of surrender developing in us. So from interest to commitment to surrender can be one way of explaining progress.

Now, surrender is a term which many people are afraid of. They think that it is a loss of freedom. Often we find people asking us–even yesterday we had some questions, whether could we go to pictures, could we attend music parties, things of that sort. Now there are innate tendencies in us which have to be expressed until they are cleaned out. So, it is reasonable to expect that until the cleaning process has reached its completion, at least one small tiny portion of our samskara must find expression, must find expression in our external life, and that is permissible. But as Master emphasizes in his works, if we look at the flowers and admire their beauty and praise the Almighty Lord who created it, it is not wrong. But if you look at it a second time, if you look at it a third time and create in yourselves an attachment to its beauty which breeds in you a desire to possess it–which perhaps tempts you to cut off the flower and take it home–then you commit an act of theft. That is the problem. So these trivial worldly things, we should not pay much attention to. Master says it is only necessary to divert the mind, and automatically it will take care of itself. So, what Master is teaching us is not a denudation of our lawful ways of life. We have to live in this world. Whatever we may do or not do, our existence is something over which we have no control; I mean the physical existence. But surely we have control over our spiritual experience, when we surrender ourselves to the Master. His control comes only when we give up our control to Him. That is, instead of my depending on myself, I transfer this dependence to our beloved Babuji Maharaj, and then when the dependence is surrendered it becomes a true state of surrender. That is, as Master states repeatedly, "Create in yourselves a state of dependency, and surrender will automatically come."

I thought I should exchange with you some of these ideas which my beloved Master explained to us yesterday in our preceptors' meeting, which will be circulated to all with his approval.

Darshan

There is a fixed belief in the minds of most Indians that to have *darshan* of a great soul, one advanced on the path, is in itself an act of piety which can endow substantial blessings on the person having such a darshan. This belief in the value of darshan is rampant, and has assumed the proportions of a deep-seated superstition among the people of India. It is a common sight to see thousands of persons waiting patiently to have a darshan of a person they consider to be a *sadhu* or a saint. No matter what the real inner worth of such a person may be, if he is clad in the saffron robes sanctified by centuries of custom and tradition, he is put on a pedestal, as it were, and thousands flock for his darshan so as to receive his unspoken blessings. Even ordinary persons, without any higher aspiration whatsoever, rush for such darshan if they hear of a sadhu or a saint in their vicinity.

Does such a darshan have any real value? Can it confer anything of a higher approach on the people who flock for it? Master answers this question in his own inimitable and profound manner in *Voice Real*. Master writes, "It is good that you like to have darshan of the Mahapurushas [saints], better would it be to have the darshan of your self alone." Master implies that the real darshan is of the Self.

In our *sanstha* too, this craze for darshan is quite obvious. Abhyasis who do not even practise meditation as taught by Master spend hours waiting to have a brief glimpse of his form. As Master remarks quite often, such hours wasted in waiting to see him for the purpose of darshan could be much more profitably used in sadhana. It is not for nothing that Master has remarked again and again, "Many come to see me, but no one really sees me." This cryptic comment by the Master is pregnant with a wealth of spiri-

Reprinted from Shri Ramchandraji Maharaj's Birthday Souvenir, Malaysia, 1981.

tual meaning. To see a great saint's physical eyes has nothing to do with having his darshan. It is only an act of corporeal vision, something which even animals do when they look at a saint; it is only looking at him, not having his darshan. When we see Master with our physical eyes, and gaze, however fondly, at merely his physical person, we do nothing more than what an animal does when it looks at a saint, or anyone else for that matter.

What then, is the meaning of darshan? Darshan means 'to see'. It is obvious that normal seeing has nothing to do with this. Therefore *darshana* really means to go beyond the physical person and see the inner condition of the person one is looking at. The next stage would be to go beyond the condition to the essence of the person seen. And the final stage, as far as my thinking goes, is to go beyond the essence to the Reality pervading the essence.

Our Master gives us a hint about this, again in *Voice Real*. Master says, "I have had so far numerous coverings one after the other. But the present one which I now have, if observed minutely, will be found to be only a covering of nakedness which is the last, and which when cast off shall not be replaced by another." As a further pointer to our own goal in our sadhana, Master adds, "I wish you all to be clad in the same covering of nakedness." Then, as if to give us a gentle hint as to how one should really try to have his darshan, Master continues, "That is not possible so long as one remains entangled within the charms and attractions of this outer covering, the physical body."

It is a selfish desire for material fulfilment and a comfortable, disease-free existence that makes most people rush to have the darshan of a yogi or saint. There is no inner craving for higher approach. There is no desire for spiritual well-being. There is not even the idea of a goal to be achieved. Of those who have stepped into the field of spirituality, it may be said that if this hankering for darshan of the Master still persists in them, then the past tendencies are still having their sway. There may perhaps be a few persons in whose hearts some love for the Master may have begun to develop. Perhaps they want to have the darshan of the Master, but if they are satisfied with the physical aspect alone, they continue to perpetuate the former error.

When true love for the Master develops, and when one has sufficiently advanced on the spiritual path, a time comes, when the abhyasi sits in meditation he finds the form of the Master coming to his vision naturally and automatically. I consider this to be the beginning of the true darshan of the Master. The form one sees in the heart resembles the physical appearance of the Master, but is no longer the physical form that one sees with the physical eyes. It is but a reflection of that presence. I may say that it is the inner presence of the Master in one's own heart that one sees now. To my mind, this is the first real darshan of the Master, and it is now appropriate to take up meditation on the Master's form. If meditation is continued along proper lines, a stage comes when the form of the Master fades away even from the inner vision of the abhyasi. The essence comes to one's vision–or I may say that the Master now benevolently blesses the deserving abhyasi with the second stage of his darshan, His essence. In the final stages of one's spiritual pursuit, one comes into the condition where one finds the Master in His essence, spread out throughout the universe. This, I believe, is the culmination of one's sadhana.

Love for the Master alone makes a proper beginning possible. Love for the Master alone makes it possible for the abhyasi to continue along the right lines of the sadhana prescribed. In the process, love itself grows. And this growth of love for the Master, to an extent where nothing other than the Master comes before the abhyasi's gaze, makes the final darshan of the Master possible. May Master bless all on the path who seek Him with sincerity and love and devotion.

The Principles of Sahaj Marg

Volume 3

Balanced Existence

I am going to speak about the difficulty of Sahaj Marg; because I find all my brothers and sisters and the ultimate Master himself always saying that everything is simple. Of course, for Master nothing is difficult, "How to do this?" "Concentrate!" "How to change?" "Transmit!" "How to achieve God?" "Turn your head from here to here, and He is there." So for about twenty years I have been bombarded with the simplicity of Sahaj Marg. But for every moment of those twenty years I have been facing the biggest problems: "How to change, how to do, how to transmit, how to correct–ourselves first, others later?"

As in everything in life, there is a similarity between one end and the other end. In between, everything is different. The child is simple; the child is innocent; it does not have to speak; by just looking at its mother or weeping a little, it gets everything it wants. The old man also gets the same treatment. In between, we have to fight for everything that we have to get. Similarly, in our abhyas, particularly in our Sahaj Marg abhyas, when we start our sadhana– I won't say it is deceptively simple–but the simplicity deceives us. Master used to say, "It is my simplicity that deceives." And when we come in with our enthusiasm, with some idea of the goal–we delude ourselves that it is the goal. In most cases it is not the goal at all! We feel everything is simple; our preceptors advise us it is very simple; Master adds to our problem by saying everything is so simple; and we are very happy. We say, "But if it is so simple, why not we try and get?" And then Master says, "Someone achieved in seven years, Lalaji achieved in seven months." So we say, "Between seven years and seven months we should have."

The first problem comes when he says he took twenty-two and a half years for his own perfection! Then we say, "What is this?

Talk at Raichur celebration on 9 October 1983 morning.

The Grand Master took seven months, someone took seven years under the Master, but the Master himself took twenty-two and a half years." This seems to be some sort of a contradiction that the Master should take more time than the abhyasi! When you ask him, he says, "It is very simple. You know I have to do this, I have to do that, but it is very simple I am telling you!" We say, "All right, the Master himself has said, so it must be simple."

When we sit in meditation we find we are not really meditating. We are thinking of something else. As someone said, when we sit in meditation the mind is in the office. When we are in the office, some abhyasi comes and we are talking of meditation. We run to our preceptor: "Sahib, how to meditate?" He says, "Brother, don't you read the instructions in that small list–one sheet we give you? There are only three things to do. Sit with your eyes closed; imagine there is a Divine Light in the heart (it is a mere suggestion); just put your mind over it. It is so simple." We are reassured. We come back and say, "Brother...has said, and so-and-so has said, Master has also confirmed, that it is really simple." "I am a fool, you see, because I have been struggling and I am not able to meditate." We do for three to four days, again we are not able to do something; rush to the preceptors. Patient people. Our preceptors are to be praised for their patience, for their dedication. Instead of spending half an hour, he spends two hours, and tells us how simple meditation is: "What, there is nothing else! It is the merest suggestion. Can we not even make the suggestion that there is light in the heart, and put our mind on it?" We say, "Yes sir, it is very simple. I must have been doing something wrong." He says, "Yes. Go and try again." We go home, reinforced by the simplicity of Sahaj Marg. Either we do it or we don't do it, some walk out, some few are fighting it all their lives. Some few who had the good fortune to have been associated very closely, in a very integrated way with the organization (that means brothers and sisters, preceptors, Master himself), in spite of their sadhana they develop.

If I am convinced of one thing, after twenty years of Sahaj Marg practice, it is that we develop in spite of ourselves, in spite of the sadhana that we are supposed to be doing because, with my hand on my heart I can tell you, I cannot claim to be a sadhak of

Sahaj Marg at all. It is Babuji's grace. This creates a second problem: "Sir, if it is possible by Babuji's grace, why should we undergo this torture of meditation, cleaning, night prayer? Can he not give it to us also, if he can give you, if He can give it to the big people who have assembled here before us?"

It is only grace. Babuji himself has said, "Sadhana does not confer on you any right to development." It is only something we indulge in, with faith, with devotion, with humility, to attract his gaze towards us. Only he whom He wants will achieve. Second complication: "I am a devoted abhyasi, Sir. I am doing meditation, I am doing cleaning, my preceptor also says that my condition is lighter, there is a glow in the heart. Yet Babuji looked at me like this and turned away! Why?" Preceptor says: "Grace must come. You see, there is no right conferred on anybody; least of all, us." How to get over this dilemma, of a practice which is supposed to lead us to the goal, but which at no stage (in the words of the Master himself) confers on you the right to reality or realisation. It has to come at His choice. It is a very difficult problem.

Along with this problem, we have the associated problems–this concept of the two wings of the bird. The materially poor abhyasis look at the millionaire abhyasis and say, "Sir, I am a very faithful, devoted abhyasi. I don't get thirty rupees a month. If my spiritual wing is being strengthened, should not my material wing also be strengthened?" For instance, someone used the *upamanam* [example] of the tank, levelling of the level of the water–it is a misleading conception. It does not mean that a saint will become a millionaire or that a millionaire will become a saint. But when we read about it, when we hear about the two wings of the bird, there is a certain amount of self-deception. (Mind you, I am saying self-deception–it is not the deception of the theory or the practice or the Master.) We deceive ourselves into thinking that here is a system which preaches and which promises equality in spiritual and material attainments. It does not do anything of that sort. It only tells us what to do. It says attend to both halves of your life–the spiritual half of your life and the material half of your life. Don't ignore one side for the other. Don't ignore spirituality for material life, don't ignore the material life for the sake of spirituality. You attend to both. You will get what he wishes you to get, in both the spheres. If he wants you to be a saint and also a millionaire, you will become one. If He wants you to become a saint and remain a pauper, you will remain so. But your attention should be on both sides.

This I find very few people have understood. They are always looking to better endowed people, comparing their own poor selves and saying, "Why am I not like him? He flies, I have to walk. He sits in the air-conditioned office, I am sweating it out in the fields. He is made a preceptor, I am not." So many problems; and you evaluate all these problems, and then equate it with the need for material life, and the 'apparent need' to devote more time to material life than spiritual life: "Sir, after all, if I have to look to my material life, if I have to look after my wife and family, I have to work eight hours in the office." Accepted. "It means I have to get up, have my shave, my bath, that takes one hour." Okay. "Evening when I come back I have to spend some time with my children, eat with them." Accepted. But where has Master said, "You spend twelve hours of the day in spirituality and twelve hours of the day in materiality?" Master has only said: "One hour in the morning, half an hour in the evening, ten minutes at bedtime."

So this one hour and forty minutes, that is hundred minutes total out of the whole day, is able to keep us in a balanced situation, as far as balancing the two halves of our lives is concerned. We mislead ourselves into thinking that Master has said that we should meditate all our lives forgetting the material life. He has not said so anywhere. So we find most abhyasis coming and saying, "Sir, I have no time." If you cannot find hundred minutes in twenty-four hours just to maintain a balance, when are we ever going to find time?

So, this again is our own self-deception, that a balance means apportionment of equal time; it does not mean anything like that. A thinker thinks for half a minute and he solves a problem, which solution an architect or builder puts into effect over probably eight months or one year.

Then comes the problem, why one progresses, another does not. This I have already told you in the beginning. Master has said, only he whom He wishes will get. "Why am I not the person whom He wishes for?" This question we are all asking ourselves. See, years ago, when we were reading through the Gita, we found that in that situation of the Mahabharat, there were several categories of people associated with Lord Krishna. Some took him only as a human being. Some took him purely as the Divine. Neither achieved the Ultimate. It was only Arjuna who loved Krishna at the human level, and who revered him in the Divine level after he revealed himself to him. He accepted him in both levels, he could love him in all his levels of existence–transcendence, ultimacy–he got.

Similarly, in our Mission we find many people approach Master as a human being, forgetting his divinity; they remain stagnant. There are also, unfortunately, abhyasis who have taken him only as the Divine, forgetting his human levels of existence. I don't think they have also proceeded much beyond the others. And what is it that makes you accept one individual both at the human and Divine level? It can only be love! If you love him as a human being, love leads to reverence. Whereas if you accept him only as Divinity, there may be fear associated with your acceptance; an awe you see, the distance you create–"You see, He is God and I am man, there is always going to be a separation between us!" But if I treat him only as a man and forget he is God, then I am going to have the problem of proximity, familiarity breeding contempt–"After all he is an old man, toothless, walking with a walking stick!"

So when we sort of dissect Master into his two halves, of his material and his divine existence, we fall into this error. It is the happy few–I don't know how many there are, perhaps there are many, I am not able to say–but it is those brothers and sisters of our satsangh who have been able to merge the Divinity of Master into his humanity or vice versa, who have been able to go to some extent by his grace. And if Master favours them, or apparently favours them (because Master has said in *Voice Real* such a Personality has no friend or foe; for him there is no friend or foe; he cannot have partiality towards one and not towards the other; there can be no selectivity in his approach; he cannot say, "To him I will give, to her I will not give,"–such an attitude cannot belong to our Master–it is in his own words! Yet, apparently he has favoured) then in our human minds we think he has favoured so-and-so, he has not favoured so-and-so.

"It is precisely because this man–he adores me at the human level, serves me at the human level, he loves me as a human being, as a father–he also has accepted and recognized my Divinity. I am for him a complete Personality. I am the Purnathva"–so one who accepts Master as the Purnathva, the Purnathva has to accept him– I mean, the Ultimate has no choice! This is why I said that sadhana can be an impediment if it is going to make us think of Him only as a man or only as a God. As we have to evolve from mere human beings, full of samskaras, ridden by samskaras to the bestial levels–if we have to evolve from that to the ultimate level which Master is holding up as our true *lakshya* (goal), it means that we in our lives have to encompass in our progress, 'The Two Ends'–the lowest karma–samskara-ridden, diseased imagination, diseased mind, diseased activities–from that level, we have to go to the ultimate Godhead, where you can say this man has been divinised, he is now like–in every attribute–the Divine itself!

We have to encompass this whole spectrum of development from the grossest to the subtlest, and we have before us the Master who has done it in his lifetime, and who has come here precisely to show us what is possible. Now, what is the purpose of a Master coming here? Can he not do it sitting in his *vaikunta* or whatever it is? After all, he says, "Sitting in Shahjahanpur I can transmit wherever you are. I can transmit to Venus, I can transmit to Neptune." Such a Personality is spread out throughout the universe. Why did he not do it? Precisely to tell us, that a God can become a human being without losing any single attribute of Divinity–to show us the way how we as humans (with every single dirty human attribute) can become like him, divinised. He comes in a human form precisely to show us, "I am This that you have been seeking! In me you will find everything that you should seek. I am the way. I am the instrument of that progress from yourself to what I am. See me, accept me, follow me, emulate me with wisdom, and you shall become like me." This is the message of his existence.

If in this message of his existence, we accept his example of a human life on this earth segmented into parts, taking one but not the other, we have lost our goal, we have lost the thread of our sadhana, we have lost the purpose of our existence. Otherwise, his existence is meaningless. Why on earth should a person like him come to earth and suffer all that he had suffered? A brother told you with much emotion how much Master suffered in the last year of his life. What was the purpose of his suffering? It too has a meaning. It only shows us: "Don't think that a divinised person when he comes here is free of suffering." You see, this is the promise he has made in his literature: "A saint is the target of the world's sorrows." We read it and we are happy! Why are we happy? Not because he is the target of the world's sorrows, but because we hope, in some inner recess of our minds, that we will not have to share in those sorrows! "Baba, He is there to take care of all those sorrows, let me be happy." This is our petty human mind which is willing to give all sorrows, miseries, sickness, disease, pain and frustration to the Master and we go to him and beg for ourselves happiness, wealth, education and a good life!

The Master in his life has exemplified, has illustrated–physically and perceptibly to every single one of his abhyasis–what a human being can rise to, how it can be the Ultimate itself, and even–after having achieved it in the human frame, if you are worth the salt you are eating, and if you are worthy of being called an abhyasi, you have got to be prepared to face every single sorrow, every single obstruction, every single pain that the Master himself has faced and suffered. This is the real meaning of the two wings of the bird. I cannot look for happiness and avoid sorrow. I cannot look for success and avoid failure. I cannot look for pleasure and avoid pain. Am I willing to accept a life which–precisely because it is life–has within it everything that life holds?

We have the twins of existence–the *dvandvas* as we call them. One who wants only one half and not the other half is unfit for sadhana. And a dedicated abhyasi, a devoted abhyasi who wants to be like the Master in every way, must also be willing to suffer everything that the Master has suffered; undergo every torture that the Master has undergone. See, it is a very facile explanation to say that it is all *maya*, it is a drama that he is playing for us. I say "Nonsense." Every second, every multisecond of the Master's life was filled with Reality. His sufferings were real. His joys were real. His achievements were real. How can there be unreality in Reality? Has he come to fool us and to deceive us?

So, when we want to pretend that we have pain without having pain, we are negating the value of his existence–of his teaching. On the contrary, our prayer should be: "Babuji, if you want to give me pain, give it to me in a concentrated dose." I remember once some Western abhyasis had come to Master and were complaining to him of their problems, miseries, sorrows–so many problems. Master says, "You will excuse me if I say one thing. In India we have had saints who have prayed 'Let the pain and misery and the sorrow of the whole universe come to me.' Now you please compare yourself with such saints."

See, we pride ourselves in coming from a great nation–from a great land hoary with tradition, filled with mystics. Throughout the history, there have been avatars and saints who have been born only on this *bhumi* of ours–Bharat Varsha. And yet we are the children of such a wonderful, noble, highly spiritual heritage, sons of rishis! You ask any fool on the street, "What is your Gotra?" "Vishwamitra Gotra, Kasyapa Gotra, Vasishta Gotra", and then we are like this *chuchunder* [newborn mouse which cannot see] which goes, trying to avoid, trying to evade; and all the time we are talking from platforms, "Master wants lions but not sheep." Everyone who speaks imagines that he is the lion, all the rest are sheep! This is the tragedy of Sahaj Marg–that there is no introspection, there is no self-examination.

The second tragedy of Sahaj Marg is that people who know– people who have achieved–they are unable to speak about it, because it will not bear expression, it cannot be told about, it cannot be talked about. It is not that there is anything secret. There are no words to express it. Those that have but book-learning are able to talk glibly about all these things and mislead us more and more: "Everything is simple; everything is nice; Babuji is here; Babuji is there; Babuji is spread out throughout the universe." I would like to know how many of us have seen Him in our hearts! I would like to know if even one of us has seen Him spread out throughout the universe. I would like to know how many of us have known him when he was materially present before us in a living, pulsating, suffering body. Which of us have known him? Which of us have known his inside? Which of us knew what he was suffering from? He was ever smiling! He was a Kalyana Purusha! Have you ever seen him weeping? Have you ever seen him in pain? And those who have had the opportunity (to see him in pain) come out and say, "No, no sir, this is all maya [illusion]. You know, it is a drama. How can the Divine suffer? How can the Divine have pain?" Yes, but then, why the needles and the pins? And the second, very facile, and very acceptable and very nice explanation is that, "He has taken our samskaras, and therefore he is suffering."

I say it is a shame that we should think like this; that we can go on misbehaving, go on with our corrupt attitudes and thoughts and actions, and leave that poor old man of eighty-three to suffer for us. Do you think it is right? Do you think it is love? Any mere mother is able to suffer for her child; any mere wife is able to suffer for her husband. Please forgive me if I say 'mere' because the women are supposed to be the weaker sex! It is a misconception. They are the stronger sex. They are able to suffer for the child. They are able to suffer for the husband. They suffer every moment of their lives–the poor women of India. And we, the lions of Sahaj Marg, the men, the preceptors, shame I say on us, that we are able to accept even intellectually the idea that he is suffering for us! If I have contributed to one moment of his suffering, I don't deserve to exist; not now. I should not have existed in the past, I don't deserve a future existence.

Forgive me, I am speaking with a little force. But Sahaj Marg has been made too simple, for too long, by too many people, all arising out of the misconception that we have very little to do and that He has to do everything for us. It is an utter misconception to think that I can get anything for nothing. Sahaj Marg is simple–as I told you–when we begin, and when we achieve mastery. In between it is full of frustrations, of loss, of misery, of problems, and loose talk of brotherhood. In this brotherhood there are many problems, you see. We expect the ultimate brotherhood to come at one stroke; that there shall be peace and plenty on earth, there will be Rama-Rajya, there shall be no hatred, that there shall be no *abipraya-bedas* [differences of opinion]. Is it possible?

What does brotherhood mean? See, this is the simplest idea of Sahaj Marg that we are all men and women, and we are brothers and sisters. What is brotherhood? What is sisterhood? How are we going to become one? I say that our differences are precisely what highlights our brotherhood! You see, when two people can have differences of opinion, differences of outlook, differences of goal (perhaps!) and still remain together, is it not a sign of brotherhood? I am sure that every one of you here has something in which you differ from me; yet we are together. Why is this togetherness coming about? Because we love and adore Him who is common to all of us. We are not bound by individual love of each other. We are bound because we love Him, from whom we are all suspended like puppets on a string! And that is the beauty of Master's message: "Love Him who loves all." If you ever try to love each other, is it ever possible in a world, I don't know, with about four billion population? Can we love three people in this world with proper love? Can we love one? I have been asking myself "Which husband loves his wife with that love? Which wife loves her husband with that love?" And we talk glibly of brotherhood where there shall be no differences of opinion, there shall be no frustration, it should all be Rama-Rajya. It is impossible. This brotherhood can come only when you love the Master so much that everybody you see appears as the Master, and therefore there can be no loss of virtue, no loss of anything, everybody is perfect in themselves; not because they are perfect, but because your eyes see nothing but the perfection.

When a brother was reading from the prepared speech there was a reference to brotherhood. The idea came to me that we admire some of these superbly beautiful girls who have a beauty spot here on the cheek. It is the beauty spot which heightens the beauty. Without that they will be just plain painted dummies! Similarly it is our diversity–diversity of culture, language, colour, opinions– this is what binds us together. If we should all think alike, feel alike, talk alike, walk alike, what are we trying–is it a society of robots that we are trying to build? Kindly try to understand what brotherhood really means, and how it can be achieved only by loving Him who loves all. There is no other way. It is impossible for us to go around loving. I am sure here itself, the abhyasis cannot love each other in that perfect way, because it is a lifetime's task to love one person; and if that one person happens to be Master, you have achieved what you have to do. You know that Puranic story about Siva, who said: "Who goes round the world three times first will get;" and this poor elephant god had the wit to walk around his father and mother and get it. Master: if I adore Him, if I obey Him, if I am faithful to Him, I have achieved the goal in every respect that Master wants us to achieve. I have achieved brotherhood. I have achieved mastery. I have achieved, most of all, His love. So these are the things.

Let us deliberate, let us think, let us not be satisfied with what we hear from platforms. Let us read the books of the Master. There is nothing that which our speakers can tell which is not in the books. Because, in Sahaj Marg, the creation of the philosophy, of the theory, has been perfected by the Master. Does it mean that it is an end in itself? No! What does it mean? That means anything worth saying has been said by the Master. We expand it, like the great Karikas of the past. (You see somebody wrote an Upanishad in twelve sutras, and one man wrote six hundred pages of Karikas on it!–obliterating all the original meaning and sense of the original. Let us stick to the original.

You see, Master was always concerned that the pristine purity of the practice and the philosophy of our system should be maintained for eternity. It is not for today or tomorrow. And how are we going to do it, if in the very first generation of abhyasis, we start distorting it, moulding it to our own intellectual fancies, predilections? Is it possible to preserve it? My advice to you brothers and sisters is, "Read the literature of the Master again and again; understand it. It is unnecessary to ask questions." Master has given us the hint, the practice: "Question your heart, the heart will reveal." "Whom should I love?" "Ask your hearts."

You know it is a tragedy of Master's life and of his passing away, that I am flooded with letters: "Sir, who is the Master? On whom should we meditate?" People who have not been able to achieve meditation on the form of the Master in his lifetime, are asking now after his form has become invisible. You see already the allegiance is being transferred, in the process of transfer. People are in a quandary. Why? Because it is a selfish approach to the Master. "How will I get?" is their question, not "What should I do?" On whom should I meditate? "Meditate on your Master." Who? "Your Master, with whom you have been associated all your sadhana years." You see, this is not a society, where we have two marriages and three marriages, least of all in spirituality! We have only one marriage–the Master is eternal. Saints know no death. With the result that there is chaos, there is confusion, and there is this unnecessary talk about this and that, so much of political nonsense. He whose heart is straight oriented towards the Master will have no questions about the past, the present, or the future.

The only advice I have to offer you is: "Please do your sadhana without fail." The abhyasi is not supposed to judge his own progress. I know, because many people have asked Master, "What is your condition?" and Master said, "Only Lalaji knows." If the Master could not know his condition, I am sure we are not going to know our condition. Let us leave it to our betters, our preceptors, to decide what is our condition, whether we are progressing or not. The second biggest (I should say) breach of faith, lack of faith, is to question the idea of progress: "Am I progressing?" It is a question, "Is Master worthy of being called a Master or not?" How on earth can he be a Master and you not progress? Every time an abhyasi asks, "Sir, am I progressing?" he is exhibiting his lack of faith in the Master.

You see, take a train. Trains may stop at stations, trains may stop at signals, trains may stop for the engine to take water. We don't know about all these–why is the train stopping? Will I reach the destination? You have got into the train; leave it to the administration to take you to the destination. Secondly, if you are concerned only with your progress, it means you have no love for the Master; you are still wedded to your self–my progress, my evolution, my realisation, my spiritualisation. He who loves the Master does not think of progress. So why worry about progress, why worry about this, that and the other, bring semantics into it, big philosophical questions?

"Sir, can I go to the Master in the morning and temple in the evening?" See, this sort of question means that there is still a desire in your mind, there is still a bifurcation in your mind between two ideals. If I go to the Master and ask, "Babuji, is it permitted to drink in Sahaj Marg?", it only means I have still a desire for drinking. If I go to him and say, "Babuji, can I eat meat?", it only indicates that there is still a desire for meat-eating. No questions come except based on desire. If desires are lost, questions are lost.

So I would suggest that if you want to see an abhyasi who has developed, look for a silent one and you will find him.

The Purpose of Existence

Most human beings do not know their goal. Even educated ones, even sophisticated ones, they do not know. I have been wondering why this should be so. When we compare the animal kingdom with the human kingdom–the animal life, bird life, the insect life, they come with some sort of a pre-programmed existence–to use computer terminology, they are pre-programmed. They do not have a choice. They come with a programmed existence which they meticulously follow, by means of what we call "instinct", when we relate it to what our Master said about human beings living as animals. It is because when we come here, we are also to some extent (why to some extent?–to a very large extent) pre-programmed by our samskaras. It is one of my convictions that no human being has any freedom–of choice, of action–until and unless he is able to eradicate, to erase, the programming which his samskaras have imposed upon him.

This is precisely the need to seek an external guide, an external superior force, a yogic force which can do that very vital job for us, of erasing the programme, and substituting another programme for us–which starts with the idea of a goal towards which we aspire. So when people ask, particularly in the West, "Master, can I not do this by myself? Am I not capable? I am a PhD, I am a doctor, I am an engineer, or what have you," it is very difficult to convince them in today's world of 'do-it-yourself' activity, here is one line of pursuit–the yogic pursuit–which you cannot do without external assistance, for this very vital reason that you have no ability or power to change your programming by yourself.

People who are handling tape recorders know that it cannot erase by itself, you have to erase it; or by recording something

Talk at Raichur celebration, 9 October 1983 evening.

superimposing on it, the old one is removed, the new one is imposed. This is the first function of a spiritually enlightened person to open our eyes to our goal by imposing–it is not an imposition of will, it is an imposition of knowledge or *jnana*–and say, "My dear friend, you are suffering from this. This is your samskara. As long as your samskaras exist, you have no choice. When you have no choice your mind will not work in the proper way. When it does not work in the proper way, what idea can you have of your goal? And when you have no goal, towards what are you going to live, to exist for?" This is a very vital point which a brother has rightly stressed.

In the next important idea of the necessity to read Master's books, I will tell you from my own experience. When I first came into the Mission, and I was given a copy of *Reality at Dawn*, I read it through in about thirty-five or forty minutes, and I literally threw it away saying: "What is there in this that we have not known before? There is nothing new." One year later, having nothing else to read, I read *Reality at Dawn*, and I was surprised to find a wealth of meaning! Now, every time I re-read it, a new meaning comes up. It is a theory of mine that such books, which we call eternal books (written by the greatest personalities of this world–in themselves whether they contain any knowledge or not is not the question) seem to reflect our growth, our development, very much like a mirror which, remaining what it is, shows very much the change in my stature, in my face, in my physiognomy. As I change, the mirror reflects. So the books are very vital, because as our understanding of the contents of the book changes, it seems to give me an idea of my own growth. They are spiritual mirrors. We turn to the mirror every morning for shaving, but unfortunately we do not turn to these Divine spiritual mirrors for our spiritual enlightenment, which we should do.

"Anything new in Sahaj Marg?" Well, if you read our ancient literature, you find that every saint had held out the same goal– Divinisation; you must be like God, you must aspire to be God. But one interesting and important point is that the very idea of Divinity seems to evolve into something new as we develop. You know, if you study the history of religion, you start with things like worship of the crudest sort: worship of animals, worship of birds, worship of trees; then going into worship of the forces of Nature which produced these things: worship of the rain, worship of the wind, worship of the sun; then evolving into the idea of the trinity: the triumvirate, the creator, the destroyer and the preserver; the coming into monistic worship of there being only One who manifests as the three. Is it God who has changed? It is we who have changed. And as we develop, our idea of the Ultimate develops.

That is why our Master has beautifully put a title for his book: *Towards Infinity*; because the goal seems to recede as we approach. The goal seems to show itself in a different way as we approach: "Subtler and subtler, yet subtler." Master can do nothing except explain in his *Towards Infinity*, when you start from point one and go to the thirteenth, he says, "This condition is yet subtler than the previous one." Unless we experience, we are not able to know what it is. It cannot be explained. But, is it the sins of the past that they were not able to do it? It only reflects the level of development of the human mind at that stage, which could posit before it only the level of Divinity up to which it was capable of perceiving. Today, the human being has changed in its ability to conceive of the Godhead itself in a different way. There comes the Master who says "Well, go beyond!" And then, he gives the brilliant, very ununderstandable and very confusing idea of 'nothingness'. Now, this is something we have all to ponder over.

Then, coming to transmission, we have had the explanations by many, what transmission really does? Master said, "It is the utilisation of the Divine energy for the transformation of man." But how does it work? Because, as Master himself has said, there are cases where even the transmission is reflected back from the man who comes to take the transmission. It is as if it cannot penetrate. So, the important thing, even prior to receiving the transmission, seems to be the need to accept the Master. One who does not accept the Master does not seem capable of receiving the very transmission which is designed to transform him. And when does this acceptance of the Master begin? When we see him, when we move with him, when we are associated with him, we grow to love him, to cherish him, to adore him, and the desire comes to be like

Him. "In every aspect of His existence, I want to be like Him"–this sort of attitude.

There seems to be a progressively increasing ability in the transmission of the Master to transform us as we go further and further ahead on our spiritual path. In the beginning it is very difficult; in later stages very easy. At the final stages, as Master said, it is like taking something from here and putting it there; it is so easy, ridiculously easy.

So the creation of craving by setting an example (to the man who comes to the preceptor)–it is not only the Master's duty to set an example–it is the duty of every preceptor. I would extend it and say it is the duty of every abhyasi of the Mission to create an example, by his actions, by his thoughts, by his deeds, by the way he behaves in society, in his house. People should look at him and say "What is it that you are, that you have become like this? What are you doing?" So, the first need of all of us who are abhyasis of the Mission is to become living examples of the Master's teachings– even before this transformation can take place–by acquiring this craving; by creating in ourselves this craving to be like Him; because, that is the first step in becoming like Him.

There was some reference to restlessness. I remember Master's usual way of defining restlessness–very humorous, very penetrating, profound in its meaning. He said, "Restlessness *se* less-ness *nikal do, tho* rest *hai*" [Remove 'less-ness' from restlessness, and what remains is 'rest']! How is it applicable in my practical life? We are always feeling 'less-ness': "I don't have enough of this; I don't have enough of that; I don't know enough; I have not enough wealth." Who is it that feels? It is "I"! That means, all of us. When we feel lacking we become restless. Now, how to overcome this feeling of lack? Of course there are the traditional ways, saying, "Be content with what you have, take it as God's gift." *Theek hai.* That is all okay. But when we start getting this transmission, which removes our samskaras first, and puts the power of the Almighty in us through the Master's grace, in some mysterious intangible manner it progressively removes this 'less-ness' from us, and brings us to a peace, to a state of balance. It is not so much a state of peace as a state of balance; because restlessness is really an imbalanced state. So this thought I wanted to share with you.

Then talking of *Tat Twam Asi*, we have been to some extent guilty like the other great religions of the world. "Tat Twam Asi" [That thou art]–the finger pointing somewhere else! It is said that there are two approaches. One is where we see God externally somewhere in heaven (which some of the major religions of the world do). "God is somewhere in heaven and there is a journey towards Him;" which they interpret very wrongly as a physical journey, over time and space. To some extent this "Tat Twam Asi"–it is called one of the *mahavakyas*–seems to be guilty of the very same thought. I would rather say "This you are." You are **This,** and when have I a right to say this? When, That which was talked of by the Master as Divinity, has been permitted to enshrine and enthrone itself in our hearts; and instead of looking outwards, we look in and say "He is here," because what is inside me, I am. If I have money in my pocket, I am a rich man. If I have knowledge in my head, I am an educated man, a wise man. If I have God in my heart, I am a divine person.

I recently read somewhere, I think it is a quotation from the famous American philosopher Ralph Waldo Emerson, where he says: "That which remains, when everything that we have learnt has been lost, is education." I am not offering this as a mere definition of education. It has a profundity of meaning associated with Master's own teachings: "Destroy your creation and His creation comes into existence." The first thing we learn when we come into Sahaj Marg, much to our sorrow, much to our regret, is this. (Very often we put our hand on our head and say, "Is this what I bargained for when I came into this *sanstha*?") We are told to unlearn everything that we have learnt; because that is also part of our samskara–the ego associated with knowledge; the wrong conceptions arising out of wrong knowledge, misinterpretation of knowledge; all this has to be lost; and when all this is lost, the essence remains, which (Master very kindly says) is your true education. Therefore, the immense stress laid by the Master to dissolve our creation, to destroy our creation, so that His creation can come into effect.

About Patanjali, a brother told us, between him and today some three thousand years have elapsed, and yet this very tenacious clinging to this Ashtanga Yoga, which few people understood and few people follow. This is an indication of human aversion to change. "What has been said by the past–the Masters of the past–is true, for ever and ever, true for eternity." If there is a need for avataras to come again and again, if there is a need for *mahapurushas* to come again and again, it only means that there is a tendency in the human being to go backwards when he is imagining he is going forward; and he has to be pulled every now and then periodically, and shown the right path. Now, there comes this inertia–this aversion to change–which has to be overcome. This we find in our traditional *panthathis* of worship, *puja karmas*, temple-going, *pithru karmas*, all these associated facts–whether it is Hindu, Christian or Muslim, it is immaterial–because the same fixity, the same solidness is there. In fact, the English word is 'petrifaction'–that which has become stone-like. So systems tend to petrify because of the misplaced veneration for something which is past, which is old, which is hoary with age. We seem to think or evaluate spiritual systems, very much as we evaluate antique objects–by their age rather than their efficacy.

In the Ten Maxims, a brother has delightfully told us, how unlike other religious systems, we are not told what to do, and what not to do. Do's and Dont's do not exist in our system. In fact, many Westerners have asked Master, "Babuji, don't you give us the Ten Maxims which are similar to Christianity, for instance? 'Thou shalt not covet thy neighbour's goods, Thou shalt worship no God but me.' Master said, "I do not distinguish between good samskaras and bad samskaras. Samskara is samskara. As long as there is samskara, you are going to come back here. Bad samskara means a worse life, good samskara means a better life; no samskara means no return."

So in his immense wisdom, Babuji has given us a system which (as its primary purpose) rids us of all feelings of guilt. Because, when you are given specific instructions like, "Thou shalt not covet thy neighbour's goods," and we do covet, and we are unable not to covet, we are guilt-ridden, adding one more guilt. In fact, Master has told us this very very solemnly, I should say. Once I asked him, "Babuji, why don't you give us direct instructions?" He gave me two reasons. He said, "Lalaji never gave direct instructions; I am following His way." I asked, "What is the second?" He said, "If I give direct instructions and the abhyasi does not obey, I impose upon him the sin of disobedience of the Master. I do not wish to do it." So we are given 'Guidelines', and I accept that it seems almost impossible to follow even one of those Ten Maxims. The first one seems particularly difficult in modern times, that is: "wake up before sunrise and do your sadhana"! We have fallen into this Western curse of loving our beds too much! And on Sundays we want to sleep even later than on other days, so that on Sunday satsangh we find half the people missing! Here precisely comes Babuji's wisdom, and more importantly, Babuji's grace, Babuji's benignity, his benign love for us–that he only proposes, he does not order! He places before us something for our acceptance, and says, "If you want this, do this." There is no implication of sin or virtue, there is no implication of punishment, therefore we do not feel this guilt associated with non-performance of the Ten Maxims–though sometimes I feel it is desirable we should do so, at least to goad us to pursue them!

A very important thing in Sahaj Marg is–it goes from inside out–the centrifugal working. You see, it is such a simple thing that most people do not seem to be able to understand. A tree does not grow from outside, it grows from inside. When you put it into the earth, cover it up, it is from inside the life force springs as a sapling, throwing aside the shell that is imprisoning it. This is the natural way. And in the process of growth it sheds its *avaranas* as we call them in Sanskrit–this is one way of shaking off the [sheaths or] avaranas in us, because when we grow from inside, the avaranas have to fall, like the bark which falls off the tree which is growing. The trunk is expanding, the bark is falling; it acquires another rind, that also goes. Whereas if you try to impose growth from outside, it affects neither the outside, nor the inside, it can only whitewash (like whitewashing the walls) hiding all the sins and blemishes behind them.

Karma, gnana, bhakti–a beautiful example of the unification of the three principles, and in exemplification thereof, that only by doing we can know, only by knowing we can love, only by loving we can achieve or become. Master's oft-quoted statement is: "Everybody comes to see me, but nobody really sees me." It is a tragedy of our historical, spiritual heritage that we are taught more to look with the outside vision. We are always talking of *anthar gnana* [inner knowledge], *antharyoga* [inner yoga] and politically *antharrashtriya*, things like that which do not mean the same thing. But as long as we restrict our perception to the gross perception with our physical eyes and other sensory apparatus at our command, we are never really going to know anything. Now, how do we know here at all? By doing we can know better–how? Precisely because when we turn our gaze from the outside to the inside in the act of meditation–it is a reversal of the gaze, turning away from the outer to inner–to the chamber of the heart, where we are asked to imagine the presence of the Divine Light (*divya prakasham*). Thus, the ability is nurtured in us to turn away from the external universe to the internal one, which (Master assures us) is incomparably vaster to the mere external, physical universe, however immense it may be. It has no relationship at all!

But this act of turning our vision from the outer to the inner– closing our eyes and learning to perceive with closed eyes what is in–gives us the ability to go inside, whatever it be. Such a person is able to see the heart of the individual, when he comes and sits in front of him. Such a person is able to go to the heart of the matter (as we say in the English language) whatever be the subject matter under perusal or under examination or under inspection. This ability, if I may say so, is valid not only for spiritual existence and growth; it is vital even for our material growth. Because, how often have we not struggled with problems, with personality problems among individuals, with growth problems in industries, with educational problems with students–because we are not able to intuitively perceive the inner condition of this thing or person or event?

I am highlighting the importance of this, because people foolishly imagine that spiritual knowledge–spiritual science, spiritual growth, spiritual ability–is restricted only to the spiritual life. On the contrary, only a truly spiritual person can be an effective person, in any walk of life. It is said in the Gita: "*Yogah karmasu kausalam.*" He becomes a perfectionist in every aspect of his approach, whether it is external or internal. Therefore, by following this idea of "karma leading to gnana leading to bhakti," we find that we can have command over two realms of existence: the physical and the spiritual, the material and the spiritual. If for nothing else except success in our material life, this is a very valid point worth remembering. And this also perhaps shows, "*Bahunaam janmanaam anthe gnanavaan maam prapadyanthe*"–why not? Why does Krishna say, "A gnanavaan takes so many janmas to come to Me"? I would suggest it is precisely because those gnanis restricted their gnana [wisdom] to the external, and did not penetrate inside.

I have one thought to offer in conclusion. Very often abhyasis mistake the spiritual pursuit, the spiritual goal, as something for their personal edification, for their personal possession, for their personal aggrandisement, whatever have you, you see. I would say that the more we get, the less we give; because as Master once told me: "God does not waste His time on you, my dear friend, for **your** purpose. If God is going to take an interest in you, and makes a saint of you or a perfect human being of you, it is for **his** purpose that He takes you; not for your purpose." I would like to caution abhyasis, because very often we think that a saint becomes a saint for himself; a gnani becomes a gnani for himself or herself. No! One who grows and betrays the purpose of the Master will lose that growth. One who grows and betrays the Purpose of the Master (in the Master's mercy, if he keeps that growth, what he has attained up till that moment) he will grow no further. There is always the possibility that Nature can intervene and take away that growth from us.

It is very much like a banyan tree, which as it grows, puts down adventitious roots for its support. The adventitious roots of the banyan tree are not meant for the growth of the root itself! They are there to form pillars of that which is growing above! In our case, it is the Master's supreme spiritual reign for the next few thousands of years–or maybe even longer. I do not know, I am not competent to say that. Unless and until we contribute to His purpose, to the fulfilment of His plans, for which He came, and subscribe to His views and ideas wholeheartedly, and understand that I am practising Sahaj Marg, not to become a saint, not to achieve human perfection, not even for *layavastha* which is so touted about as the ultimate purpose of life even by the Master–unless and until we realise this, my dear brothers and sisters, spirituality has no meaning for us.

Thank you for your patient hearing.

Spiritual Growth and Development

My Divine Master has bestowed upon us the task of continuing the work of spiritual development of mankind. The responsibility for this auspicious work may perhaps be considered to be that of His representative alone. The work has, however, to be shared by one and all. This is fair and just, because each one of us, in performing the task allotted to us by my Master, is working upon himself or herself and that, too, for one's own spiritual growth and development up to the highest level of Divinisation.

What is the reward for this work? It is not a crown; one does not work for honour or glory or recognition. My Master worked for results and results alone. This, if one ponders over it for a minute, is what work is really undertaken for. When we work for recognition or glory or other things like that, we miss the real result that work should be blessed with, namely progress and growth.

Growth involves change. Can there ever be progress without change? Can a baby become an adult without changing? Can a seed become a tree, and yield fruit, without change? Change is thus perceived to be an integral part of the growth process. In fact it is change which brings about the desired result, and what we really work for is to bring about such change. My Master has stated categorically that there can be no progress without change.

When things cease to change, a stage sets in which can be justifiably called death. Looked at in this way, death can be said to be a cessation of the process of change. That is, death is the cessation of growth.

Spiritual progress, spiritual growth, involves change. Progress, after all, is nothing but a change for the better in our condition. The sadhana is the process created by my Master to bring about continuing change for our spiritual betterment, from moment to mo-

First Message given at Yogashram, Hyderabad, 29 December 1983.

Spiritual Growth and Development

ment. If we ponder over it, we shall see that a resistance to change is a resistance to our own growth and progress. Can we stop change? Is there anyone capable of arresting change? No! Change is inevitable. It is a law of Nature that things must change, must evolve. Change is thus seen to be inescapable. My Master has said that the only permanent thing in the universe is change. We must be grateful for this because if it were not so, progress, all growth, would cease.

When we accept change, we accept the Master's will. When we accept it totally and unreservedly, with the faith that it is essential for all progress, the stage of surrender sets in. Surrender, looked at in this way, is a humble submission to the process of change that my Master initiates in us, for our growth to the highest levels of spirituality available to mankind.

Resistance to change is caused by fear and prejudice. Prejudice is the resistance to a change in values. We resist the change in others; rather, we refuse to perceive such change. Since our views become fixed, our own progress is adversely affected. My Master has cautioned us that prejudice is one of the most harmful things on the spiritual path. Why is this so? It is because prejudice is a mental phenomenon. The power of the mind, thought power, is the highest power, the most potent power, available to man. When we use this power in a negative way to oppose change in others or ourselves, that is, when we yield to prejudice, we are using the power of thought in the wrong way. The greatest alertness is therefore necessary to avoid prejudice.

My Master has made available to us, most graciously and benevolently, the Sahaj Marg sadhana to bring about spiritual change in each and every one to help us to attain the goal. It is our solemn duty to practise it assiduously with faith, and love for all, so that our goal can be achieved in the shortest possible time, which, as my Master has emphasised, should be within one's own lifetime.

May His benediction ever be upon humanity. May His divine grace ever flow to one and all through eternity. May He bless us eternally with His divine presence.   Amen!

Continuity of a Tradition

Once I was travelling with my Master, Shri Babuji Maharaj. On the way to Delhi from Europe, Master was very preoccupied for about half an hour. Afterwards, when he relaxed a little and became his normal human self, I suggested to him, in an inquisitive way, that he had been doing some spiritual work. He said, "Yes, I was doing some spiritual work; please study and let me know what I was doing." I smiled foolishly, and said, "How can I see what you are doing?" He replied, "When our preceptors are given some work, they immediately think they cannot do it! I insist that you do it." So I tried my best to study what he was doing, and said, "Babuji, I think you were working in the future." Master said, "Very good! You have done something which few preceptors can do." As I did not do much, and had thought over it only for a few minutes, I asked him, "How is that?" He said, "To know whether I am working in the past, present or future is itself a great achievement, you see. You have answered correctly that it is in the future. Tell me now, how far into the future?" I had to put on the thinking cap again and told him, "To me it appears that it is very far into the future; it may be many thousands or tens of thousands of years." Sitting next to me, he hugged me and said, "Few people could have assessed my work in this fashion. Shall I tell you what I was doing?" I said, "Please, Babuji." He said, "You know there will be a Personality who will come at the time of *mahapralaya* for the dissolution of the universe. I had some idle time on my hands, and so I laid the foundation for that Personality's work!" I said, "Babuji, according to the calculations of mystics, that is something like four hundred and thirty-two million years into the future!" He said, "How does it matter? four hundred and thirty-two million or forty-three thousand million makes no difference. I was free, the work was

Talk at the Founder's Day celebration at Madras, 1 January 1984.

there and it was done. Poor fellow! Whoever has to come at that time should not suffer! So I laid the foundation for his work."

I have told you this story not to give you the impression that I am very good at reading Master's work or anything like that–that is incidental. The exercise of what little I was able to do gave me the knowledge of Master's true Divinity. We should never confuse Master's temporal existence in his physical frame, in his weak physical body and its unfortunate, unforeseen and sudden end, i.e., Master's temporality, with the manifested Divinity or eternity of the Master. The temporal self was impermanent; his eternal Self, his divine Self is eternal.

The concept of a Master, therefore, is not limited to a person or a place in time. If the Master ever existed in the past, he will continue to exist in the future till the end of time. This is the same as what they say about the soul–that which was created will certainly cease to exist, because a created thing means that it has a span of existence which can come to an end. That which was and is, shall ever be–is another concept. Now Masters take their authority, they derive their power, they exist solely for and on behalf of the Divine, for the Divine, by the Divine. Divinity is a concept which one cannot say began with time and ends with mahapralaya. The Divine is **not** going to have a brief span of existence–even though that briefness may last the lives of ten thousand Brahmas, which is yet brief.

In the place of eternity, the life of ten thousand Brahmas is like a mere second for us. So, the one who derives His authority, who draws His power, who gets His wisdom, who is allotted His work and who emerges from the Divine cannot cease to exist at any moment in time or space.

This small episode I related to you was, to me, a first-hand proof of Master's Divinity and, therefore, his eternity. So even to think whether the Master is existing today or tomorrow is foolish. It is like saying whether Lalaji Maharaj has ceased to exist or not. Unfortunately, nobody likes to project backwards and think of Lalaji Maharaj. People ask, "Was Lalaji the true Master or was Master the true Master? Who was the Special Personality–Lalaji or Babuji?"

I am not prepared to answer that question, because it is a foolish question. If my grandfather was not alive, my father would not have been born, and if my father was not born, married, lived a family life, I would not be here! So it is a continuing stream of consciousness which Master has labelled the Divine Consciousness. It seeks for itself a conduit through which it can flow. A conduit serves only to permit the channelisation of the Divine energy, the Divine resourcefulness, the Divine powers, to flow through itself. The Divine itself becomes a conduit and works as a conduit for its own work. It is as if a man should suddenly become a pipe, his energy flow through that pipe and at the end of the pipe, become himself again–the form changes.

I am reminded of a beautiful story in the *Bhagawatam*. Jhambavan, a devotee of Rama, meets Lord Krishna but refuses to accept Him [as the Master]. Krishna tries to persuade him saying, "No doubt you are a *Rama-bhakta* [devotee of Rama] but brother, I am the same!"

Jhambavan persists, "You? How can you be Rama, that famous Lord, my Lord, my Master whom I adored and whom I served? You are a *ducha* [crook] etc." He argues against Krishna in so many ways. Then Krishna suddenly reveals Himself in the form of Rama, and Jhambavan falls and worships at His feet! That may have been necessary to convert Jhambavan to His way of thinking.

I remember a stage when one abhyasi went to Master and said, "Babuji, you know so-and-so transformed such-and-such a person. For instance, Krishna revealed to Arjuna the Viswaroopa Darsana [the vision of His universal form]. Can you do it for me?" Master very humbly said, "You may be Arjuna, but I am not Krishna."

So it is the prerogative and privilege of the Master as to when, why and where He should reveal Himself, if at all. It is very difficult to decide. As Master has often said, "All these difficulties crop up because we use our rational mind instead of our heart."

Yesterday, you might have seen on the television a story of the cinema wherein a father told his little daughter that her mother died because he threw her out of the house. Later, the child was unwilling to accept the mother when she came back, saying, "No, no! My mother is dead. You cannot be my mother." Now, how can the poor mother change or transform herself and prove to the child that she is the mother? But when an accident or crisis arrives, the child comes weeping, running to the mother and recognizes its mother. Likewise, often it is the unfortunate fact of human existence that we seem to need crises to guide us in the right direction, just as the bull is pricked with a spur to goad it on in the right direction.

People ask, "Can he be what he claims to be?" This is a good question because if the Master's representative should claim anything for himself, he does not deserve to be there! They ask the next question, "Can he be what the Master says he is?" It is the height of impertinence to ask this question, not because it affects me personally but because our philosophy of Sahaj Marg teaches us to unquestioningly obey the Master once you have accepted Him. But you have the privilege of not accepting Him also. As you see, nobody compels us to accept the Master. We came voluntarily, stayed voluntarily and we grew to love Him. It is, therefore, incumbent upon the continuation of our love for the Master that what the Master says continues to exist in our hearts. It is only our idea that we are temporal, physically limited, spatially limited and restricted persons that brings about these questions and doubts. Forgive me for saying that any controversy on the subject of His representative is a direct attack on the Master's supremacy, His Divinity and His Ultimacy.

Change always comes, as somebody rightly said. In Lalaji's time, Lalaji passed away and there were several groups. Some created new sansthas [spiritual organizations], of which one is still flourishing today. In Fatehgarh itself there is one organization claiming a membership of lakhs. We, who claim to be the true branch of spirituality under Shri Ramchandraji Maharaj of Shahjahanpur, have hardly touched one tenth of a lakh in membership. Now what is it that attracted people there in such large numbers, where they only have a picture of Lalaji Maharaj, some *bhajans* and talks?

You have all seen so-and-so here who belongs to that organization. He knew nothing about transmission, and did not offer to give us a sitting. He came like a visitor, spoke like a visitor and went away like a visitor and he was a direct associate of Lalaji whom he had contact with for eight long years! All that he could say was a bit of a charitable speech when he said, "I am glad Ram Chandra has done so much in spreading this Mission abroad. We are all doing Lalaji's work together." He was able to take from Shri Ram Chandra Mission a part of its achievement and glorify himself. But a hundred thousand people are there in that organization, or perhaps more.

So what attracts people or what does not? As one of our brothers spoke, the wise are few. But it is not a reason to be unhappy about, because in Sahaj Marg even wisdom is not required! Master has never said that he wanted wise abhyasis. He has said, "I do not need wisdom." Intellect is only a bar. What is wisdom? It is a tool for evaluation, synthesising mentally and taking decisions. If any abhyasi claims that he has surrendered to Master, he does not need wisdom, as it is the Master who is guiding him. Why should I have wisdom? Why should I have power? Why should I have strength and courage? I do not need any of these things. All these attributes–whether they be *shodasha lakshanas* [sixteen attributes] or *ashta eishwaryas* [eight types of wealth] or whatever they may be–belong still to the humanly divinised plane where God is still thought of as an extraordinary human being.

But one who has surrendered, and claims to be a mere tool in the hands of the Master, needs nothing–because a tool by itself has nothing. When you take up a hammer it does not hammer by itself! It is used by the hand of the Master who uses it as a hammer. If it is a knife, by itself it can do nothing! A knife lying in the drawer is useless–somebody has to take it and use it.

So the beauty of the Sahaj Marg system–I should say the absolute and utter beauty and simplicity–is that an abhyasi is not required to have anything at all! That is, if an abhyasi can start with no attributes at all, I think he can be transformed by the Master the moment he came into the sight of Master–because he is jumping from one state of nothingness into the other state of Nothingness; from a finite state of nothingness to the infinite state of Nothingness; from a temporally limited state of nothingness to an infinitely unlimited, exuberant state of Nothingness.

I would, therefore, like to caution our brothers and sisters to be ever alert against the dictates of their wisdom. Those who have read *My Master* know that I made that mistake myself when I went to see the Master for the first time. He was lying there like a baby curled up in bed, and I literally put my hand on my head thinking, "Is it for this that I had undertaken such a long journey?" It may be justified that it should happen to every one of us in the beginning, but if it should stay with us till the end, it will be a tragedy. These things happen only because we use our mind, our intellect, our eyes, ears and nose far too much! We try to smell out the representative! His representative is not a piece of trash that can be smelt a mile away. He is not something unique in that your eyes can perceive what he is. He is not going to say something which no one has ever said before, that with our ears we can conclude that he is the true representative of the Master. His form and figure are nothing new–it is a human form and figure–that you can touch him or face him and say, "This is the Master–Master's Representative!"

So how can one judge? There is unfortunately no way. It is, therefore, unfortunate and a little contemptuous on the part of the Master to have left a document–contemptuous of us because Lalaji left no such document in the utter confidence that his representative would be accepted at his own words. Master [Babuji] had to think of leaving a document behind, because he knew in his own wisdom, that his tribe is not going to accept him so easily. I do not know what the next generation of abhyasis are going to be -- we may have to carve a document on stone pillars that so-and-so is the next representative! Such a time should not come. It is not a laughing matter and you know I have a way of looking at things differently. To me it is a little shameful that Master thought so little of us, so poorly of us, that he had so little confidence in our trust and faith in him, that he had to put down in writing which Lalaji left in the atmosphere.

So, brothers and sisters, it is my earnest hope that we will throw away all these mundane, merely human, attributes, whatever they may signify. To be intelligent is thought of as a great thing–people admire intelligence. We fall a prey to that admiration and, therefore, we try to become more intelligent. People admire power and so we seek more power. Unfortunately, people cannot see spirituality, so nobody admires us for our spirituality and, therefore, we fall–because we only respond to admiration, adulation and praise. We seek that in ourselves, for which we are admired by others! Any fool can see your wealth, your strength and your intellect, but there are few today who can recognise a spiritual man if he is walking on the road. This is the greatest danger to us because nobody admires us for our inner growth, for our inner benediction that Master is showering upon us. We may think or even feel that we are less than others and, therefore, try to go on the other path of power, money, fame and so many other things, and forget that which is 'inside'–and one day it will disappear. This is the greatest danger.

I should, therefore, caution you all today to forget you are human beings and imagine that you are mere instruments in the hands of the Master–to be wielded by him at his purpose. When he wants a chisel, he takes a chisel; when he wants a saw, he takes a saw; when he wants a mallet, he takes a mallet. It is not the knife's fault that it is sharp, or the saw's fault that it has teeth. It is for the Master to use the instrument which he feels appropriate to the time.

We have all been ranting from platforms that it is the need of the time, and Lalaji was an epitome of Nature. I say that it is arrogant pride to attribute it to Lalaji and deny it to the Master. If Lalaji could fashion his own instrument in his own time saying it is the need of time and Nature, surely you do not intend to say that Babuji was something less and, therefore, could not fashion his own instrument as he chose. It may not meet with our approval. If the Master wants a cutting instrument, who are we to deny him that? If he wants fire to burn, who are we to deny him fire? If He wants water to wet us with, who are we to deny him water? It is our arrogance, our pride, our lack of humility, our anger and, mostly, our lack of faith in the Master which make us demand the type of person we wish rather than the type of instrument He wishes to leave for us. To my mind, this, more than anything else, is the tragedy of the present situation.

I earnestly pray to the Master to release us from the bondage of the senses, of the intellect, of our efforts to judge. We cannot see a tiny seed grow, and here we are trying to judge a man, a personality, the Divine itself who is laying the foundation for mahapralaya. We measure our life by years (which may stretch up to ninety at the most) which is not even equivalent to a hair's breadth in eternity and we are playing with His wish, His will. We are also saying from platforms that Master has said that Sahaj Marg will continue for several thousands of years, forgetting that it is in our hands to see whether it will continue at all or not. It is like a family where if the first child dies, the family may very well stop there. Only the parents know the tragedy. Therefore, they hurry up to make a second child, and then pray intensely that the second child be spared.

Continuity is a function of every instant of time. There is nothing that begins which can go on forever except an inanimate body moving in the universe obeying the laws of Newton. Inanimate bodies are spared the function of human arrogance, human ignorance and human pride. Once set in motion, they go on forever. They are, by and large, more mercifully treated by the Almighty. They are not subject to our constraints and restraints of ignorance and foolishness. It is by far better to be a lump of rock out there in the universe, going on forever towards the source. It may take millions of years, no matter we have taken millions of years, if the theory of evolution is to be believed. We have already taken something like five thousand million years (which is the age of the earth) but we are still where we are! How are we any better than a lump of stone flying in space, unimpeded by anything under the touch of the Divine hand? And here, every second of our existence in spirituality is fraught with dangers and stumbling blocks.

We must remember that nothing continues unless we allow it to continue. The Divine Will may work by finding another channel for its purpose–that is beyond the scope of our discussion here. What the Divine can do and cannot do, we are hardly in a position to judge. Whether **we** will be in the scheme of things, whether **we** will be part and parcel of the Divine plan that He has made is very much in **our** hands. Please remember this.

The Task Ahead

We are all gathered here today to celebrate the auspicious and holy Birth Day of our beloved Master, Samarth Guru Mahatma Shri Ram Chandraji Maharaj, Founder President of Shri Ram Chandra Mission, Shahjahanpur, to whom we all belong, body and soul. The Mission is the spiritual organization which he has created with his loving hands to shelter and succour us. His Divine teachings, and the efficacious, practical system of sadhana, the system of Sahaj Marg, perfected by our divine Master, is there for our spiritual benefit, to enable us to reach the spiritual goal of human perfection, and divinisation to the highest level ever open to humanity. It is his sublime grace and Divine love that has made available to us such an easy method of practice which can lead us to that goal safely and speedily. It becomes our bounden duty to practise it assiduously, with one-pointed devotion, with our hearts full of "Love for Him who loves all," with unswerving faith, to enable him, our beloved Master, to lead us up to Himself!

We are all co-travellers on this divine journey to the Ultimate. Our journey will be made all the easier for us if we undertake it in a spirit of total co-operation and mutual brotherhood, in a spirit of service to all our brothers and sisters, together with a surrendering willingness and preparedness to make any, and every, sacrifice that may become necessary to reach our destination. The Master's assurance of the ready and permanent availability of His Divine help and guidance is there to encourage us on the way to the destination.

The special Personality, our great and benevolent Master, graciously descended to this misery-filled and strife-torn world only to help suffering humanity. He has perfected the system of sadhana, and removed all the thorns, impediments and lurking dangers that

---

Message given on the occasion of Shri Ram Chandraji's Birth Anniversary celebration at Madras, 30 April 1984.

beset earlier generations of spiritual aspirants. His holy lotus feet have converted a jungle path into a broad, smooth and direct highway to the Ultimate, for us to walk upon on our spiritual *yatra*–our journey–to the goal!

Was the goal ever so easily achievable? Was such Divine assistance and guidance ever available to human beings burdened with the cares and responsibilities of a human existence? It is our solemn duty to ponder over this deeply, and to keep the highway to the Lord, our benevolent Master, in good repair, so that it may remain open to the coming generations of humanity that must, and shall, follow His Divine way in ever increasing numbers in the future. His Divine dream was to make this world itself into a "Way to the Ultimate", and our part in it, however humble it may be, has to be played with a sense of dedication to this duty that our participation in this yatra itself lays upon us.

The task shall be fulfilled because it is **His will**. Our part in it is no doubt there, for us to play. But when? Only when we do not allow ourselves to be diverted by the glamour of this earthly existence, and by the selfish loves and hates that dominate it, keeping our eyes fixed upon Him and Him alone, the goal of our yatra, who is the Divine vessel of our love, and the supreme guide to Himself.

Whatever will be, will be! That is absolutely certain! Alongside with this is the inevitability of **change**! Master has stated that the only permanent thing in the universe is change. This inevitability of change is the foundation for all our hopes and aspirations. At the lowest level our hopes are for a betterment in the human condition; at the highest level it is an aspiration for spiritual evolution to the Highest! Whatever our hopes may be for, hope is founded upon the possibility of change. The truth of this will appear if we but ponder over it for a second. Upon what do we base our hopes? How does hope exist at all? Hope exists in our hearts only because we naturally and intuitively perceive the inevitability of change, which gives us the understanding that under no circumstances can the present continue as it is. It must change into something else!

It is this aspiration for change that is reflected in our hearts as a hope for the future. Without change, therefore, there can be no

The Task Ahead

future. It is this perception of the process of change, and its promise for the future, which makes us strive to bring about change in ourselves, in our condition of existence. We strive to become something which we are not! Change alone holds out the possibility of progress. It is change that offers us the promise of growth, and the certainty of becoming what our Divine Master wishes us to become. Viewed in this way, change is the process of becoming! The Divine Personality, our benevolent Master, has come down only for effecting such change, to enable us to become what He wants us to become. Our beloved Master is thus seen to be a Divine agent of change! Can we oppose change? Do we have the power to prevent change? If we oppose change, we are really opposing His Will! Our duty clearly lies in speeding up the process of change by dedicated sadhana, so that our journey to the destination, our Original Home, is accelerated.

What is dedication? Dedication is the state in which our commitment to an ideal becomes total. In the beginning a sense of commitment is lacking. As we progress along the path, the sense of involvement increases and becomes a commitment to the effort, to the fulfilment of the purpose. We begin to remember the purpose of this existence. We begin to remember our Original Home. We begin to remember Him more and more, and as our commitment increases, or rather as it deepens, the remembrance becomes more and more frequent, until it culminates in what our Divine Master has called **constant remembrance**. It is thus seen that dedication is reflected in constant remembrance. The greater the degree of remembrance, the greater the degree of dedication it reveals!

What do we work for? We work for those things that we love. We work for our children. Why do we work for them? Because we love them! Why do we love them? Because they are ours! So we find that we love everything that we feel to be ours. We work for those whom we love. Dedication increases because our remembrance of those whom we love keeps our nose to the grinding wheel, as the saying goes! The greater the dedication, the greater the effort. The greater the effort, the greater the success. I may say that constant remembrance becomes possible only when we take the Master as our very own, without any reservation, and love Him with all our heart and soul. The way then becomes smooth and easy, and the goal is reached in the shortest possible time.

Every traveller has a responsibility to see that the way is secure; that it is maintained in good repair; that our brotherly love and affection is freely available to all those who are accompanying us; and that our services are unreservedly offered to all those who may need it, without considerations of any nature such as caste, creed, colour, etc.–such as have unfortunately served to divide humanity in the past–coming in the way. All our differences must be firmly set aside. "Unity in diversity" is the law of nature! The thread which unifies us all, the love for Him which binds us together in our aspiration, in our endeavour, must be strengthened. The teachings of our great Master must not merely be followed by us for our own personal benefit, but must be preserved intact, in their pristine purity and holiness, for posterity. It is our sacred inheritance, to be used, and then passed on to those others who shall come after us in innumerable numbers.

Our Master has stated that His teachings will serve the spiritual needs of humanity for thousands and thousands of years to come! The spiritual heritage entrusted to us is, therefore, a sacred trust, to be held and passed on from generation to generation of spiritual aspirants all over the world, in its pure and unalloyed form. What we have inherited from our Master is, therefore, this sacred trusteeship of his method, his teachings, casting upon us a solemn duty which each and every one of us must strive to fulfill. It may not be an exaggeration to state that the spiritual future of humanity, its very destiny, lies in the frail hands of the present generation of our Master's devotees! It is an awesome responsibility. We have to ponder over the ways and means of fulfilling this task, and justifying the faith that he has so lovingly reposed in us. We must pray to him to grant us the wisdom and the strength necessary to fulfill this great and noble task that lies ahead of us.

The trust that our beloved Master reposed in us must not be betrayed. The love that he has so freely showered upon us must be offered at his lotus feet, multiplied a million-fold. The foundation that he has laid must be built upon. The work that he has done must

The Task Ahead

bear fruit, over and over again, season after season. The way that he has trodden, and made smooth and perfect for humanity to tread upon, must be trodden by the untiring feet of the multitudes of the future. The goal that he has set before us must be reached, ever more easily, by the sons and daughters of the Original Abode who have unwittingly strayed down to this world of ours. This was the Divine dream that he dreamt, and to make it a reality is our duty. To make all this possible is the task that lies before us. In its fulfilment lies the fulfilment of the Divine and loving aspiration of our benevolent Master. Let us heed the clarion call to "Arise! Awake! And rest not till this Divinely endowed task is completed to His satisfaction!"

May His benevolent grace, His Divine love, His eternal presence, serve to keep our feet firmly planted on the path. May His merciful guidance assist us in fulfilling our duty to Him who is our ALL AND EVERYTHING!

Call Of Conscience

I came to the feet of my Master, Samarth Guru Mahatma Ramchandraji Maharaj of Shahjahanpur, in the early part of March 1964, not knowing what was spirituality and having, through an exposure to religion, tradition and culture, veered away from those traditions, more emotionally than intellectually. Because whatever association I had till then, with formal modes of worship, rituals, our traditional forms, had in some way, created a feeling of, initially disappointment, subsequently frustration and finally, I should say, (I may confess to you) a feeling of disgust!

Fortunately or unfortunately the major part of my life has been spent in North India, and at one stage I had to live in Benaras, where I graduated from, and the goings-on there among the religious community–among the temples, the cheating, the hypocrisy, the way suffering humanity is dealt with in the citadel of God–were shocking experiences. And when I discussed these things with my so called *acharya* of the South–I belong to the Vaishnava community and we had our own traditional acharyas–when I discussed with them, all they could say was, "You have to tolerate. God's ways are mysterious. By evil comes good; from darkness comes light."–all these sorts of funny things. None of them could really give me an answer. And having been blessed with sincerity or cursed with sincerity, I used to do all the rituals that I had to do, because I lost my mother at the age of five, and the annual *shraddha*, I used to do with utmost sincerity, with meticulous observance to the *niyama* and all these things such as the early morning bath, not drinking even water. And when I found how the *purohits*–who were to come and administer the puja and the rites–behaved, I was horrified.

Talk at Ahmedabad, 21 October 1984.

On one occasion, I had the misfortune to be away from Madras and I had to perform the shraddha ceremony. The purohit who was supposed to come at nine o'clock, didn't turn up. I sent a boy and the boy in his innocence came back and blurted out, "He has performed shraddha in another house, and he is eating the *pitru-bhojan* [the food-offering to the departed soul] you see, and when he is finished with that, he will come here." Now, the Shastra says that when you do *pitru-tarpana* or *pitru-shraddha*, that purohit should not eat for the preceding three days. It is a *prayaschitta* [act of repentance]. But he was eating there, after performing a shraddha and coming to me to help me perform my mother's shraddha! This was the ultimate 'straw on the camel's back'. And on that day, if I may use that phrase, I broke with traditional religion as it is understood. I just said, "This is over." This was a few years before I came to the feet of my Master.

Then, without guidance, I used to do some forms of the *hatha yoga*, do some *asanas*, do some *pranayama* and ultimately, I should say, my destiny led me to my Master Shri Ramchandraji Maharaj and, if you permit me to say, his training was a series of shocks. I can assure you from personal experience, nothing works like a shock. You know even in common life when a man is on the point of losing his job and the boss calls him and says, "Well, either you quit or ...", it is a shock. We become aware. When there is a market crash, there is a shock. So these shocks are very essential to shake us out of our complacency, of our passive acceptance of everything that has been said, done in the past, of an intellectual blindness to the teachings of the past. None of us is willing to read for himself and understand for himself. It is easier to listen to some pandit or purohit who is conducting a *pravachan*. We have no patience, we have no interest to confirm what he reads and what he says by a second reading for ourselves. What he says goes because we have no interest in it. All that we want to do is to listen and walk out, and by the time we are out of the gate, that is forgotten!

So shocks are essential to shake us out of these inner complacencies which, if I may say so, have brought the Indian society to the degraded levels in which we are seeing it today, of which we are all part, you and I and all of us here. My Master administered these shocks progressively because he had no qualms about shocking us. The first shock was when he said, "Religion is utter nonsense!"

I asked Him, "What do you mean? Religion is supposed to be the thing from which we draw our succour and by which we have come from the past, and into which we are going in the future, if tradition is to be believed."

He said, "It is the kindergarten school where, at best, you are taught something of ethics, something of morality, and some idea of what is called Divinity or God is given to you. Beyond that, religion can do nothing." And he chose his own personal example and said that, as his mother was a very pious lady, he started doing the traditional puja. He said, "I found no benefit in it."

I said, "How long did you do it?"

He said, "It is immaterial. I don't have to do a thing all my life to find out whether it is useful or useless! Suppose a blade doesn't shave properly, you don't shave with it all your life before you discard it. When a pot of rice is boiling, if you take out one grain of rice and press it in your hand, you know whether the whole pot is cooked or not. You don't take it one by one and say, 'this is cooked', 'this is cooked', 'this is cooked'; you will have no rice left to eat!"

It was an argument I had to accept! So that was the first shock– Religion at best is a kindergarten school where some idea of ethics, some idea of morality and some idea, a very very vague idea or the concept of something called Divinity or God, exists.

I said, "What next?"

He said, "Well, I started hatha yoga. I did some asanas and pranayamas and I did for a few days, few months maybe, and I found out that was also not beneficial!"

I said, "Surely, Babuji! One would expect a little more time to be given to hatha yoga."

He said, "No, if a thing has benefit, it must have benefit from the beginning. I cannot get into a wrong bus, and expect it to go to my destination after three hours! It is wrong from the moment I stepped into it. Nothing can become right when it is wrong, whether more time is given or less time is given."

That again was a very logical argument, you see. I cannot get on to a wrong bus and say, by virtue of moving in it over an extended period of time it can ever possibly take me to the right destination! His logic was unbeatable!! So he gave up hatha yoga.

Then he started pranayama. He found psychic disturbances, problems arising in his sleep. So he said, "*Use bhi humne chhod diya.*" [I left that also.]

Then I said, "Babuji! What did you do after that?"

He said, "Nothing! I waited patiently, I prayed to God to send me a Master. And after a few years, I went to Fatehgarh and found my Master!" This is what he said to me. I said, "In between you did nothing?" He said, "It is better to do nothing than to do what is wrong."

It was confusing to me because we have been taught that to do something is better than to do nothing. Here was a man who was preaching me, "To do nothing is better than to do something which is wrong." Well, palpably it was wisdom of the highest order. Like our boys (children) when they study, if they have nothing else to read, they read comics or they read the trash literature that we get today and we are happy. *"Arre bhai! Kuch nahin to kuch to padh raha hai woh!"* [Brother! At least he is reading something!] You see, this habit has ruined our conception of what is good and what is bad, that to do something is better than to do nothing, whereas my Master taught me, "When you do not know what is right, or what you should do, **do nothing.**" And that was the highest wisdom he taught me, in the third shock.

Then I said, "What happened when you came to your Master?"

He said, "When I looked at Him, I found **That** which I sought and my eyes never turned elsewhere, I saw and I fell."

Now we are familiar with the other quotation, "I came, I saw, I conquered." That was the idea of conquest, of victory, of power. Here was the summation of surrender! "I saw, I fell, I never rose again!" People often ask, "What is surrender?" you see, I think those three short words–"See, fall and do not rise"–these epitomise the value of surrender.

So like this, I was administered shock after shock. Then I said, "What is this spirituality of which you are teaching about?"

He said, "*Dekho isme kai baten hoti hain. Log samaj nahi pate.*" [See! There are many things in this (spirituality). People are unable to understand.]

I said, "*Aap to samjha sakte hain?*" [You can teach me?]

He said, "People confuse religion for spirituality. They are called spiritual discourses, when they are nothing more than religious discourses! You cannot change the content of a bottle of water by calling it wine. It will not become wine. But these people are cheating the public by calling them spiritual discourses. The poor people don't know the difference between religion and spirituality."

I said, "*Aap to hamen samjhayiye?*" [Please let me understand.]

He said, "Religion deals with dogma, tradition, ritualistic worship–only three things."

I said, "What about *moksha tatva*? What about after-life? I am supposed to be lifted up to realisation."

He said, "*Bekaar hai*! [Useless!] No religion can do it!"

I said, "Babuji! Surely you are not denying the efficacy of the Sanatana Dharma of which so much has been written!"

He said, "If you have eyes, you can see for yourself. There have never been more temples in India than there are today. And there has never been more degradation! There has never been more moral decrepitude! There has never been more corruption! There has never been more dishonesty, viciousness, lust!"

I said, "Surely–you don't attribute it to temples?"

He said, "I don't attribute it to temples. But the existence of the temples is the direct index of the fall in society of moral standards and values."

I said, "Surely Babuji! I am not able to understand this idea that when there are more temples it shows more moral degradation"

He said, *"Bhaiya, socho, kisi nagar me jahan ek haspatal tha, wahan bees haspatal ho gaye* [Brother! Suppose that in a city which had only one hospital, there are twenty hospitals now], what will you think?"

I said, *"Vahaan beemari jyada hai."* [Sickness has increased there.*] "Ab dekho jahan mandir jyada hote vahaan kya hota hai?"* [See, now, what happens when there are more temples?]

I said, "Guilty conscience *jyada hai."* [There is more of guilty conscience.]

"To tumhare muhse tumhi ne iska jawab de diya!" [So you have yourself answered your question.]

And again it was an unbeatable argument -- the more the temples, the more the moral degradation; the more the fall in values, the more the corruption.

He said, "You know, religion deals with you in an external way, whatever good may have existed in it in the past. Undeniably there were values in it when the founders started it; there is no denying that. But through generations they have become corrupted, today it is a money making machine."

I said, "All right, what about spirituality?"

He said, "In spirituality we deal with the essence. That which is here inside you."

I said, "Is it the soul?"

He said, *"Haan* [yes] *'Soul' keh sakte ho. Lekin woh soul bhi nahin hai."* [Yes, you can call it the soul but it is not the soul either!]

I said, *"Soul bhi nahin hai*? [It is not the soul either?] But I thought we deal only with the *atma*. The *sharir* [body] and the *atma* [soul], are the two *tatvas* [substances] we have been taught about."

He said, "*Vaise tatvon to bahut hote hain, lekin hum essence ke bare mein apko batana chahte hain.*" [That way there are many tatvas, but I want to tell you about essence.]

I said, "What is this essence?"

He said, "That which sustains **you** through eternity."

I said, "Is it not the soul?"

He said, "No."

This was the next shock. Because we have been taught to understand that the soul goes, you know, by transmigration from body to body, lives from the beginning to the end, it is incorruptible, it is not created.

He said, "As the body lives by the soul, the soul also lives by something and that is this Divine transmission which we call–*pranahuti*, which the guru pours into the heart of the disciple, which is the food for the atma itself. Therefore, the atma is a living breathing thing, it can be destroyed."

I said, "Any proof of this?"

He said, "Today's existence! Most people are soul-less!!"

I said, "Surely there is something, some remnant left."

He said, "Yes, it is like a balloon without any air in it. It has to be inflated again."

So the whole Sahaj Marg *siddhanth* [philosophy], rests on the fundamental assumption that while the body exists by the soul, the soul **has** to exist by something else, which has to be infused into it by a guru who has command over the powers of Nature and is therefore called a saint. The guru by virtue of his connection with the Ultimate, what you call *Brahmalaya* in Sanskrit, is able to transmit that energy into the heart, recoup the soul and make it flower again. And this you have found in yogic terminology as the *adho mukhi* [downward facing] lotus, which becomes *oordhwa mukhi* [upward facing] and then opens and flowers and then falls the nectar into this. So the references in yoga are not false. I said, "Then what has happened to these references, Babuji? You yourself are saying these are correct and it did exist in the past."

He said, "Seventy-two generations before Raja Dasharath, the system of transmission existed. It was lost."

"How was it lost?"

He said, "You know the Indians are a peculiar race. Everything that was valuable, everything that was sacred, they made it secret and the person would not transmit it even to his *chelas* and when he died, it died with him."

And this is true not only of spiritual values, spiritual methods, spiritual disciplines, but also of arts and crafts and so many other traditions you know, like making even pickles, medicines! There have been medicines for snakebites, simple things, but for which they make a mystical nonsense out of it and say that "You have got to have *upadesh* [instruction]. Then only it will work." Medicine works not by upadesh, it works because it is a medicine!

So by mystifying, by cultifying, all with the idea of *nakar*, our traditions have been corrupted, the originality has been lost, the reality has been diffused into nothingness, and we are left today with false values, ephemeral values, lies, cheats. And we go to them for spiritual succour, when we are troubled and all that they are able to do is to give us some *vibhooti* [sacred ash] or some prasad and say, *"Beta, tum theek ho jaaoge."* [Son, you will be all right.] I said, "Babuji! What about this vibhooti? People go to gurus for vibhooti!"

He said, "You know, you go to gurus for reality and they give you ashes!" So we are left with the ashes of reality! And my Master, by progressive shocks administered one after another like this, was able to infuse reality into us. It is not something which you can explain over a half an hour talk. It took me twenty years. It is a thing which you learn through eternity. It is something which is an eternal pursuit. We can **start** at one moment of time, but it never ends. So spirituality is that which deals with the essence not with the body, not with the soul, not with the *panchatatvas* [five substances] or the *gunas* [their properties] or anything of that sort. I wish to stress this because many people say, "Sir! He is spiritual. But his behaviour has not changed." Now a behaviour is treated by psychology as a subject called 'behavioural psychology'.

A man may have a very good character, but his behaviour may not be congenial as far as you are aware. See, I have a good barber who, whenever he is shaving, goes on talking and I don't like it. It is his behaviour. But he is the best barber in town. You go to a cloth shop, and the best salesman is an irritant. He says, "What money have you brought? What are you going to buy?" But he is the best salesman. Otherwise he wouldn't be employed there. We want not the thing itself but we want the wrapping. You know modern packaging technology survives on this foolishness of the human being, that the thing which is inside is not so much valued, as the outer packaging in which it is wrapped. Therefore you see the trash sold in so-called book shops with lascivious pictures printed on top, which both the sixty-five-year-old and sixteen-year-old want, on the basis of the picture. When they read it through, they are disappointed because there is nothing inside which the picture displays outside.

Religion does the same thing—*swarna rathas* [gold chariots], gold covering for the *vigraha* [idol]. Is that idol going to perform less of a service to you had it been just mere stone? Why should it be covered with gold? Why should lakhs and millions of rupees be spent on gold rathas, and *acharyas* made much of. You see the publicity they give them in the press. Is a gold god more than a silver god, or is a stone god less than an ivory god? Does that mean that god has to be measured in terms of tola content of gold? We have corrupted God Himself. Our temples are a living testimony to the corruption that even God suffers at our hands. We besmirch His name, we falsify His generosity, we deny His love, when we go and put prasad and ten rupees in the *hundi,* and say, "God, take this ten rupees and raise my salary by one thousand rupees!" "God! Take this ten rupees and make me managing director of the company; now I am only an executive director." "God! Take this ten rupees, I am a civil court judge, make me a supreme court judge." For ten rupees, *hum sauda karne ko taiyaar hain Ishwar ke saath.* [For ten rupees we are ready to clinch a deal with God.] And this religion we are quoting from every platform *Satyameva jayate,* the most shameful thing in the Indian tradition, that you have to put this slogan on your national emblem! It is a testimony to the lying character of the Indian, not from today but from the time of Vedas.

From the Vedic rishis' time we have been told *satyam vadah, satyam vadah, satyam vadah* [tell the truth, tell the truth, tell the truth]. Now in no society have you to be told to tell the truth, if you are already telling the truth! When we read in railway coaches, 'Do not spit', what is the conclusion we come to? That people spit. "Keep latrines clean. Flush after use." The Westerner sees this and is amused. He says, "Don't your people flush the toilet after use, Chari, that you have to put up a notice?" The unfortunate conclusion is that they don't! Satyam vadah means what? We have been liars since eternity. *Is desh jisme Ganga behati hai*! [This country where the holy Ganga river is flowing.]–You see this, the great flaunting tradition that we fool ourselves with and are trying to fool the rest of the world with, that we are a nation of saints, we are a nation of incorruptibles–"See! Satyam vadah." This is what the ancient tradition says, and the Westerner and the Easterner both laugh and say, "Fool! Have you to **say** 'speak the truth', if you have been speaking the truth?"

So gentlemen, ladies, brothers and sisters, this is the state of affairs. Things will not change by whitewashing them. You have a mud wall which is being eaten away by rains, by weather, by white-ants. Whitewashing it, will not make it sound. It has to be broken down and a cement and brick wall put up in its place. It is left to the present generation of human beings, to correct the mistakes of the past and leave a better heritage for the future. This is the destiny. It is an important duty of the present generation. We are signally failing in this because out of our selfishness we are only concerned with ourselves. No parent is today worried about where his child goes; no parent today is worried about what his children's marks are. So long as they go to school, the mother is happy that the children are away and she can cook in peace for her loving husband who is in the club, dancing with somebody else. The father is happy that the mother is busy cooking so dutifully even if he is cheating her and fooling her; the child is happy that neither is attending to it, so it can do what it likes. Triple selfishness! And we are talking, we are bewailing, we are condoling with each other on the fate of society, what is going to happen in the future, when **we** make that future ourselves.

So there is no government, there is no society, there is no God. Even God cannot save a humanity which seeks to condemn itself by its selfishness, by its lustful pursuits, its avarice, all centred on the self. "I must have this, this and this." "What about your children?" "*Arre*, for what am I earning?" Very pious, you know! "It is only for my children!" And thirty years later the child says, "My father was a damn fool. If he had not left me this wealth, I would not have gone to dogs like this. I would have earned an honest living with my two hands. He has corrupted my existence." He has no love for you because when he is old enough to understand what you have been doing, he sees what all practices we have indulged in, in building up the so-called wealth for him, which he dislikes, which he hates, which frustrates him, which denies him his humanity, his manliness, everything. It emasculates him. We have had this lesson from the West in the so-called, you know, the hippie movement, when they deny their parents, when they condemn their parents for destroying the heritage of the past–which should have been handed over to them as a sacred inheritance to be passed on from one generation to the other. The only heritage which we are passing on, I am sorry to say is the 'HUF account' carefully garnered, nurtured and passed on!

So you will excuse me if I am a little harsh, but my guru shocked me. It is my duty to shock you into some awareness that "things are not all that good in the state of Denmark." (It is a Shakespearean quotation–All is not well in the state of Denmark.) Here we have been fooling each other on the political front, on the religious front, on the moral front. We are all happy, because we all know we are all liars and cheats, by mutual recognition and mutual back patting, "*Shu karvanu Saheb*." [What to do, Sir?] This has become the standard phrase in Gujarati, its translation the standard phrase in all languages! There is a lot to be done. 'Shu karvanu' means, do this, this and this. The way is available. Change yourself. By changing yourself you change your family environment, your children grow up better, they become moral when they see their parents are truth-loving. Unfortunately you know, we start teaching our children to tell lies from the age of three. Bell rings, somebody comes, "*Bol do papa nahin hai ghar mein.*" [Tell the caller that Dad is not at home.] And then later on when he tells lies to you, you beat him. Poor fellow, **you** have taught him to tell lies! He says, "Papa, how is it different when you told me you are not at home and now you are beating me for saying–'I am not at home'." "*Jhoot nahin bolna sach bolna.*" [Don't tell lies, tell truth.] The child is bewildered, you see. You are at double standards yourself, which, in your adult stature, adult wisdom you are able to handle. Like we handle two accounts, three accounts, we are able to handle two sets of moral values, multiple sets of moral values, but the child has only one set, his parents' behaviour. There begins children's indiscipline which goes on in the school, which goes on in the college, which creates communism, which creates goondaism of the streets, a rampant destruction let loose by a cry of the heart against parents, against society. They cannot destroy their parents, thank heavens, our children cannot destroy us! They don't have the courage. They love us too much! But we have the love which destroys our children!

So spirituality teaches us what is the real meaning of love. Love protects; love does not violate; love nurtures. If you put a chimney around a lamp and immediately the lamp is blown out, what would you think of the chimney? It is after all to protect it from the winds and to keep that tiny flame alight. So we have to learn what is love, what is morality, what is ethics. *Yahaan "Shu karvanu che" se kaam nahin chalega*! [Nothing can be accomplished here with 'Shu karvanu'.] There is a lot to be done. The beginning is now, here.

So those of you who have the courage to say, "Yes, brother, I wish to do this sincerely because when I change, I change a part of the universe; and when I change a part of universe, the totality **has** to change;" there is no question about this. Every individual change is reflected throughout the universe. It is said that not a leaf falls in the universe that He does not know about. And this, you know, we create. There are self-helping arguments, "What can we do Sir, society is like this," conveniently forgetting that the whole of the society is sick, we want to be healthy. Everybody is begging, we want to live and eat *sandesh* and *garam masala* [sweet and savouries]. Everybody is foolish and paying taxes, we want to be in the citadel of tax evasion. There we have no choice you know– 'I', 'It is for my benefit!' But when you say you change, the society will change, then we would prefer to wait! We would prefer to evade payment of our railway fare when everybody pays, forgetting that in everybody, I am also part of it. Isn't it? I mean if you question yourselves, your hearts, nobody can deny the truth of what is being said here, whether we are willing to accept it, face ourselves with it and do something about it.

Well, my prayer to my Master is that he give us the courage, because it needs courage. It is very easy to forget or, I would say, it is even more easy to remember that anything we do might destroy these false edifices, citadels that we have built of a false security, of a false wealth, of a false social eminence, nurtured by nothing more than ill-gotten money, where a man is great because he has ten lakhs, another man is greater because he has fifteen, and he is the greatest because he has seven crores! What is his education? "*Kai vandho nathi saheb, tran karod to chej tyan?*" [No difficulty, Sir! He has three crores rupees there!]

So, this is our society! You see, we have forgotten values. Today we have no respect for teachers, we have no respect for aged people. Why? Because they are a drain on us. Every old father has to be supported by his sons. In our selfishness you know we grudge the thirty or forty rupees that the poor fellow eats–it is a mere pittance of the tax that we have to pay -- pittance! It doesn't even pay for the paper on which we write our false accounts! But we are, you know, denying the old man because he is not contributing. Today is the day of productivity! Contribution!! So old people are relegated to a dungeon, in a beautifully built house with a puja room conveniently allotted to them, to continue to perpetuate the paucity on themselves and pray for wealth to us.

So brothers and sisters, I have to humbly and very forcefully request to you to re-examine yourselves. It is all right, every man has a right to destroy himself, but he has no right to destroy his inside, much less his family, which is all we are doing. And it is said that God, in His Ultimate wisdom, is giving us sufficient leash, sufficient time, with immense patience, with immense mercy. He says, "*Theek hai* [all right], let me see how far can he go in this play of corruption and ill-gotten gains and stupidity and vices!" But we have to remember that a time will come when we have to answer for it. This is what He says. Let us not worry about what He says, but let us worry about what this [pointing to his heart] says, which is more immediate. My heart says, "Do this and don't do this," let us obey it. You call it God, the conscience, let us obey it so that the tiniest voice can become the most powerful. One day 'I' will be its servant, instead of it being my servant.

Thank you!

Revelations

We have come to the concluding part of our Founder's Day celebrations. I think this has been a very well attended and, thanks to the co-operation between Salem and Coimbatore centres, a well conducted celebration. We have also had the pleasure of listening to a uniformly good standard of lectures. All our brothers and sisters who spoke have given us some very valuable thoughts and, knowingly or unknowingly, they have exposed the truths of the various principles of Sahaj Marg. Some of them, I am sure, did not know what they have spoken about. As is usual with Divine things, the speaker himself does not know what he says, why he says it, and what is the truth behind what he is saying. When we become totally merged with the subject (and perhaps it may be a little incorrect to say that Master is the subject of our meditation or the subject of our thoughts, He **is** that!), we can only speak what he speaks, what he would have spoken, and the truth that he would have revealed.

My Master did not reveal the truths in the traditional sense saying, "I am going to tell you one truth! This is it! Note it down!" He spoke, and every word that came out of his mouth was the truth. We have been conditioned by education, by society, and by the fallen moral and ethical standards to expect to find only certain things as truth embedded in a mass of verbiage. This is the unfortunate training we have gone through, so much so that when a great man speaks, or Master speaks, we want to pick out some of the words or some of the thoughts and say, "This was the truth," as if the rest could not have been the truth! I think this is one of the greatest humiliations to which we subject our Master in assigning grades of truth to what he says, such as, "Some are absolute truths, some are relative truths and the rest are for common consumption!" It is said that when a Master breathes, he breathes out infinity; when he breathes in, he breathes in infinity. So it is the play of infinity upon infinity, and everything is the truth even if he says mundane things like "You are Ramaswamy!" That is also the truth. Just because he addresses Ramaswamy as Ramaswamy, it does not cease to be the truth–it is very much the truth. So let us learn, let us accept the fact that we do not have to search for the truth when Master speaks. All is truth, and nothing but the truth can come out of Him!

Now what are the truths that our brothers and sisters have unwittingly revealed to us today? I think one of the most remarkable ones was the one about Karna [one of the characters appearing in the Mahabharata] that he had to surrender even his *dharma* [the effect of good deeds] as it is said. It may sound a little unfair that the Lord Himself should come to His own devotee and say, "Give me all the dharma you have performed, so that I can take your life." But this is only the vindication of the truths of the Vedas that we have to rise above both *punyam* [virtue] and *papam* [vice]. If papam has no value, punyam has no value either. It is **our** human intelligence, **our** human understanding, which has assigned a different set of values to the papams and a different set of values to the punyams. This makes us hold on to one and release the other, not knowing that where we hold on to one, we have to hold on to the other also whether we like it or not. You cannot have only one side of a coin, you have to take both. So also one who holds on to punyam, holds on to papam, too, whether he likes it or not. And this was the truth that Krishna had to teach Karna at the moment of his death, as if saying, "Fool! Part with it because with it you cannot reach me."

This is what our Master says–good samskara is as bad as bad samskara, because with samskaras you are going to be reborn if not as a saint, a sinner, and if not as a sinner, a saint. But you have to be reborn. So this was perhaps the greatest truth.

As for the *Viswaroopa Darsana* [vision of the cosmic form] it was a foolish thing to have indulged in, because as Master said in his Munich message, "Divinity is a PLAY and Divine the way". So

Krishna was playing with Arjuna like a cat playing with a mouse—with due apologies to those of you who are very keenly bent on the orthodox traditions—it was just a play! It was a *tamasha* [a joke] showing Himself with a thousand heads and thousands of hands. No true *bhakta* [devotee] of the Lord could have been more misguided! He should have said, "Krishna! Come on and stop playing the fool with me. What is this nonsense you are indulging in? Am I a child to be frightened by your thousand heads and thousands of hands? They are no more real than I am, because you can change forms like a chameleon and show me this and that. For heaven's sake, don't treat me like a *bacha* [child]. You say I am your bhakta and have not shown this vision to any rishis or *munis*. Are you playing with me? Are you cheating me? Are you lying to me?" These are the questions that a devotee of the Lord could have asked the Lord Himself! Instead of that, that poor fellow got frightened and cried out, "Please assume your ordinary form," as if that was more real! If tradition is to be believed, we must remember that that form of the Lord was also cremated!

So the Bhagavad Gita has to be taken with a pinch of salt! Not every revelation is a valuable revelation because what is revealed must be the Truth, must be the Reality, must be the Ultimate. Therefore, I think Master has said (he has written about it in very guarded terms) that the Viswaroopa Darsana, **after all** pertains only to the Brahmanda Mandal. It is nothing very wonderful because He showed what He could, and called it the 'Virat Swaroop'. Now, whether God shows Himself to be an atom, or as the Ultimate cosmic form, both are forms. What is the reality behind the forms? I don't think Krishna showed, or Arjuna saw, what That was. This seems to be the tragedy of most thinkers that, even at the last moment, they are halted by a form being presented to them which is either beautiful or delightful or attractive or fearful. And with that they are satisfied! To me the chapter on Viswaroopa Darsana is a travesty of the truth; it is a play with Arjuna as if Krishna is testing, "Let me see if this fellow is happy with the Cosmic form, let me see if he goes beyond that." Now, if that was the truth, the Gita should have stopped with that chapter. He need not have gone on to the eighteenth chapter and said, *"Sarva Dharmaan Parithyajya* *mamekam saranam vraja."* [Give up all dharmas and surrender to me alone.]

Why on earth should the Lord show Himself in His absoluteness and **then** teach him to surrender all over again? It becomes redundant to do so. So this is the message of the Gita that I have tried to piece together from whatever Master has taught me of Sahaj Marg. I think Krishna did a greater service to Karna than He ever did to Arjuna, and we call Him Karna's enemy! As one of the speakers said, "He showed Himself to the embodiment of sin, i.e., Duryodhana, for one reason. He showed Himself to Arjuna for another reason. He showed Himself to Karna for a third reason." Which was the transcendental reason of all? I think it was to Karna that He gave the maximum grace and removed the last impediment from his way, i.e., his holding on to *punya phalam* [fruits of virtue]. You know in Telugu they say, *"Tholinu Chachinna Puja Phalamu,"* meaning fruits of worship are what are holding us earthbound here and making us beggars, life after life for more punyam. One of the Alwars [leading devotees of Vaishnava cult], I think, said that he would like to be reborn again and again to serve the Lord! Master laughed when the story was told to him and said in Hindi, *"Eisi Bevakufi Kahan hogi?"* [Where can you find such great foolishness?]

So this was the interlinked message of the Gita two of our speakers presented, and the inner *tatwa* [philosophy] is that which we have always got to penetrate. You see, even when a great man speaks, even when a saint speaks, what we understand is what we understand. No more! So it is necessary that we seek to enlarge our understanding. How to do this? Not by referring to dictionaries nor by learning languages nor by studying the original texts. They are all meaningless excursions into the fields of knowledge–the more you learn, you realise that the more you have got to learn because that is an endless quest. The thirst for knowledge is as misleading, as evanescent, and as ephemeral as the search for pleasure, for instance. It is another samskara. I do not differentiate between the thirst for pleasure and the thirst for knowledge because both are leading you on and on like the carrot in front of the donkey's nose.

There is no limit to them. If one is a desire, the other is also a desire. Desire for knowledge is no more sacred or holy than the desire for pleasure. So what is the difference between one desire and another desire? No difference–obviously!

We have therefore to follow a path; we have to follow a Master who will not indulge in all these trickeries and childish by-plays showing us forms, showing us manifestations of Himself. And then, I do not know whom He fooled–Himself or Arjuna more! For a person who comes patently to guide humanity back to Himself– that was His own statement in the Gita, "I come again and again to rescue *dharma*, to punish the evil-doers, to re-establish this and that, and protect the doer of the good, etc." -- that is all He did, with due apologies to the Lord of the Universe, or the *Yuga Purusha* as He is called. He achieved nothing more than re-establishing dharma, killing Kamsa and protecting a few doers of the good -- some rishis here and some pundits there! What did He do as a Cosmic purpose? You call Him a cosmic being! What cosmic purpose did He fulfil? Either it is hidden from us or it is not stated in the Gita, or the unfortunate, and perhaps irreverent, conclusion is that He did not do anything more than that.

This brings us to the point, "What has my Master done about which we are so happy here?" As they say in the Vedas, we can only describe it in the negative. "Neti, Neti" meaning "not this, not this." He did **not** fool people. He did **not** show forms. He did not entice us with promises that if you do this, I will do that for you. He lived a simple, absolutely blameless and, I would even say, meritless life because, if it were a meritorious life, it again falls into the category of having one description attached to it, an adjective attached to it and a meritorious life would lead him also back to this earth. So his was an existence balanced on the knife edge between two opposites–neither sick nor healthy, neither rich nor poor, neither educated nor uneducated, neither wise nor foolish, neither tall nor short. He conformed to the 'Neti, Neti' truth of the Vedanta. You could not say of the Master he was a kind man; you could not also say that he was unkind. What was his kindness in feeding some people, in feeding abhyasis, in giving away a shawl? Well, he himself said, "If you consider human beings as your brothers, it is your duty and not kindness." So to throw back Master's own words at the Master, by giving away your own shawl to a man who is shivering in the cold, it does not become an act of kindness. It was his duty to humanity. He was the embodiment of duty, he could not but give it away! So where is the kindness?

I believe he was very kind to us in teaching us not to set values, artificial values, exaggerated values, inflated values, taught to us by society, by religious heritage, by social custom. Do not set false values on the actions of human beings. Do not apportion false values to the thoughts of human beings. Going beyond this, do not even seek to give credit to Divinity itself if it manifests to you with a form, talks to you with a mouth, frightens you, threatens you, entices you, tempts you and goads you into action–which It does for Its benefit as Lord Krishna very correctly says. But He comes for **your** benefit, to take you unto Himself, to make you as formless as He is in His essence, to make you as quality-less as he is in His essence, to make you as existenceless as He is in His essence; because, of such a person, you cannot say that he exists, you can neither say that he does not exist. That is the great truth which the Master himself pointed out from *Naasadiya Sukta*, "You cannot say that he exists, you cannot say that he does not exist either! He is at the mid-point. He transcends both existence and non-existence."

So these few truths–Viswaroopa Darsana, Karna, etc., it is amazing how our speakers are able to reveal truths unknown to themselves–because of the grace of the Master who speaks through them. And they have also been shattered to hear the explanation of their own words to themselves! That is what dependence on the Master brings. This is what dedication to his work brings. This is what following him brings. As somebody very beautifully said, "It is not central region or this region or that region which should be our goal, though many people still hanker after and aspire for regions, states and conditions." Master has very clearly said: "It must be the stateless state, it must be the conditionless condition." And what can that be but what He was, what He is and what He shall always be. The beingless Being, the conditionless Condition, a personality-less Person–all these opposing attributes which seem to have no meaning for us, unless we actually experience them in our own lives.

Lastly, I would like to end with that reference to science by one of the brothers here. It is said in science that there are two or three categories of forces–the strong force, known as the sub-nuclear force which holds the neutrons and the protons together in the nucleus. It is called the strong force but it can act only over the distances prevailing inside a nucleus. It has no strength to draw something six feet away or a hundred feet away. It acts within its own limits of the nucleus itself. Whereas gravity is called the weak force but it acts over enormous distances, cosmic distances, distances measured in light years, millions of light years. The weak force acts over a distance, the strong force acts only within the nucleus, within the boundaries of only sub-nuclear distances involved within the minuscule atom. Now this must give us reason to think over two principles: (i) that of invertendo–that the strong does not act as well as the weak and the weak acts farther and longer than the strong; this is one aspect; (ii) that of love–which has no force at all.

So you extrapolate this truth and bring it to that force which Master used to call the 'forceless force', which he called the transmission which I say is only his love for us because he was only transmitting love. It is not a force; it is not anything else. *Tatvavadis* [philosophers] who like to mystify things, like to say it is His essence; some people say it is Life, some others say it is *pranasya prana* [life of life]; but I prefer to believe and have reason to believe that it is his love which was being poured into our hearts which we call the transmission, which we call *pranahuti*. Being forceless, it will act, not only over infinite distances to the very borders of Infinity (the cosmic infinity, the physical infinity) but also through eternity of time. Love alone can act, breaking the barriers of space and time. No other force exists which can do it. Gravity needs bodies to act upon. If you are a spirit, gravity cannot act upon it. If you are a mere soul without a body, gravity cannot act upon it. You need at least that much matter as exists in light, in a photon of light, because it has been proved that light can be deviated by gravitational force. But love can act whether you have a body or not. Even when you are just a soul, it can act upon you because that is how Master guarantees our further progress even after we leave this body (as we are bound to do one day). We are not going to live eternally in this body. This is a brief existence upon earth for Him to come to us, for us to cherish Him, to love Him, for us to establish an association so that when His body disappears and my body too, we can yet react and interact and love each other and progress hand in hand, to the very Ultimate end!

So these are a few lessons which we have been told today, some of which I have tried to amplify for your sake. Now it is time for those who have to leave. So I say we part only to meet again wherever it may be next time.

Thank you.

Accept Him In His Essence

I regret not being able to speak to you all in Telugu, because I don't have any proficiency. But having been able to understand something of what our brothers and sisters have spoken today and yesterday, starting with Dr. Kuppuswami Garu, and having been listening to so many people, so many years in Sahaj Marg, starting with my Master at the top, down to the lowliest, mere beginners of Sahaj Marg, one thing I have observed–I cannot say it is a discovery–when we put on red glasses we see the world as red, when we put on green glasses we see it as green. In the reverse way also it operates. What we say reveals what we are, what we do reveals what we are, what we think reveals what we are. So these barriers, these filters, work both ways–the one who sees, sees the coloured world, and the one who is outside, looks through that window into the interior, he also sees the other person as coloured. So I have found it necessary to caution my brothers and sisters, not to set too much store by what people say or do because we can hardly know what they are by just judging them from what they say and what they do, as they cannot judge us by what we say and what we do.

So our actions, our thoughts–they are impediments to mutual understanding from both sides of the fence. From my neighbour's house if they throw rubbish into my garden I get annoyed. But when I throw rubbish over the very same fence from my garden, I think I am cleaning my house. So this sort of 'across-the-fence' attitude–it breeds animosities, it breed dissensions, it is the cause for wars; whether it be inter-personal, international, inter-religious, it makes no difference. Because where there is a barrier, where there is a fence put up between two entities, whether they be individual or political entities or even two religions, there is going to be trouble across the border sooner or later.

Talk at Tirupati, 30 December 1984.

Accept Him in His Essence

And the only person whom we could see–we have all seen that–where this barrier did not exist, was the Master himself, because he did not wear coloured glasses at all. People have said much about his generosity, about his kindness, about his love, all of which I have questioned at various times with considerable logic, spiritual logic, too. That I shall explain later. But when he did not have coloured glasses he saw us as what we are. He didn't judge us by our speech and by our actions.

It shows we could see him without any barriers interposed by him to our understanding of him. So we could see the Master, in some measure differently from what we see in each other. That we could not see him fully was not his fault, because we still had our coloured glasses on our eyes. You see, it takes two to play this game of clear vision, clear understanding, perfect understanding; it is not enough if I remove the glasses from my eyes and have transparent ones. You should also do it. Otherwise you are still impeded in your understanding. I am making bold enough to say this, even though I am faced with a galaxy of academic luminaries in Tirupati. Such an assembly used to make me very nervous in the first few days when I came to Tirupati to see Dr. Varadachari, in the good old days, in the golden days of my youth in Sahaj Marg. I benefited very considerably from Dr. Varadachari's association, and it may not be much of a secret to you all, to know that it was Master's orders that I should go to him at least once a month, which brought me here. He was one of those rare persons who also never judged things like that; and it is one of my personal sadnesses and it is one of the losses to the Mission that he passed away so early. But the point I am coming to is, in those days with all this galaxy of academic luminaries present, I never looked upon Dr. Varadachari as a doctor. He was a doctor among doctors, but his behaviour, his love, his attachment to the abhyasis whom he may have cursed left and right for half an hour and then with the utmost compassionate look, loving look he would say "Yes, look here my dear friend, let us sit and meditate." And that dissolved away all the half an hour or one hour of lectures he used to give in a very bullet firing manner.

So, we have to be doctors and make sure that the other man does not feel that we are doctors. Therein lies the dignity of the professional teaching that he would teach without being a teacher, that we are able to be a Master without being a Master. I remember my Master once told me, "I am the servant of humanity."

So, it was precisely because he was able to serve us and we were able to appreciate that service that he was doing for us continuously with every living breath of his body, that we were able to experience this miracle of transformation within ourselves, that we perceived the one who was serving us as a Master. In service alone lies mastery. In mastery lies the slavery. One who wants to be a Master must be a slave. One who is prepared to be a slave becomes a Master.

I am reminded of something, you know, in the military sense because my friend Capt. Murthy is thrusting upon me his military samskaras; it is an axiom of the army that "He alone can command who has learnt to obey." One who has never learnt to obey, one who has never obeyed, can never command, because he doesn't know what to do. So my humble request–let us not colour our views, let us not put barriers to the inputs that we are receiving from outside whether they be sensory, whether they be through the medium of the mind, whether they be even intuitive, let us not colour them by the glasses that we wear and then ruin our own spiritual future. You know, one of the great religious traditions of the West has constantly cautioned its practicants that a day may come when you may hear the divine voice, but be ever alert that it is not the voice of the devil.

Now I can't conceive of a situation in the Sahaj Marg system where an abhyasi can rise to the level of direct communion with the Ultimate and then has to be cautioned "Beware, it could be the devil." Such a thing cannot exist. Because at the highest level of spiritual evolution where there is all wisdom, all humaneness, all compassion, all love, how can such things as devilish voices, if they do exist, how can they ever intrude into my consciousness? I once queried Master in relation to an abhyasi whom we introduced into the satsangh and later found was not morally adequate to be

Accept Him in His Essence

introduced into our satsangh, and to whom Master had given three sittings, and whom Master was praising. I asked him, "Babuji, how is it that you didn't know all these?" He said, "My vision does not descend to lower levels."

So it is no use talking about the Master, my beloved Master, my beloved Babuji, "You are this, you are that." You see, we are all liars every time we praise him and we refuse to emulate his divine way of looking at things, his compassionate way of dealing with people, his merciful way of solving human situations of morality, his most generous way of doling out his immense spiritual fortune to every deserving or undeserving beggar who crosses the streets; if we just mouth these empty terms, I am sorry to say that 99,999 out of one lakh times, it is empty phraseology. For instance, when one of our preceptors in America gave an introductory talk and praised Master to the skies: "He is the Divine incarnate. We see today on the stage of America, the divine personality enthroned in a merely human body, this that and the other," Master beckoned me and said, "Ask him to stop this nonsense." I said, 'Babuji, why are you objecting. He is only saying what you are." He said, "Until he knows me as I am, if he says I am this and that, he is telling lies. You have a right to say I am Divine, you have a right to say I am the Ultimate, you have a right to say I am Perfect when you in your experience have seen these things in me. Till then you are a liar." These are my Master's words. And excuse me, if I sometimes appear to talk less than what I should of my Master, it is because I don't wish to tell lies. I only say what I have seen, I have only written what I have felt and experienced myself in his company and that is the truth.

I request this from you also–let us not flatter that old man, because all flattery is false–it is an axiom of the English language that flattery is falsehood. We stand up every time and mouth empty phrases like Divine, and this, that and the other, and now more so than ever, in the confidence that the old man no longer can hear what we are saying. I beg your pardon, because in his presence we have told him lies, in his presence we have by empty eulogies denigrated him.

When we praise something without knowing what it is, it is ridiculous. You know, once I entered a drawing room and one of my friends was with me and at a distance there was a beautiful vase of flowers, and my friend was all eulogy for those flowers. He said, "What lovely flowers, what divine flowers, what glorious colours." The whole tirade, I can only call it, of eulogizing was shattered by the wife of my friend, who said that they are plastic flowers from Hong Kong [laughing]. So when we praise something without knowing what we are praising, without knowing the qualities we wish to praise, we are falling into the old ritualistic, ridiculous nonsense of this *Sahasra Nama Archana, Ashtottara Sahasra Nama, Ashtottara Sahasra Sankya*–all this foolishness, we don't know what we are praising and we say–"*Twameva mata cha pita twameva.*" When did you ever see him as the mother, or the father or God? So let us not perpetuate lies.

You see, it is said in Latin "*De Martris Nirnisi bonum*"–"of the dead, speak nothing but the good." I am at variance with that wisdom, I would say–of the dead, speak nothing but the truth. The greatest offering is not the floral offering that you put up to Master's picture. The greatest *archana* that we can wash his feet with are the tears of love and the words of truth that we can speak about him at any, every and each of the occasions.

I am telling this to you very bluntly. You know, when my book *Garden of Hearts* was published, it was published after approval by Master. He had read most of it. I asked him before it was printed "Babuji, there are many things here I have related which the public might view as being derogatory to your august personality." He said, "Such as what?" I said, "Such as your physical weakness, your occasional lapses of memory, your confusion sometimes." He said, "You are only telling the truth." I said, "Yes, Babuji, but you know, people may not like the truth." He said, "That is not your business. You tell the truth about me as you have seen it. That is enough."

Now, I am ashamed to say that some people want us to present Babuji as a six foot six monster with an eighty-four inch chest, you know, and I think that is one of the reasons why we put upon poor

Lord Krishna, the Yuga Purusha as we call him, also the husbandhood of sixteen thousand wives. Because man measures the strength of his Master by his own manifestations of strength. If I am virile I think my Master should be virile, if I am intelligent I think my Master should be intelligent, if I am a frog I think my Master should be a frog, if I am rich my Master should be rich. This is again the same story of the coloured glasses before the eyes. An academician, he wants a PhD as his Master. But the precise and the very obvious lesson that our Master has taught us was that he was nothing. Up from nothingness he came, into nothingness he went, and during his life, he manifested that nothingness.

You could not say of him that he was educated, you could not say that he was a fool. He was not rich; he was not poor; he was never sick; he was never healthy. He was on that knife-edge of balance between the two extremes, what they call the 'golden mean', but which I call the 'suffering mean' because at that mean it is all suffering. Like a tightrope walker, he was ever on the balance. He cannot afford to swing this way, he cannot afford to swing that way. Go over a little towards poverty and the blessedness, the so-called blessedness of poverty, of renunciation, of suffering, the mortificatory ways of a ritualistic sadhana, put on a *koupeenam* [loin cloth], go with a begging bowl, sleep on a bed of nails, chant Aham Brahmasmi–this attracts us. You go to the other side, swing a little, you see the air-conditioned bungalow, the powerful cars, the radios, the television sets, the transistors, what have you–that attracts us. Then you are told Janaka was a Raja Rishi who was a king, who had his wives, and what not. And we say, why shouldn't I also be a rishi like that, with a palace, with beautiful wives, with horses, palanquins? The greatest temptation is for the Masters. It is not for fun that we hear in all the *charitras* [history] of the great ones that they had moments of temptation; that Christ was tempted on the mount by Satan, that Nachiketa was tempted by Yama. You see, it is a test. "Are you what you claim to be?" Well, in Sahaj Marg, we have this peculiar phenomenon that there are no tests. That was after all what my Master told me. He said, "In Sahaj Marg there is no test because the Ultimate is not a fool to have to test its raw materials. It knows what you are when you come here.

Where is the need to test you?" But yet we find there are situations in our life, when we feel we are tested, when we feel we are being pushed through the mill, as one man put it recently, and the secret is, as some of our speakers this morning have pointed out, we ask for things!

Now do we make mistakes in asking for things? I don't know. I wouldn't dare to say that we are making mistakes. But if you think again, you see, I am trying to pinpoint the lies we have been telling, the ones I have come across during the last twenty years of my association. I don't know how many years you have been associated with the Master–on one side we say He is 'Sarvagnya', 'Sarvavyapi', 'Sarvasva', He is all-knowing, this, that, X, Y, Z. On the other side we have the temerity, we have the cheek, we have the impudence, we have gone to manifest our disbelief in all those qualities by saying, "Master, I lack food, I lack clothing, my daughter is to be married, will you permit me to pass the examinations?" And some have gone to the extent of writing their roll numbers to him–"my roll number is 999."

So, my dear brothers and sisters, are you aware of what you are doing? Are you aware of what you are speaking? Are you aware of what you are thinking? You have to come back to the Vedic exhortation which is printed in every one of our Patrika issues also: *Uthishta, Jagrata, prapya varannibhodhatha.* Whether we be the merest tyro, or we be the highest advanced, we are still to learn what is the truth of Sahaj Marg, what is the truth of the Master. We are PhDs in various disciplines, we consider ourselves truthful, moral; but what is most needed is this basic humility of approaching my Master with the truth of what he is, and accepting him as such. I consider this to be a manifestation of every abhyasi's ego, that we were not satisfied with Babuji as we found him, and in trying to satisfy our own ego that our Master should be like this, or our Master should be like that, we created a fantasy of a guru, which fantastic or fantasy-ridden personality we are trying to put upon the Master and say, "He is this, he is that," and we want to perpetuate that fantasy now. And now it is even more easy because the coming generations have no idea of what Babuji was, leave alone what Lalaji was. None of us here, I make bold to say, has ever seen

Accept Him in His Essence

Lalaji. Some of us here may not have even seen Babuji; I am sorry for their unfortunate condition. This Divine personality was here, he breathed among us, he lived amongst us, he suffered amongst us–and alas some few of us were not able to see him.

Now what I want you to do, is to think "does it mean that the coming generations of humanity are damned or condemned?" To the contrary, we have the divine promises of my Master who said that this system will be the sole system in the world. When? In the coming ten years; that was one promise. The second promise was, it shall last for thousands of years. The third promise, a saint never dies. He knows no death. Fourth: His oft-repeated words that, "Lalaji is with me, I am with Him, we are one." You must use your wonted, much wonted, much flaunted, much shown-off intelligence in going to the core of things, not in superficial triviality, like the form, name, etc. Either my Master is a truth-sayer or he is a liar. There cannot be a medium path. And if Sahaj Marg is going to last, well then Sahaj Marg is a way. You know, it is like the national highway from Kanyakumari to Delhi, say National Highway No. 7, the way is there always. The road is resurfaced, sometimes the bridges have to be rebuilt, but can you say the road has changed? It is a *marga*. There is the marga, there is the *marga-darshaka*; there is one who treads on that–the *musafir*. The musafir is ever changing. You are but only a traveller on the path; well, there are thousands going ahead of you, there are thousands going to follow you; but the road is the same, whether you go on it today or you go on it tomorrow; Sahaj Marg will not change. So I won't like to say too much about this question, because it can be twisted, interpreted in various ways. But you know, we have to use our sense.

There is a principle; there is at the same time the thing that the principle represents. If I say give me gold, you can give me a necklace, you can give me a coin, you can give me a ring, you can give me a lump without form. If I say give me a necklace, you can give it to me in metal, you can give it to me in plastic, you can give it to me in anything. If I say give me a golden necklace, there are two specifications now. It shall be of gold and it shall be also a necklace. If I say give me a gold necklace, worth 1,75,000 rupees–now it has to have a value fixed to it. But, the world of name and form–

this concept, this bondage has prevented us from seeing the Master when he was amongst us. I make bold to say that those who have not seen the essence of Babuji when he was here with us physically, may perchance have a better chance of knowing him today without that barrier of his body. His body was divine, it was adorable, it was beautiful beyond compare, but yet, it was a barrier. I say this because from the day that Master fell sick and he was unconscious, it has been the universal experience of the abhyasis all over the world that the sittings were most powerful, that the transmission was more persistent and people felt his presence, even those who have never felt his presence before. The simple explanation is when he was alive at Shahjahanpur our minds automatically located him at Shahjahanpur and created a distance between him and ourselves.

Now there is, as the mathematicians say, no locus; we have to locate him. His presence is felt, and it is not anything new that his presence is manifesting itself today. It was there always. I make bold to say it was there even before he was born. But the birth of such great people is precisely to say, "my dear friend, I come so that you can use me as a point on which to fix, learn to love me, learn to cherish me, learn to believe in me, learn to have faith in me, learn ultimately to surrender to me, so that the connection between us will be internal and then you don't need the name, the form. I may manifest myself in another form, I may not; the connection is yours."

So in denying this possibility, we not only deny the principles of Sahaj Marg, we deny the entire Hindu heritage. "*Yada yada hi dharmasya glanir bhavati,*" becomes a lie, because Krishna says very very emphatically that He taught this yoga to Manu long ago you see, and to many people before that. "Arjuna, you don't know but I know all my lives of the past, and the lives of the future also. You are bound by time, you are bound by form, you are bound by name." And when Krishna was gracious enough to show Himself in His *Viswaroopa Darsana*, and Arjuna, you know, had nothing but fear as a response. He says, "Please come back to your form which I love so much." Now, I pray that no abhyasi of Sahaj Marg should be such a fool, excuse me for using that word, that my Master will one day manifest Himself in His Ultimacy and we should cringe and cower before Him and say, "Lord, please push back to your normal form, let me see you as you are." He will say, "Fool, is it for this you come to me? I came to you in a form which you could touch, smell, love, to teach you how to love me in my true essence, as one day I hoped that I shall manifest myself to you."

"It was for a preparation and you want me to ever remain a child because you could not love me as an adult. As you could not love me as God Himself, should I be a child?" This is Balakrishna worship. We can't stand Him as an adult God and we can't stand Him as a Viswaroopi, we can't stand Him as a Yuga Purusha. Why? Because if he comes crawling, mouthing silly nonsense, you want to hug him and cuddle him and kiss him, but in His ultimate form we have to cringe before Him, we don't know what we are, and we are ashamed, we are sin-ridden, we are ridden with the guilt of ages and ages of life. There again we are denying him, because in one form, we think, he cannot do anything to us, he cannot punish us, he cannot correct us, he is after all Balakrishna–lovable, soft, tender, but when He comes as God we are afraid of Him. So what do we really want? Are we in abhyas for reality or are we in abhyas to think soft things to cuddle with? We are not teddy bears!

So let us make very sure, brothers and sisters–all of you, the learned, the literate, the highly educated–it is time you see that education is only a veneer. The basic intelligence of all is guaranteed. God does not play tricks with human beings. He has given us *pancha indriyas*. The sensitivity may be lacking. That is because we have put on coloured glasses. Remove them, which is being done for you every day by our devoted preceptors, who are giving you the cleaning again and again which we destroy–the effects of which we destroy by taking the glasses again and putting them on.

All this talk of Prarabdha, Sanchita, it is all, you know, so much trivial trash to be consigned to the waste paper basket. I have the Divine at my service, and I make bold to say that He is there, and He says "With a glance Lalaji could have transformed and could have liberated, it required but a glance from His eyes." These are the words which Babuji used. I have known Babuji doing it himself too. So when you come to this aspect and we still keep harping on samskaras, and tendencies, and intelligence and lack of it, I am only sorry to say that we are now not only carrying the burdens of our education, the burdens of our wealth, the burdens of our culture, but we have, in some intangible way become proud of them.

So let us shake off the pride first, so that we may get rid of the burdens, because only then shall we see them as bondages to our understanding, as limitations to our understanding; because we see a biologist talks of God in the biological way, a scientist talks in the way of science, an artist takes pictures of Him. What is it that is the reality behind all these?

I remember Dr. Varadachari once said the sloka *sarva dharmaan parityajya* should be read as *sarva adharmaan parityajya mam ekam saranam vraja*. And what are the *adharmas*? The basic adharma is on one side we pretend to love God, to have faith in Him, to have surrendered to Him, when with every breath of our existence we are only showing that we love ourselves, have faith in ourselves, and surrender only to ourselves! This thing we have got to shake off. We have got to, as Master said, "Change your vision from here to here and God is there before you." These three things which we are capable of doing to ourselves, let us just take them out and invert them toward Him, and the goal is achieved. So the moral of all that I have got to say is, clear your vision before you try to clear others' vision. Remove the glasses from your eyes before you want to remove them from other people's eyes. Correct your wisdom; make sure it functions properly notwithstanding the degrees that are appended to your names before you have the cheek, the temerity and the courage to interfere with another man's understanding and his intelligence. And then the victory is won; we shall all travel together on this path. Let us not worry who is the Master, who is the guide, who is the goal; our hearts know it. And as Babuji ever said–his clarion call to humanity I would say, his most valid advice, his most important advice through ages–"When in doubt, consult your heart."

So I would say, brothers and sisters, the time is before you to consult your heart and having wasted so much time let us not waste further time, but make sure we go towards Him who is ever with us, who is not only in front of us or behind us, and the Vedas say

Accept Him in His Essence

that He is all around us, and He is inside too! We don't have to seek Him anywhere. So let us refer to Him in our hearts, forsaking this idea, forsaking this weakness, forsaking this despondency, that He has left and gone, that we are left bereft of guidance, of assistance, of help. I am often fond of saying that–there is a song, devotional song, in Hindi: *Andhe ki lakdi tu hai.* He calls Him the walking-stick of the blind man. Surdas I think, but I am not sure. But why the need for a walking-stick? If the blind man has such transcendental confidence in the Divinity whom he is addressing that, "you are the walking-stick in the hands of the blind," he should throw away the stick and walk. Let us not have the walking-stick; these are props to misunderstanding, to self-deception, to misery.

Let us throw away all props, props of wealth, props of intelligence, props of understanding, props of even sadhana. Because, you know, I once had the impudence to question the effect, the need for and efficacy of the Sahaj Marg system. Babuji said, "What do you mean?" I said, "Babuji, I am convinced these are unnecessary things." He said, "Why?" I said, "You are yourself quoting to me often the Vedic precept *'emevaisha vrunute tena labhyaha'*– 'whatever you may do, however well you may do it, with whatever great degree of devotion you may do it, until He wishes, you cannot achieve it.' This is a fact. This is the truth. If this be so what is the fun in wasting my time upon sadhana?" He said, "What would you do?" I said, "Leave that to me. After all the victor knows how he is going to conquer. Why should he tell the secret in advance?" Then he smiled. At that time, I had in mind the story of Sahadeva who went to Lord Krishna before the Mahabharata Yuddha was to begin, and he said, "Lord Krishna, you are the culprit behind this whole nonsense. You are going to destroy the Kauravas and Pandavas and I am going to stop it. If you don't stop it, I am going to stop it." Krishna of course became, for a moment, non-plussed. He told Sahadeva arrogantly, "You...stop me? Do you know who I am? Do you know my plans are already laid?" Sahadeva said, "Yes, Lord. But I can nevertheless stop." Krishna asked "Sahadeva, how would you do it?" Sahadeva said, "Lord, I meditate upon you, put you in my heart and bind you up. You cannot move your little finger even!" Krishna came to his senses. You see that was the power of the lover, you know, of the true sadhak. Krishna pleaded, "Sahadeva, please, you will spoil my entire plan, Nature's plan will be spoiled. Don't do this for my sake." Sahadeva said, "What will you do for my sake?" Krishna replied, "Anything you ask," and he asked "The Pandavas and Draupadi should come out of this war unharmed." Krishna agreed. Sahadeva went home.

See, this is the power of love! Enthrone Him in your heart, enshrine Him there, pray to Him silently. Let us not eulogize in public. I am ashamed to hear so many things of Master from so many insincere lips, pardon me for using harsh words. I made bold to say on one occasion where I was garlanded–I said, "every garland that you put on the neck of a man without affection for him, it is like the noose of the hangman." It is a bondage. What makes such bondages acceptable is the love behind it.

So I would rather a man call the Master a fool with love, than praise him with insincerity. The time for insincerity has long passed. Let us not insult that poor old man even after his physical end has come. Because He is ever with us. Let me assure you, He knows precisely what we are doing, what we are seeing, what we are speaking, even now at this moment. And I am sure He is smiling along [pointing towards the heart]. So let us not insult Him, insult His divinity, insult His magnificent generosity by continuing to tell lies about Him, about His work. We have a right to speak only of that which we know, no more no less.

So, with this humble request to all of you, I thank you for listening to me. Thank you.

Interiorize Him

I am really happy to participate on such auspicious occasions. It is neither a duty for me nor a privilege for me. It is something that I have to do, so I do it. But I am nevertheless grateful to you for calling me and permitting me to be here with you all. Because it is the Master's work that we are doing and in which you are as much participating as I am. And in spiritual work you cannot say, this is only the preceptor's work or only the abhyasi's work, it is all mutual co-operation. And if you ask who benefits, I would like to say that perhaps even God Himself benefits, because otherwise there is no point in His creating the world and creating human beings and then sending a Master to them. Because I consider in a way, that the creation that God made at the time of creation was something which is not complete. This may go against the theological arguments. But it was something He made and then sent human beings down to perfect it, because He had no mind.

So, all that the energies of God could do, when they came out of the first *kshob*, was to progressively solidify until there is the material creation. The way back had to be found, and for this the guru comes, again an *amsa* of the Divine, but he is able to do what God could not do. God could send us down but a guru has to take us up again, back to Himself.

I don't think people will consider this to be blasphemy because our own Shastras say the same thing...*Guru Brahma Guru Vishnu*...all that sort of thing. And without the guru, God cannot be achieved. This is one of the most crucial points of all the systems of practice in India; our whole life, our whole spiritual approach, our aspiration, is based on this fact that a guru is necessary.

So when we honour the memory of such a great man, such a great personality, who founded this system for us at his personal

Concluding talk at Tirupati, 30 December 1984.

level, brought it down for us, whatever may have been the mechanics of that, our heart beats with gratitude for him, for his work, for the opportunity he has given us to go back to our original home as he called it, and in this expression of our gratitude, in the sharing of the *marga* for our mutual benefit, because we are all proceeding towards the same goal; otherwise we wouldn't be here. This makes us co-passengers, and it is our duty to mutually support each other, love each other, help each other, cherish each other, and in that activity of mutual trust, support, and love, there should be no conception of any differences of position or power or things like that.

A preceptor is a person who is to serve the abhyasis. He has no other position. He has no other claims upon the abhyasis, what shall I say–respect, regard, even love. Because what the preceptor must get is the result for the work which the Master guarantees provided he does his work. Master has said time and again that when you do something right you cannot have a wrong result. That is against the Laws of Nature. So right action must be followed by right results; right action must be preceded by right thought; right thought must result in right endeavours to the proper orientation of the goal. And in such a person, with such powers, with a marga like this, which our Master has given us tailor-made–everything has been made for us–he has left the way for us. He has tailor-made the system for us. The literature exists for us. The preceptors are there for our service. Therefore, the word 'failure' should be erased from the dictionary of spirituality, at least as far as Sahaj Marg goes. The very idea of failure is repugnant. It cannot be, because it casts aspersions for the effectiveness of the way, the abilities of the Master and the effectiveness of the powers that he has used in creating these things for us.

So, any lack of faith is only a lack of faith in ourselves. We cannot by any means, by any stretch of imagination, have lack of faith in the Master. It only means we have no faith in ourselves; and essentially it is also the same spiritually, because when you say, "He is in my heart," and I don't believe in myself, I don't believe in Him, too. So this is another aspect of the situation that I would like to place before you all, that whenever we doubt somebody else, we are really doubting ourselves. So let us make up our minds that this way shall exist for ever. It is for the Master to promise; it is for us to make that promise come true. As every seed has within it the promise of life, of unfoldment of that life, of fruition of the possibilities contained in that seed, but yet if that seed is not planted, well watered and looked after until it is a tree and it can give fruit, the promise remains a mere promise. So I don't believe in some of the sententious statements that Master has said so and therefore it will be. Master has said so–therefore it can be. The realisation of these possibilities, the actualization of Master's promise to us, the achievement of the goals, of the levels of 'being' that he has outlined for us, is very much in our hands. Please don't misunderstand me as saying that there is something lacking in the Master's efforts.

We buy a packet of seeds from a shop, if you let it rot in the ground or if you keep it in your drawer of the table, it remains as mere seed. Somebody in the succeeding generation might have the good fortune to find that packet of seeds and sow it and reap the harvest; it will not be us. If you ask why there have been gaps in the spiritual regeneration of mankind, in the spiritual advancement of mankind, my humble opinion is, it is precisely because the seeds of spiritual growth, the seeds of spiritual aspiration, the seeds of spiritual possibilities, have been left dormant until another agriculturist in the form of a guru came and said, "Don't waste the seeds, they are for you. Sow them. This is how it is done. This is the first harvest. I have shown you what to do with it. Now continue the good work," and he goes back. And we lapse back into our old lethargy, to our old lack of faith and we say, "How can this tiny seed become such a big *vriksha* [tree]?"–not having the faith, the patience, or lacking the efforts to put it in the ground and see whether it grows or not. That is all that we are expected to do. No man can claim that he creates agriculture. We are only sowing the seed and reaping the fruit.

So I think it is with some sense that the word *krishi* has been used in yogic literature; *Vyavasaya* has been used in the Bhagavad Gita because it is very much an agricultural activity; you can say this is an activity of soul culture where the seed of divinisation sown into us by His grace, must find suitable soil in the environment of our hearts, must be watered with our love, must be nurtured by our faith in Him, by our devotion in Him, until one day the seed has flowered into Him. The seed that was His seed becomes Him and then we find that He is occupying our entire self–not because we did anything wonderful. We allowed Him to sow the seed and saw to it that it was not destroyed.

So abhyasa confers no distinction on us. We are not doing anything. All that we are doing is not to go against His wishes; not to oppose His will; not to place impediments to the work of His powers but to accept them passively, docilely, with faith, with love, that anything that He does for us is for our good. Because some of our speakers have said that we must ask, we must get. You see, when a child is born in the family, we think it is a good thing; this is traditional; big hullabulloo is made, cakes are bought, candles are bought, birthday party celebrated. Some years later we regret having had that child because we have no means to support it and it is running like a stray waif on the streets, adding one more *goonda* to the existing gangs of goondas.

So what is good or what is bad, only the end can show. Beginning can never show. Cyclones come; trees are destroyed. Ten days later you find the city is much cleaner, all the dead-wood has been thrown out, all the rubbish has been cleared away. It was a necessary evil. To say that it was a necessary evil even, is wrong. It was something which we interpreted as evil, but which ultimately we found is good. So in the course of our existence we find things happen to us. Something is lost which we think is a loss. Something is gained which we think is a gain. Days after, weeks after, we find what we thought was a gain is really a loss, and what we thought was a loss is really a gain! So time alone can tell us in what way, in what form, a seed is going to grow and what it is going to become.

So, the fact that people whose lives are going on well, trouble-free, smooth, that they have faith in the Master, is something to be amused about, because there is no faith in it. They are not having faith in the Master. They are having satisfaction of the fact that their life is going smoothly according to their desire. I want a child, my child is born; I want my daughter to be married, she gets a good alliance. Some people go to the extent of buying lottery tickets, promising twenty percent of the profit to Master, as if Master had to give me a lakh of rupees to get a mere pittance of 20,000 rupees for himself. If he could give a lakh of rupees, he could surely get that himself if he wants it. And this we see epitomized to the ultimate level of stupidity and perfection here up in the hills. And this is the *kshetra* where financial corruption even to the god-hood has been perfected organizationally and in every other way.

So let us not indulge in these stupidities. When I get rich I am not getting rich, riches come to me; when I am getting poor, I am not becoming poor, my money is taken away from me. So it is like, you know, some thin people go on eating like anything and they cannot get fat; some fat people are dieting all their lives and they cannot lose half a kilo. So we are not in any way competent, not empowered, not capable of interfering in our own personal life. There is some force working which is outside our control, which knows what exactly has to become of me, and under its guidance I must go on. Today I am fat, very good I am fat; tomorrow I am thin, very good I am thin. Today I have friends, excellent. Tomorrow I am hated and reviled, wonderful. It helps me to remember the Master even better. Because you will find in our Ten Maxims of the Master, we are taught to accept all these things. Miseries and all should be gifts of God; because when we are happy we never think of Him. Diwali comes, Pongal comes, Ugadi [New Year Day] comes, we only think of ourselves, our children, of the *payasam* and *vadai* [kinds of sweet and savoury] that we make, and of the stray friends who visit us. But let there be an illness in the family, God forbid–a death, then comes the thought of the Master.

So without having to go to extremes there is a wisdom in God which makes Him keep us on the negative side of the situation; a little poverty, a little ill-health, a little misery. It is always good for us, because it has several benefits. If a man is a little below the optimum health levels, he doesn't do all the things that a healthy man does. That arrogance of the health, that pride in the health, that I can do anything and get away with it, he will not indulge. Indulgence is the word. When a man gets ninety-nine rupees where he needs one hundred rupees, he is careful with the money. Let him get rupees 101/- and he is a debtor.

So it is not for nothing that Master or Lalaji has outlined the three principles, the three very great requirements for a person to be a saint–permanent poverty, permanent illness, and permanent *ninda* [criticism]. They have very great benefits in keeping us within our limits, within our limits of arrogance, within our limits of pride, within our limits of misuse of the body, the mind, the intellect; they endow us with humility, they endow us with sensible attitudes towards physical life, mental life, moral life, and therefore they guide us through the channels into that path which can ultimately lead to perfection which Master calls 'the saintly path'.

So it is only a fool who will want happiness, and a bigger fool who will refuse miseries. The wise man always accepts. For him there is no distinction, because what comes from the lover is a love letter. It is not the contents of the letter which makes a love letter. When a lover writes a letter, it is a love letter. But we want it to start with, you know, XXX representing twenty kisses, and ending with forty XXX's representing forty kisses, with all the lies that a lover can tell his beloved in between.

We are happy with lies, with false promises and with flatteries. But when the Master writes and says "Dear Brother, I find your condition is a little less than what I expected, and I am praying for you," the first sentence annoys us, the second sentence shakes our faith. Because, we say, "Well, you know, my condition is good. He told me last time. Now how he is writing like this. I don't know what is wrong with the Master." The second sentence where he says, "I am praying for your improvement," we say, "Well, Master himself has to pray. What sort of a Master can he be?"

We should know that when a doctor operates surgically on us, it is not for satisfaction that he is giving us pain. It is to rid us of the disease, to cure us of the disease, to make us whole, well. If a mere doctor can be like that, how much more must be the Master? How much he must weep internally to move even the smallest thing against our wishes? But yet, it has to be done; because otherwise he would be going against the integrity of his own existence.

So I can assure every one of you that if the Master permits us as abhyasis, to undergo certain samskaras which are painful, which are troublesome, which may demean us, which may make us lose those whom we love, whom we cherish, he weeps much more for us than we could ever weep for ourselves. But we don't see the tears in his eyes. We don't see, as we say in Tamil, putting of *muttakku* over his head. So we think he is happy and he is testing us. It is not a test, because, as I told you this morning He needs to test nothing, he needs to test no one, least of all himself. He knows his powers better than anyone can know, because he is the Master of his powers.

So let us believe that whatever happens to us is for our immediate good, for our ultimate good. There can be nothing which comes from the Master which is even capable of remotely being against our existence. If we are able to realise this, to understand it with our hearts, not the intellect, then the realisation of the maxims will come, that we will truly, not only accept miseries as gifts, we will pray for miseries, because then it opens up the possibility of our progress being accelerated. Now we are co-operating. Acceptance is one thing; co-operation is another.

So when do we really co-operate? I personally believe that some day somebody may have to formulate another set of maxims, where Master will not stop at saying "Accept miseries as gifts," but add "Pray for miseries as gifts." Because don't we do everything that will accelerate our progress in the material world? Should we not similarly do everything that is essential to accelerate our progress in the spiritual world? So this is the dawning of divine wisdom for which we have all to pray.

We pray "Oh Master! Thou art the real goal of human life"– but nobody knows who is the Master, nobody knows what is human life, nobody knows what is the goal, leave alone the real goal.

"Our wishes are putting bar to our advancement"–we are repeating it day in and day out and yet we wish for progress, we wish for this, we wish for that, everything is a wish.

"Thou art the only God and power to bring us up to that stage"– we deny Him when we question His powers, when we deny again

His magnanimity, we deny His wisdom, and most of all we deny His right over us.

In today's law, a mere husband has so many rights over his wife. A father has so many rights over his son. An employer has so many rights over his employees. A mere passenger has rights over the transportation. And if you read the newspapers, a tragedy which took place in Bhopal has attracted all the vultures of the West, American lawyers, who have suddenly become interested in the fate of these poor people of Bhopal and are filing suits on their behalf. Where were they so long? Why this sudden interest in the people of Bhopal, in the Bhopal tragedy by these American lawyers? I am told that it is because the suits are worth probably one hundred billion dollars and they will get forty percent if they win it. But this is welcome as a sign of sudden awakening of interest towards the Indian community by the American community.

This is the sort of mentality we have, not knowing that our interest lies not in importing foreign goods, not in importing foreign technicians, but in helping ourselves. And this, only spirituality does. Because the Master by being first foreign to us, enters our hearts, becomes us in every sense of the word, and now we become self-dependent, self-reliant, self-growing, self-evolving systems. The Master from outside is guiding us, helping us, enabling us to realise that He is within us, so that we co-operate with 'this' rather than with 'that'. Because as I said somewhere else once, the external Master will disappear some day. The physical form will go. Then if you are dependent on the physical form, your spiritual journey stops there.

So the whole secret of yoga, is in bringing that Master–his subtle essence, his spiritual self, which he is putting into us in every transmission–into our heart, accepting it in the heart, making it grow there, so that when he leaves the physical self, he is still here for eternity with us, wherever he may be, however he may be, in whatever situation he may be.

So, the only possibility of eternal guidance, eternal help, eternal support, is from within, not from the external world, not even from the Master of the external world. If we don't permit Him to come into our heart and interiorize Himself, we may as well never have had a Master.

So this is why we meditate on the heart and we do this cleaning and so many things which Dr. Kuppuswamy also explained. When we invite the Master, naturally we want the place to be cleaned. So that is only an aspect, it is an aspect of etiquette, more than anything else, that the place should be cleaned when a great man comes. When ministers visit Tirupati, the streets are cleaned up. It is not for the public good. It is not a sudden awakening of the need for public health or the consciousness of the welfare of the people of Tirupati that enters into the minister's mind. It is the minions who wish to show a good Tirupati before the minister whose constituency it is. We do the same, recognising that He is the Master of this constituency. He is not elected. It is His, by right of creation. He has created it, it is His. We did not create our hearts, we did not create even our bodies. So, we are only respectfully, lovingly, humbly handing over something to its creator which foolishly, arrogantly, pridefully, we had accepted as ours; we had imagined it to be ours. Now we say, "Lord, take it, it is yours, do what you will with it." This symbolizes what the spiritual life is. This is all that surrender means.

I had this tape recorder to look after for him. To me it was a burden; because I was responsible. Because when it didn't work, I was upset. Why? Because somebody has kept something with me and I am responsible for its right protection, right preservation, right functioning.

So we are answerable to Him for the right performance of this organization, for its right and effective functioning, for its right movement towards Him and one day when He comes and says, "Render unto me thy account."

You say, "Here it is. You look for yourself."

"What is it you have done with it?"

"I don't know."

"Why did you do it?"

"That too, I don't know. But such as it is I render unto you. Now Lord, take thine."

So, this is all that is surrender. People imagine that they are giving themselves up and that they are going to lose their identities. This idea is very common in the West, that we will lose our individuality. What is your individuality? Who said you have any individuality? Just because you have a name and a form, you think you are an individual. So is a grain of rice, if you could give a name to it or number to it. There is nothing which distinguishes the human individual from an animal or from a grain of sand. In fact, there are millions more, many billions more, grains of sand than there ever will be human beings on this planet. So this is one aspect of the arrogance, the ego, the pride which says, "I am so-and-so. How can I surrender and give up my existence?" It never was yours! It was a momentary aberration of your emotions, of your intellect, that you thought you are something separate, you are always of Me as a piece of property. Today you have to account for it, give it back.

Whenever we die, this is what is going to happen to our bodies. We cannot carry it with us. Happily or regretfully, healthfully or sick, this body has to be surrendered to this planet. It belongs to this planet because it is constituted of five *bhutas*, as we call them and there it belongs. So whatever has come, from wherever it has come, to that it returns. That which is eternal, goes back to that which is eternal, in whose custody it belongs, who created it, to whom it must inevitably return, whether we like it or not. So, whenever we strive to express our own wishes, our own will, our own desire, and to manifest what we call our individuality, our independence, our right of action, we are going against the will of Nature and therefore we can never succeed. Therefore, such a man's life is full of miseries, full of disaffections, full of troubles, illnesses, losses, calamities, and he says, "If God is all merciful, why does He penalize me like this?" It is not God who is penalizing you. You have turned your face away from the sun and you see nothing but the shadows in front. And you are afraid of your own shadow. Turn towards the sun and the shadow is left behind, the darkness is left behind.

I had one thought a few days back during meditation which I exchanged with some of my friends: that we see light and shade, light and darkness, because we are rotating. Sometimes we are facing the sun, sometimes we are against the sun. But what does the sun see? It sees the changing face of the same planets around it. It doesn't see light and darkness. One moment it is seeing Africa, then it is seeing Asia, then it is seeing Europe, and it goes on. So you see, depending upon where you are looking from, you see different things. If you look from the aspects of the self, everything is a tragedy. If you look from the aspect of the higher 'Self', everything is growing, everything is going unto Him. It is a progressively evolutionary path. For him there is no misery, he is ever smiling. And He says, "Yes, you are coming, whether you are falling a few feet or not. You are still rising to me because that is inevitable." So in giving up our desires, in giving up our foolish wishes, prejudices and things like that, we are only going up without impediments which we create ourselves.

So spirituality has to be understood in very fundamental terms, that I am spiritual whether I like it or not. There is no such thing as progress; there is only a returning to the starting point from where I set out. I still remain what I am. In His mercy if He says, "My son, you are divine even if you set out," that is His grace. But if I am a son, whether I am a fool or a wise man, whether I am rich or poor, whether I am sick or healthy, if I go back, He has to take me back. Because I am no less His than He is mine, once that relationship is there.

So it is only the foolish human mind which says, "Sir, I am unfit. How can I come to you unclean?" Clean or dirty or whatever it is, 'go back'. You know, when a child comes out of the street, having played all day, stinking, filthy, mother doesn't shout at it. On the contrary the dirtier it is, the more she hugs it, quickly bathes it, quickly changes its clothes; that is her function. So to keep us clean, to keep us strong, to keep us healthy, to keep us wise, as befitting His children, that is His business, so long as we are in His domain, which is our home. When we are outside we have to look after ourselves. When we are in the house, He looks after us. So let us make sure that He looks after us in every possible way by getting back to where we belong, becoming His charge rather than being independent and having this big tragedy of having to look after ourselves and our problems.

Discipline

One way of problem solving, or rather the only way of problem solving, is to first recognize that the problem exists. In our sanstha we are too prone to think that we are already saints, that everything is as it should be and that the brotherhood which exists, if at all it exists, need exist only in a small closed circle like at this moment as it is here.

I have often commented on this even at Basant Utsav, that during those three or four days the two thousand, three thousand, four thousand abhyasis live very amicably, very harmoniously; we meet each other, respect each other. But on the fifth morning when the Utsav is over, indiscipline starts even while boarding the bus for departure. People rush in for the front seat, people rush in to put their beds and feverishly position their luggage, so that they can take them out easily at the railway station; people rush into the train and occupy even the reserved seats and then quarrel with others, I mean among our own brothers and sisters. And then on top of all this indiscipline, the people who are not disciplined will themselves comment, "What is this brotherhood that we talk of, if twenty-seven people who have reserved seats cannot adjust or accommodate twenty-two of us who have the misfortune of not having reservations?" They conveniently forget that the railway rules require that the reserved seats should be occupied by only those who have reserved the seats. They further forget that we have no rights to distribute the seats among ourselves. Reservations are not transferable. They forget that the poor fellows had made the reservations perhaps thirty days or forty days in advance, only so that they could travel back in comfort. And all this they expect, at the cost of the comfort of those who had made advance reservations, who had foresight to do so and who are now being blamed for lack of broth-

Talk at Chittoor on 31 December 1984.

erhood, that one-for-one adjustment was not made. And then they suddenly turn round and see the General Secretary sitting in another seat and they start blushing, even then not because of shame but because of their being caught.

This has happened so many times. I am ashamed to say that once, after a Basant Celebration, after three days stay at Ashram, Babuji was going back home in a rickshaw, instead of in a car, and there were thirty or forty abhyasis going on the road. They looked up, saw Babuji, they didn't even care to stop or even respectfully bow before him or fold their hands, not even this; they pretended not to have noticed him and turned away. I commented to Master, "This is the sort of discipline we seem to have brought about in the Mission, that even when you are going on the street when you are outside the Ashram, they believe as if your mastery, your high position, spiritual authority, your elevation in spiritual realm, everything is left behind in your cottage and here you are only Ram Chandra of Shahjahanpur."

This is nothing new. In fact we have to talk about discipline in the East, in the West, in the North and in the South. It is very painful that even in the smallest of our behaviour pattern, interpersonal relationship, we have not been able to change ourselves, regulate our behaviour, conduct ourselves as we should. I have had occasion to discuss this with Master, particularly when we were in Europe, where you know people don't mind what we talk–I am left in total freedom with the Master. I asked him once, "You take Christianity. That religion is known for brotherhood, for compassion. It is not hypocritical, it is not something which is just a veneer polish on the outside, it exists. You can see it in the way the fathers, the lay-brothers, the church people, behave. You see it in the Buddhists, you see it everywhere where you say there is no inner spiritual development. You see it in the Muslim brotherhood, how they exuberantly meet each other, how they respect the Kazi, how they are prepared to sacrifice their lives if it is needed, how they respect the calls of prayer at the appropriate time, how they are disciplined. Have you seen the photographs of Mecca during the Haj–line by line there are hundreds of thousands of Muslims sitting, and when they bow, it is like one wave of that. Whereas in our sanstha, satsangh at 6:30 means arrivals will go on till 7.

We used to have an abhyasi in Madras. On Sunday morning we have generally satsangh from 7:30 A.M. to 8:00, 8:20. He was invariably coming in when we just say "That's all." There was not one Sunday on which he was present when we sat for satsangh and the explanation for late-coming was always the same, that his driver had not come. So you see there seems to be something basically wrong. I had prolonged arguments with Babuji, "Is there any law of Nature that spiritual inner development should not be balanced by the external behaviour also, modifications of the external behaviour also? Does some sense of balance in Nature require that the inner development should be at the cost of external factors?" He said, "It cannot be. On the contrary, both must go side by side." I said, "Show me one example."

I really meant it because I am yet to see one example from the highest to the lowest, where the inner and the outer are matched. If there is one example it is only the Master himself, because he was ever courteous, he was ever loving. He was prepared to give up his sweater during the cold seasons to other persons who did not bring them. He was prepared to give up his chair to somebody who had back trouble, he was prepared to go to the bathroom when everybody else had gone, eat after everybody else had eaten. And all that example we had before us, the living example–we admired, we talked about, we wrote about, but I am sorry to say nobody tried to emulate him. Have we not seen Master picking up bits of paper from the grass in Shahjahanpur and every time he bent down, people used to adore him "What a wonderful Master that he is himself stooping to pick up bits of paper from the grass!" And the man who is ready to throw away the empty cigarette packet is right there, so that on the next round Master could come and pick it up. So this was something, you know, which was very scandalizing in Sahaj Marg. It is not just something to be ashamed of, it is scandalizing. It is so bad that sometimes–you will forgive my saying it–I have questioned the efficacy of our system itself.

The inner I am not able to judge. My Master said, "He is elevated. He is in the fifth ring, you are in the third ring." That as a Master it is his privilege to commend and we accepted it. But the external we are all seeing. And where is that individual today in Sahaj Marg? Produce him before me. I wish to see one person, whether it is in India or outside India. I am still more sorry to say that the persons who Babuji said are the first examples of spiritualisation outside India ever in the history of spirituality–their behaviour is no better. So it is not restricted only to Indians. The very spiritual development that Master gives us seems in some way to tarnish our external, our conduct, our sense of responsibility, and I am still not able to understand why this is so. I am sorry to say that this was not pointed out to me yesterday. I would have set it as a research task to our academic brothers in Tirupati. I don't know if any of them are here. But this is something that we should think about and do research about. Why on earth is it possible that mountains can be moved in our inner self and a simple mole cannot be eradicated from your face? I am talking figuratively, you see.

So how to suggest ways? How to answer brother Ramamurthi's question? I really don't know, except perhaps to suggest that the very fact of spiritual development seems to confer on us certain ideas, certain assumed rights, almost like divine rights, that 'a spiritual individual need not conform to a behaviour pattern;' that 'a spiritually elevated soul is evolved above right and wrong;' that 'a spiritually evolved person is above all moral codes.' And unfortunately in the Hindu tradition we have before us very very bitter, sad, annoying examples of many of the sannyasis, the most mischievous crowd in religious history, fellows who are fanatics, who live off the land, who cheat, who are prepared to do murder and rape if necessary–and they have been the objects of our veneration.

So in some way I think the Hindu mind has been conditioned to accept misbehaviour, immorality, lying, cheating, etc., in so-called religious persons. This has gone to such an extent in our blood that we find in every cinema a sannyasin appears, there is a fellow who is *mouna* swami, who is silent and robed and dressed in yellow, who claims everything; he goes to a rich man; apple, gold, silver, everything is brought to him–and in the night he just walks off with it; it is horrible.

This is the state of affairs, perhaps, to which we have been conditioned, and this condition can be a very valid reason why in India we behave like this, why in India we associate bad behaviour with so-called religious uplift. But how can one account for such a thing in Europe where the external training, the training in ethics, the training in morality, has been deeply grounded (particularly in the Christian tradition) and where one hopes that the inner transformation will not interfere with the external transformation which is achieved so very easily? In Hinduism, yes–it has been corrupt inside, so it has been corrupt outside, all through the religious history of India.

I have often remarked with very considerable sorrow that the most faithful feature of the Indian life is this *"Satyam vada, dharmam chara,"* in the Vedas, which is a clear indication that we have been a nation of liars from the days of Vedas. And in modern life, you find "Don't spit," "Don't Damage Public Property," "Be Indian," "Buy Indian," you know, exhortations. "To be Indian," "To be Moral," "To tender the Correct Fare," "Don't Travel without Tickets." But this is a matter for us to feel ashamed, when overseas visitors who come to India see this at the airport itself. What they think of us, I don't know, I would not like to know, because what I would think of India if I were to come from outside and saw all these, I know very well in my heart.

So, morality, correct behaviour, ethical behaviour, a certain integrity to your beliefs, integrity to traditions, practising what you preach–these have never been the character of Indian life, factors of Indian life, features of Indian life. If I read my books correctly, the Indian tradition, the Hindu tradition, the Hindu culture–the more these exhortations have appeared, the more we can read into it a decline steadily from the past. And if ten thousand years ago my forefathers had to be told to tell the truth and to avoid immorality, this-that-and-the-other, I don't know if ever in the history of India there was a time when we were moral, when we were ethical. And this perhaps explains why the Indian is not quite liked abroad. Because we are masters of preaching and masters of not practising what we preach. Our preaching is all for others. We shout from the roof tops. You know, in international relationships, our Foreign Ministers are experts at this job. If somebody explodes an atom bomb we are the first to protest, but we have every right to do it ourselves. If somebody is practicing racism in South Africa we protest, but in India there is no less of it.

So in our private life, in our public life, in our religious life, there had never been in the history of India an effort to match principles and beliefs with practices and behaviour. So when our brother asked me for a solution to this problem, I can only very humbly bow before him and say, "Brother, this has been a problem for my Master even."

In spite of his divine example, personal example present before us, his activities before us, behaviour before us, his gentleness, his compassion, his ever-smiling cheerfulness, his loyalty to his Master, his loyalty to every single spoken word of Lalaji Maharaj, his immediate acceptance of orders, his implicit and total obedience—we had not been able to follow one millionth of one percent of that example. Which abhyasi can say with his hand on his heart, "I obeyed Master"? Master says "You are snoring when you are meditating." The man asks, "Why?" Master says, "Eat one roti less." And the man says, "It is a joke." Probably he ate one more to compensate for that disappointment.

So we cannot obey, you know. We can glaringly see before us: (1) We never accepted the Master; (2) We never accepted his teachings; (3) We never tried to put them into practice; (4) We have no intention of putting them into practice because they interfere with our freedom of choice, of action, which we believe to be our divine right.

So, I don't see any way by which the Indian is going to be transformed. This is not a Sahaj Marg problem. This is an Indian problem—corruption in private life, corruption in public life, corruption in every sphere of activity. Perhaps we exported it also, because twenty years back, it was not so rampant in the West and the Far East. This is a new phenomenon that in Europe there is so much corruption, in Japan there is so much corruption. Today, wherever you see, there is corruption. I see, like our language, like our art, like our tradition, we exported our corruption too during the last quarter of a century or half a century.

So, how we are going to correct? Well, it is for each individual to make up his mind: "If I don't correct myself I am inviting calamity on myself." If India is a poor country, if India is an underdeveloped country with all its vast potential of men and materials, with its immense richness of heritage, with its immense spiritual traditions and background, it is because we choose to be beggars, we choose to be liars, we choose to be cheats, as there lies a little petty money. It is so easy to cheat your neighbour and take twenty rupees from him. It is easy to tell somebody a lie and make two hundred rupees. It is easy to sell your nation and make one million dollars.

So, we are talking today of materialism and material culture corrupting our influences, corrupting our values, corrupting our very life itself and corroding it to the core. Some of our leaders have been very happy about talking of corruption, forgetting that everything flows from the top, the river flows from the top, grace flows from the top, corruption also comes from the top. It is not a grass-root phenomenon! The more the people in the top want to make money, the more the people in the bottom have to make money, to pay to those who are at the top. Where will they pay it from? So you see, this is something so widespread that we have to perhaps only pray for it, but even prayer does not seem to work today, because in prayer also we are corrupt. We are not able to pray.

You know, it is said in the Christian tradition that the ultimate point of despair, the ultimate point of denigration of the individual, the ultimate depth of his fall, is when the human soul cannot even pray. It is not when we are sick, it is not when we are unable to eat. That moment of utter despair from which perhaps no redemption is possible is the moment when a man finds, or a woman finds, that even prayer becomes impossible. I don't know how many of us are still able to pray faithfully with prayerful heart, with devotion, with belief in what we are praying, to whom we are praying. It has become another mumble-jumble ritualism, like so many of our mantras in the Hindu Brahmin tradition.

We say our prayer, "Oh Master, Thou art the real goal of human life." What is the next sentence? Ah, yes, "We are yet but slaves of wishes." Sometimes I am even tempted to think that the repetition of the prayer itself perhaps reimposes in us our slavery to wishes, by our repeating the line 'we are yet but slaves of wishes,' 'we are yet but slaves of wishes.' I am afraid of saying this because some people might think that I have intentions of changing this prayer. I am accused of changing so many things. But there is a psychological theory which says that the more you repeat a thing, the more you tend to become that. 'I am a pig, I am a pig, I am a pig'–then I become a pig. So, there is a certain psychological benefit in thinking we are already that which we should become and trying to make our way towards it. But there is also certain insanity attached to the way in which we are behaving, in believing we are that which we have to become and, therefore, we can act as we choose.

In our country this is the example set by the religious heads, by the political heads, by the heads of institutions, by the leaders of the industries, by those with money, that they believe, and have always believed, that the right of office, the right of possession of wealth, etc., become absolute rights and they can do as they like. "The king can do no wrong." But they do not remember that when they say that the king can do no wrong, it was an admonition that "if you are a king, my dear friend, you can do no wrong; please behave." Instead it has been interpreted to mean something very convenient for them that whatever they do, cannot be wrong. On the contrary, it should mean, "You can do nothing except what is right". It is unfortunate that even Master had to teach us that the freedom is only to do the right, the freedom to do the right alone is the freedom. There is no other freedom. Freedom to do a wrong thing doesn't exist. How can a man have freedom to do what is wrong? But today freedom is mixed up. The concept of freedom is totally misunderstood. East, West, North, South, wherever you go it is the same problem, that "if I am free I can do what I like. I am a free individual. Have I no right to do what I feel?" So instead of being a Sahaj Marg problem, instead of being a Hindu problem, instead of being an Indian problem, we see now it has achieved a global dimension.

Today, it is not so much a crisis of the mob or the crisis of the forthcoming–God forbid–third world war, as it is the crisis of character. And of course, the only satisfaction that people like me, who are unable to do anything in this matter, can achieve is to say that "Rome is not built in a day." But yet, all theories of change suggest that the change must come at one instant instead of ten. One doesn't progressively tell more and more truths: "Yesterday I told ninety-nine lies, today I tell ninety-eight lies, tomorrow I will tell ninety-seven lies"–we don't become masters of truth like that. The master of truth is the man who turns from lie to truth at one instant, from immorality to morality at one instant.

So how is this change going to be brought about, how is this transformation of character (which is today the basic ingredient of our life, individual, total or public) going to be brought about? Forget spirituality. I would rather prefer, like Swami Vivekananda said, "Let us have men first, people who have morality, people who have integrity, people who have faith, let them not be spiritual at all." What we need is men who have faith, even if they haven't produced a single thing which is worthwhile.

Our brother quoted Master who said, "Let us leave the world at least as we found it, if we can't better it." But the fundamental axiom or the fundamental advice should be, "Let us not die worse than we came into this world." I may not be born a saint. But let me not die a worse sinner than what I was when I came into this world. Let me not go on the path of downward degradation, ever tending further downwards, in the fond hope that every curve has to reach a trough and then come up again. Some people have this mistaken belief in a mechanical law that anything which goes downwards must come up, and anything which goes up must come down by itself. Well, any immaterial object, a thing which has no life, if you throw up, it will come down eventually. But that is only applicable to non-living matter. A living individual is supposed to condition his existence by his own volition and by his own will power using his intellect, judging what is good for himself, teaching and being taught, developing and helping others to develop, growing and helping others to grow. Instead of that, we are all now embracing each other in a mutual drama of each one deceiving the other, each one corrupting the other, each one cutting the throat of the other.

In today's life, you will find those who are praised to the skies are those who have a lot of money amassed, the rich people. You know, no rich man ever pays for anything he acquires. He goes into the best dance hall and he gets into the first row and the first row is always reserved for people like that; because his reservation is not got by paying Rs. 20/- for the seat but by buying a seat for eternity by giving Rs. 2,000/- life donation. They are very clever people. You know, he says, "If I go twenty times a year to that seat it is a matter of Rs. 400/-, at Rs. 20/- a seat." Similarly in other sabhas; and he compounds all these and he says, "What is the principle involved, how much interest have I taken. Give that as donation. That interest will take care of all these things." You buy your power, you buy your way to your office, even in spirituality people had been seeking to buy their way into the heart of the Master. You all know it. Many have commented that rich people came into the Mission and spoilt it. They are not rich people but poor people. When I say poor people, I mean the poor rich fellows; they come really hoping that in some way Master will remove their burden of guilt, their burden of sorrows at all the ways they have used to acquire the wealth, and in an endeavour to compensate for all that to mitigate the powers of evil they have created within themselves, they make a huge offering of cash donation. They didn't come with the intention of corrupting the institution or the Master.

We also have, on the other hand, the ordinary individual who gives Rs. 2/- and he expects in return liberation, realisation. You know it is a peculiar invertendo that a man who gives a million dollars does not expect anything from you except a pardon for the sins he has committed. Whereas the so-called good individual, who thinks he is moral and who thinks he is ethical, goes and gives Rs. 2/- and expects to be liberated from all bondages.

So I am really, you know, in a quandary as to the principles, because more than what my Master has given us, I don't think any human individual can codify or give rules for conduct; they are so simple to be followed. What more can be asked of the Master? You know in tasteless food the only missing ingredient is often a pinch of salt; everything has been prepared perfectly. Here, what is the missing ingredient? Our willingness, our acceptance of the fact that we have to change.

Transformation means total transformation. It doesn't mean only the inner transformation. This is a very convenient way of interpreting transformation, by saying that if the inside is transformed, it is good enough. The outside need not conform to it. Inside transformation benefits us. Outside transformation may perhaps not benefit us, which is a lurking fear in us. You see, we don't want to be straight, we don't want to be moral, we don't want to be above corruption, because we are afraid we may lose our income, we may lose our position in society.

When Master has assured inner transformation, and in his benign grace he is prepared to forgive our sins of commission and omission, day after day, why on earth should I be moral? Why on earth should I not be corrupt? This is the question each man is asking himself and finds a very convenient answer in saying, "Yes, my dear friend, go on. Babuji is ever forgiving." Therefore all these eulogizing on the public platform ... it is not you, who the speaker is trying to convince. He is trying to convince himself that the immense grace of the Master, His immense generosity, His immense forgivingness, will apply to himself because he is speaking about him in public–it is as though he says "Master, please listen to me. Don't forget me when the time comes to forgive me."

So you see, it is not that we are not aware of all the needs, the need to be straight, the need to be honest. It is not that we are not aware; it is that we hope that in some way our spiritual future having been assured, our next life having been blessed by him, let us enjoy the fruits of this life to the fullest possible extent, and beg forgiveness from him when we next go to Shahjahanpur. In some mysterious fashion, we have transported the Christian confessional into Sahaj Marg–where every Friday you know, the Catholic goes to the priest and, separated by the barrier, he confesses. And the Father says, "In the name of the Father, the Son and the Holy Ghost, I absolve you." That is that. Let us no longer live in this fool's paradise. This is because now Babuji has become merged with Lalaji and Lalaji has been a total disciplinarian, who was bold enough to write that however high a man may have reached in spirituality, whatever elevation he may have achieved, even to the highest possible extent, if he was immoral, even the breath of spirituality has not touched him. That is the statement of the Grand Master. Today when Babuji is no longer in that beautiful, compassionate, soft form of his, when he has no longer the individuality, the individual right of action to forgive us–I dare say that sort of forgiveness has gone with 19th of April 1983. I personally don't expect that in any way he can now help us. Because his mind, as somebody said yesterday, is now the total Divine mind.

If you will remember, often I have said that a guru comes only so that he has a heart and he can have compassion towards us, he could be merciful towards us. He can say "Well, you are what you are, you cannot help it and if you are still what you are, it is my fault." Babuji always used to say, "It is my fault that you are not being transformed; it is my fault that you are not grateful." In some way India has produced such giants–political people like Gandhi, who fasted for other people's errors; and spiritual people like Vivekananda, our Master, who take the blame for all that happens in the universe upon themselves. But it should not be something over which we gloat, over which we rejoice and happily go our way thinking that they are doing this for us, why on earth should we do it for ourselves now. You will carry a baby in your hand till it is able to walk. When it is able to walk, if it insists on being carried, don't you spank it?

And Babuji has written to one preceptor as long ago as 1958 that "it is my fault and I am to be blamed, that I did not have a stick in my hand. If I did not have a stick, it should at least have been a stick of flowers, so that you would have appreciated that I have something in my hand to punish with. Therefore, your temper is in this state in which it is seen today." This was written in 1958. I have a copy of that letter. Even in 1968 Master appreciated the fact that without a stick in the hand, it is going to be very difficult to control this growing organization. It was his immense mercy that he chose never to have a stick in his hand. But he perhaps didn't have it because we were children. But when we grow up, he expects us to develop a certain sense of responsibility to the organization, to ourselves, to the Master. A child of three can take a ten rupee note and put it in the fire playfully, not knowing the difference between the ordinary paper and the currency note. But if a boy of twenty puts a ten rupee note into the *chula*, what will you do with him?

So Master expected of us that we would grow out of that childish innocence and become responsible adults to whom the Mission could be entrusted, to whom their personal spiritual growth could be entrusted, to whom the transformation of the external self could be entrusted, because Babuji said, "The inner change I can bring about. The outer is your responsibility." He never undertook the responsibility for the outer change. He said, "Behaviour you have to correct; morals and ethics you have to develop. This is your work upon yourself; you know what to do. There is nothing difficult about it."

Changing the inner, nobody else can do; it needs a Master. If I expect my Master to come and shave my face every morning, is it right? Oh! He is all embracing, all loving, you know, he was prepared even to press the feet of Parthasarathi, why not shave him? My Master would have done it if I had asked him. I am sure of it because such was his nature. Such was the unbounded lowliness that he thrust upon himself. He might have done that, too. But is it right of us to ask that I should be taught to tell the truth, when I know how to tell the truth? Have I to be taught to stay away from other man's goods and properties, when I know it is wrong and not proper? These are not the things which we need to be taught. These are not the things in which we have to be trained. We all know how to do it. We still persist in not doing it because we have decided not to do it.

So, today I have no doubt in proclaiming before you all that if we are indisciplined, it is not because of ignorance, it is out of wilfulness, out of wilful disregard for the principles and practices the Master has preached to us. I make bold to say that he left twenty-five years in advance of his own sake instead of in 2006 or 2007, perhaps because of utter disgust, at himself, at his work, at the success of his work of what he has produced amongst ourselves, and said, "Well, let me take this course. If they have any sense, let them try to develop." So, when we are wilfully bound upon a certain course of action, of thought, of speech, no power on earth can change us because it is our will which is being applied. And in the spiritual field the more we progress the stronger our will becomes, and therefore we have this very unfortunate phenomenon that as we are growing, we are becoming more indisciplined, because the will power is being ever strengthened in operating more in the direction of retrogradeness, away from the principles and practices of Sahaj Marg. We are producing more and more indiscipline, more and more immorality, more and more of all these things. It is precisely because the will is being strengthened, our ideas are not being strengthened, our desire is not being strengthened in the right direction. So we are growing with this increased will power in the same way and I can only assert that if we don't change our direction and use the will to turn the direction itself in the right way, this organization, the abhyasis of this organization, are becoming or rather going to become progressively more indisciplined. There is no doubt about it. Because it is after all the Master's work. It is another manifestation of his work that the good he did for us in developing our will power is being turned against ourselves in indiscipline, in wrong activity, and we are destroying ourselves.

So ultimately who is to blame? It is the individual. The Master has no hand in this. The Master did everything. It is like you give your knife to the son and he commits suicide. In Master's own family there was this example. He had a gun in his house and one of his sons committed suicide. So it is wrong to put instruments into hands of those people who have not been trained in the use of that instrument.

But unfortunately in the Sahaj Marg system there never was and I presume there never will be, the corrective apparatus, because Master had immense faith that ultimately human beings will correct themselves. Some wisdom will dawn and we should leave it to them to accept the teaching, to follow the teaching, to practise the teaching and make themselves what he wanted them to be. He never believed in corrective apparatus. He never believed in enforced discipline. So that is the inheritance that we have derived from him that we have to continue this organization without a corrective apparatus, without externally imposed disciplinary measures, and yet pray that somehow we will all become what he wanted us to become.

I can only entreat you on this occasion, to at least start praying for it, sincerely pray for it, so that, in the not very distant future, we shall be an organization, we shall be an assembly of abhyasis of whom we can be proud and say, well at least this is what Master wanted us to become, that we are seeing before our eyes.

Thank you.

Change And Discipline

It is said that "Out of chaos cometh forth order!" In fact quite a few philosophies seem to believe that without chaos, there can be no order at all! In the system of sadhana given to the world by my Master, Samarth Guru Mahatma Shri Ram Chandraji Maharaj of Shahjahanpur, the need for chaos does not find any place. What does find a place in his system, the Sahaj Marg philosophy, is the need for bringing about change: change in the individual; in society; in customs and manners, and thus in life itself.

Where Nature brings about change, it has to resort to such means as are not considered necessary when a Master brings it about. Nature has to use means which may appear to us as being violent and destructive. A Master brings about global change by coaxing it out of the human heart. It is only when coaxing fails that other means may have to be adopted, or resorted to.

How does a Master coax human beings? He coaxes them by his Divine love, and by the offer of his unlimited services in their self-development to the highest possible level where they can become perfect human beings–which is only another way of saying that they have become divinised. This level of human development is what he offers us in return for our co-operation. Co-operation in what? It is precisely this question which we have to understand. Its import is so weighty that, as Master used to tell me, the presence of this co-operation can light up the world, and make it a place of divine harmony, peace and love, so that human existence becomes one of bliss, whereas its absence, the lack of co-operation can condemn life on this world to levels worse than that of hell itself!

What does this really mean? It means that when we accede to his wishes, and are willing to be coaxed by him to fall in line with

Message delivered on Basant Panchami Celebrations at Madras, 26 January 1985.

the scheme of self-development that he so lovingly offers us, we are really participating in a larger venture, the supreme magnitude of which we can scarcely begin to even imagine.

And what is this larger scheme in which he is interested? It is nothing other than the bringing about of change: change in individuals, then through them change in society, then in the world at large, covering eventually all humanity! The Master works thus for bringing about change on a global scale, culminating perhaps in change of such magnitude that we can never hope to even conceive of the various dimensions that such change can embrace. This, then, is his scheme.

What is our part in it? Our part in it can be covered by just one word–co-operation! But little do we realise what this single word really demands of us. It is only as we march on that we realise that this co-operation is really an all-embracing thing. We realise that no single facet of our existence can be kept apart from this co-operation. Many imagine that co-operation applies to the spiritual life only. They imagine that it applies only to the practice of the method of meditation taught by the Master. But please think over this. Can we be obedient in one aspect of life without being obedient in all the other aspects of our lives? Can we fragment our lives into bits and pieces, and claim that co-operation can apply to only one or two of them? This tragic mistake is made by most of the abhyasis who discover, as they go on, that this word 'co-operation' brooks no dismemberment. It is all, or nothing!

What is it that can make such a totality of co-operation possible? It is discipline! Discipline alone can make it possible for us to extend to him the total co-operation that he needs to make us what he wishes us to be–and then through us to bring about the vaster changes which he wishes to bring about. Discipline is the key to co-operation. Where there is no discipline, there can be no co-operation either. The two may be thought of as two sides of the same coin, as it were. It would appear as if it mattered little which way the coin falls. It would appear as if it made little difference whether we began with one of them or the other. The only difference seems to be that when we begin with co-operation, discipline begins to become established rather late, if at all. Whereas, when we begin with discipline, co-operation follows immediately of its own accord, naturally.

What is the value of discipline? It is precisely by being disciplined that without even knowing what co-operation implies, or what it even means, we are able to follow each and every wish of the Master, and to act strictly according to his instructions. That is, by being disciplined, obedience follows naturally, and makes the very thing that he wants in us establish itself without our even being aware of it. I am of course referring to co-operation!

In the other way, when we try to begin with co-operation, we are bewildered because we do not know in which area of our lives we are required to co-operate. We run the risk of making the mistake that we are at liberty to choose the areas in which we are required to co-operate, and then find out, often to our annoyance, that it was total co-operation, embracing each and every facet of our existence, that was necessary -- and that too, right from the beginning! This danger is not faced by one who is disciplined, and who is willing to obey the Master in everything, without dissecting his life into parts, and thinking that obedience is necessary only in some parts. Discipline needs no thought. Discipline needs no understanding. Discipline needs no explanation. Therefore, it is possible for all humans to be disciplined. But the very word 'discipline' seems to evoke feelings of abhorrence, implying–as it seems to do to some persons–some sort of slavery into which they will be ensnared. Can anything be farther from the truth? No. Can there be anything which can lead to one's evolution so easily and so quickly? No! A disciplined person can achieve the goal of human development most easily and most speedily. My Master defined a disciple as one who is disciplined!

We see before us the levels of degradation to which this idea of a fragmented obedience of the Master's wishes has brought us all. Such a situation has arisen only because discipline is lacking. Some persons think that they are at liberty to obey whatever they want to obey, and to ignore–or even to oppose!–the rest of his wishes. Instead of bringing about a world of harmony and peace, such misguided action is creating chaos out of prior order. This is a reversal of Master's and Nature's design. In fact, it is reversing the trend of Master's work, and giving his teachings the go-by, trying to reverse the course of events, thus negating His plans.

It is not necessary to speculate whether such efforts of undisciplined individuals can ever alter the course of events–let alone reversing them–which Master has planned for. What is important to think about is what is going to happen to the development of such misguided individuals who, out of ignorance, selfishness, or greed for other things than self-development, think that they can possibly change his will. This is what we must brood over. It concerns each and every one of us. **Do we wish to follow him upon the noble and Divine path of self-development, or do we desire to remain here, earth-bound, stagnating in this miserable existence, because of our lust for power and material advancement?** This is the question that we must ask ourselves.

His plans can never fail, because they are plans divinely ordained. Then whose will be the failure if we are undisciplined? Failure and stagnation will be the unfortunate lot of all those who, because of lack of discipline, of obedience, oppose His Will. Failure will be the share of one who seeks to impose chaos upon the state of order that he has so painstakingly created. Instead of co-operating in bringing about order out of chaos, such persons are destroying order and bringing back chaos. They are negating his wishes, and trying to negate the plans of Nature. Can they ever succeed? No!

This then, is where indiscipline leads us to. Our indiscipline can never affect his work. Our lack of co-operation can never alter his design for bringing about change. All that our indiscipline can possibly achieve–if it can be called achievement–is our own stagnation and possible fall from the levels that he has so benevolently blessed us with. Life will pass us by, leaving us grasping the toys and dolls of lesser aspiration, while those who co-operate in the magnificent venture of participating in change, will follow Him into eternity.

It is the imperative need of the hour that we understand the need for discipline, and to correct our attitude and action to ensure that the train does not go off the rails. On this auspicious occasion may He bless all with the necessary understanding and courage to follow Him with faith and fortitude.

As Above, So Below

An ancient maxim has been handed down from generation to generation; and its origin appears to be lost in the hoary past. It says, "As above, so below!" Somewhat in tune with this idea, we have another tradition from one of the great religions of the world, which says, "God made man in His own image!" These once formed the topic of discussion with my Master, Samarth Guru Mahatma Shri Ram Chandraji Maharaj of Shahjahanpur. And he cautioned me that the meaning commonly attributed to them could lead an aspirant astray, by lulling the mind into a sense of false security. He warned me that since they seem to imply that a human being is already what he ought to be, the common man may fail to take any steps for his growth. He emphasized that these two maxims have made many persons assume that they have already achieved everything that there is to be achieved, and because such an assumption is totally false, the danger lay precisely in that assumption! "Has not God made man in His own image?" they ask. "Then what is there that yet remains for us to do? He has made us as Himself." In this fashion do many persons delude themselves, and the questioner remains what he was, without even the possibility of rising to higher levels until he understands the meaning of such statements correctly.

My Master warned me, "A sense of achievement puts a bar to advancement. The person automatically stops making any efforts, and in this lies the greatest danger to one's progress." A sense of achievement or accomplishment breeds a sense of complacency in our minds, and thus puts a stop to all further effort and to progress.

What then is the truth behind the above statements handed down to us by the mystic and occult traditions of the past? Do they represent statements of fact or not? Are the statements to be taken as

Message delivered on 9 February 1985, Lucknow celebration.

eternal verities? Do they, in fact, mean what human beings of all ages have assumed them to mean, or is the meaning attributed to them merely wishful thinking on our part?

My Master was never tired of saying, "The truth is revealed to him who seeks it." It is, therefore, very clear that we have to seek out the truth, instead of passively accepting what has been said. Age alone does not confer any special merit on anything. Nor do ancient statements have to be accepted as true only because they are ancient. Their truth has to be tested again and again, generation after generation, by a fresh school of aspirants. The touchstone is the testing procedure, which alone can affirm the truth again and again. According to my Master, many things repeated in this fashion, century after century, and believed to be absolute truths, have been found to be of questionable value. If we are interested in our spiritual progress, we have to strive to realise the truth by trying to achieve, or attain, a state of being akin to what these famous and oft-repeated statements of the past say. In other words, we have to practise some method which can possibly reveal to us the truth in our own selves by creating the condition in us which alone can give us the true experience of that condition. There is no other way. This is what my Master has taught me.

In the tradition of this country, there is a famous statement which makes its earliest appearance in the Rig-Veda. It later reappears in the Katha Upanishad. It says that the immortal fig tree, representing Brahman, has its roots above, and its leaves and branches below. The Bhagavad Gita repeats this same thing in a slightly modified version. In discussion with my Master, this quotation was once the topic. Master pointed out to me that this oft-repeated, but little understood couplet gives the hint to the truth. My Master very kindly explained to me that this imagery of the fig tree, inverted in space, really shows that all things below, all life below, should draw their sustenance directly from above. If they do, so then they acquire the possibility of becoming like that which is above–the Ultimate itself!

What does 'sustenance' mean? We normally associate it with the needs of the physical body, such as food, drink, clothing, etc.

Some may be tempted to ask, "We need food and water. How can it come from above? Do we not have to strive hard to fulfil our needs of life here?" But in times of acute distress or suffering, we turn naturally to prayer, thus answering the question ourselves! We also need emotional sustenance in the form of affection and love. For the fulfilment of this need we tend to look to our friends and relatives. Here, again, some are tempted to ask, "Can God love us? Can He be affectionate towards us? He may bless us with all that we need. He may even be merciful enough to grant our prayers, but can He love us?" Such persons may even believe in one tiny corner of their heart that "God is Love"! But that He can love us, perhaps very few would be willing to believe.

In seeking for love and affection from fellow humans, many have lost sight of the true goal of human life. The desire to love, and to be loved, would appear to be far stronger than the desire for the material things and pleasure of life. In this lies the real danger in seeking for it below. Even advanced souls have not escaped from this emotional trap. In their desire for love and attention when they diverted their gaze from Him, above, to fellow humans down here, they suffered the consequences of their folly.

Many have a need, as they imagine, for money or power or position. For all these things they look below and the consequences are tragic. We delude ourselves with the idea of greatness, or power, or position, and remain here as merely human beings with the lowest of aspirations, searching for them in lowest of planes of existence.

My Master teaches: It is He, and He alone, the Master of calibre, who can grant us what we need to cross this ocean of human existence and reach the other shore safely. Therefore, it is wisdom to look to Him, and to Him alone for our needs. Our wants lead us astray. We have to distinguish between 'needs' and 'wants'. He provides our needs. We have to give up our desires which must be abandoned in our aspiration for the higher life, in our progress towards the goal.

Our experience teaches us that the desire to be loved, to be wanted, is perhaps the greatest pitfall on the path of the aspirant.

Alas! How many have tumbled and fallen because of this desire! Even advanced souls are not immune to this danger. The higher we rise, the greater the fall, and the greater the disaster. From such a fall very few are able to rise again, and for that, too, the merciful Master has to help us by pulling us up once again. My Master once very graciously elucidated this point for me. He said, "Human love has tremendous potential, but it fails because of being misdirected. Love is the greatest force. It must be humbly offered up to Him who alone is its true object–God or Master whichever you may like to call Him. You must love Him in such a way that your love knocks on the door of His heart, telling Him that the lover is waiting outside. Then He begins to love you, and when this happens, all your problems of life are solved! Love Him who loves all." This is the greatest revelation of my Divine Master.

Thanks to my beloved Master, we now begin to understand that things below are not already as It is above. But they can be as It is above, provided that the sustenance for our existence is drawn from above. Our existence, and the needs of that existence must all be derived from the source of all existence–from Him who is portrayed as being 'above'–the Divine in human form, none other than the beloved Master Himself. What can we get from here below? Food and drink? Perhaps! Clothing? Perhaps! Why perhaps? Because sometimes it may happen that a situation arises when even the breath becomes impossible without His providing the air for us to breathe. Then we realise that in our foolishness we had imagined that we could get our needs fulfilled independent of Him. Then dawns the realisation that without His sanction, even the air we breathe cannot be had. But if we look to Him for everything, then we not only have all that He is waiting to shower upon us, but because He is now sustaining us, the way opens for us to become like Him.

According to my Master, what these *mahavakyas* (as they can perhaps be called, though not in the Vedic sense of the word) really say is that a human being can aspire to become That which is the Ultimate, provided he looks only to Him for his every breath, and for his every need, for his brief existence in this world. This is what they really mean.

Discussing this idea of sustenance again: it is possible to have as many meanings for this word as there are levels of existence, levels of being. At the lowest level, it means that we should think that everything that we need in this mortal existence is coming from Him, the Divine Master. At a higher level, everything that we possess appears to us as if they are really all His possessions, the use of which is granted to us for our survival. At the next stage, the feeling arises that they are left in our charge, to be looked after by us in the role of trustees. Everything is His; we are merely trustees charged with the responsibility of looking after them meticulously and scrupulously, in the serene knowledge that one day we shall have to render account to Him. The idea of possession has left us.

At the next higher stage, even the idea of trusteeship seems to vanish. Why does it vanish? Because the very idea of doer-ship associated with the act of preserving or looking after something now bids good-bye. The idea that we do anything, or that we have the capacity to do anything, now vanishes from our mind. We are now in a state, or condition, where we have no consciousness of having anything, nor of doing anything. Yet the idea of duty remains. And this stage really seems to display all the signs of the beginning of spirituality because, while the sense of duty yet lingers on in our minds, the idea that we have to perform the duty no longer exists in our minds. The marvellous truth that we begin to perceive is that even for the proper performance of our duty we have to look up to Him for help and guidance. In fact, the stage develops into the next one by itself where we experience Him as the performer of our duty, and not ourselves.

What can be the condition of such a person at the next higher stage with which his Master is waiting to bless him? Is it possible to have a peep into it? My Master very graciously answers this question for our benefit. Master says that at the next higher stage, the devotee, having lost the sense of possession, of independent action, of action itself, and finally of the sense of duty too, now begins to lose the idea that he exists independently of Him, the

Beloved! The physical body is perceived as being His. The means for its maintenance are very graciously and lovingly provided by Him. What we thought of as being our duty is perceived to be allotted by Him. The fulfilment of the duty is also seen to be His work, and His alone. Having realised all this stage by stage, how is it possible for us to continue to have the idea of an existence which is separate from His Divine existence? So this idea, too, now bids good-bye. My Master told me that when an abhyasi, a true devotee of the Master, comes up to this level by His grace, the idea of his individual, separate existence begins to leave him. It is an indication that the next higher existence is now being conferred upon him by the Master. It is by the grace of the Almighty and Benevolent Master alone that such progress towards the goal becomes possible.

We may venture to state that only at this stage of one's spiritual progress does one begin to realise that the famous statements quoted earlier are really promises held out to mankind of what can be possible, and not statements of facts already established in the life of human beings. They are promises of what can be achieved if one adopts the proper course of life, and devotes one's time and effort to the achievement of the goal. It is very important to realise the truth of this statement, as otherwise we are liable to be misled into thinking that we are already that which we have to become!

The ancient mystics and seers intuitively perceived that human beings have to grow and evolve. This idea of growth was linked to the idea of the goal to be achieved. Then the third thing was attached to these two. What was it? It was of course the human individual. This conjoining of the three, the individual, his goal, and the process of becoming which alone could enable him to achieve the goal, was put into the beautifully condensed form: As above, so below! It was a promise that things below, life below, can be as they are above, provided we take the trouble, and make the necessary effort, to develop and establish such a state of being in ourselves.

What happens then? At this highest level, the devotee finds that there is no longer anything that can be called 'lower' or 'higher'.

All is one grand, Divine existence by the Master, for the Master, and in the Master. The devotee, the way and the Master have all become one!!

My beloved and Divine Master has shown us by his own life that such an existence is possible. In achieving the highest state, he also mastered the way, and thus is able to guide us there himself. He adopted the human form out of his divine compassion and mercy for mankind, to show us a simple and effective method for us to reach our goal–H I M! By achieving the goal in his own lifetime, he has proved to every one of us that we too can similarly achieve it in our own lifetimes. His life was nothing but an existence assumed by him to set an example for us to emulate.

I offer my humble gratitude to my Divine Master who came down to us only to lift us up to Himself. May He live forever in the hearts of all mankind!

Evolution, I

We are coming to the close of our morning session.

Brother Sarnadji, Secretary of this Mission, a scholar in his own right, one of the divine products of my Master's spiritual wonder, a man with full and onerous responsibilities, has humbly effaced himself without mentioning the fact that all the books in Kannada have come from his pen, having been translated by him. All this he has not mentioned, and rightfully so, because the jewel shining on the heart of the Lord reflects the greatness of the Almighty, not of itself. He has given us a beautiful exposition of what Sahaj Marg is, what Master's work is, the books that the Master wrote, the *paddhati*, and what it can achieve for us.

My respected sister Kasturiji, in her exposition, also dwelt on what Sahaj Marg is, some of her intimate associations with Master, intimate experiences, the value of the experience, how experiences indicate progress, *anubhav*, growth and so on. And our younger brother Kannan talked about change, and the need for change as reflecting growth and progress.

Now I have to just emphasize one point. That is, while change seems to be inevitable and is a direct indicator of growth, there comes a stage where any change can be arrested; it cannot be altogether stopped. It can be arrested, wilfully, by us. Because we find in Nature that change goes on and on. Planets go on rotating in their orbits. The sun goes on shining. The moon goes on reflecting the sun. And if there is a break in any of these systems that we see in this enormous marvellous universe outside, that would instantly put a stop to all life.

It seems as if God in His magnificent generosity, His mercy and in His desire to continue life, has been able to organize, to create and to set in motion an inanimate universe which obeys His laws impeccably, continuously, forever. The inanimate part of the universe is not a problem to the Almighty or to itself. No planet is worried for itself, it does not pray for food, it does not pray for clothing, it does not even pray for mercy; it goes about in its orbit, performing the Almighty's command, revolving around the sun and revolving around itself. If the process is stopped, perhaps even God cannot save us.

Then, we come to the animate part of the universe. There also we find that there are plants and animals–what we think in our own egoistic way (because the human being thinks that he is the culmination of the process of evolution) in our arrogance, in our egoism, we look down upon plant life and animal life, even mineral life–as something below us, something low, forgetting that they also obey God's commandments, they also obey God's laws; no change is arrested. They continue to grow.

The seed falls on the ground, it germinates, becomes a sapling, a tree, and it gives thousands of itself. Not one of you here would sow a seed if you are going to get back only one seed. I would like to imagine an agriculturist who plants one grain of rice (paddy) to get back only one grain of paddy again, or a businessman who invests one rupee in business to get back that one rupee in business; or the poultry people who keep a chicken only to get another egg out of it. The law of Nature is impeccable. It says, "Multiply." If you are only going to grow and die after fulfilling your own selfish desires, needs, wants, cravings, and all that you are going to return unto Him is what He put into you–"a handful of mud"–mud thou shalt remain. So the law of Nature is, my dear friends: growth has to be there, evolution has to be there; not because I choose it or you choose it, but because God wills it to be so. God did not create anything in this universe which just produced itself and satisfied itself, and died and said: "Almighty Lord, thank you for sustenance. I was born happy, I die happy, and you gave me life, I return this life to you." God will say, "Fie, is this for what I created you?"

In the Christian tradition there is a beautiful parable–a man and his three sons. He decided to go away as a test for his children.

He gave them one talent each, and said, "When I return I shall hold you accountable for this talent." He came back after twenty years. The eldest was a meek fellow, without any enterprise, but conscious of some sense of duty; he buried it under a tree. When father returned, he dug it out and returned it to his father and said, "Father, I return to you the one talent." The second son lent it out. When the father came back, instead of one, he was able to return two hundred. It had multiplied. The third son had invested it wisely in much business, and when the father asked him for his talent, he said, "Father, I cannot return it to you, but everything that you will see around is that–that talent. It has grown manifold, changing the environment–it is your talent." And the father said, "You have done wisely, you have used it wisely, all the talents are yours."

So, when we talk of spirituality, very often we talk of craving, we talk of need, we talk of want, as if we had any choice whether we will grow or not. This very idea of choice, whether we can participate "in my growth, in my evolution" implies that I also have the choice of not participating in it. This, to my mind, is the most foolish concept that yogic literature and religious literature have placed before us. Because I would like to tell you that we have no choice at all. Nothing which does not evolve continues to exist; it decays and dies. Those of you who are familiar with science know that there were multiple forms of existence in this world, even in this tiny world of ours–which having lost the mainstream of evolution, fell by the wayside and ceased to exist. So, that which does not obey the laws of evolution ceases to exist; it has no place, no existence, no right to exist. We blindly imagine that everyone has a right to exist; yes, so long as we obey the purpose behind that right, so long as we obey the purpose that God ordained when He created us. If we go against it, the right is liable to be withdrawn. Fortunately for us, we are never aware of it, because we go into oblivion from which there is no return. It is said in the literature that when you obey His laws you reach a situation from which there is no return! But on the other side also there is another *dhaama*, which is not *paramdhaama*; where we are eternally oblivious of the punishment that is given out to us, where we are condemned to an eternity of grossness, of darkness, of misery. Fortunately God in His mercy does not give us the consciousness to be aware of it!

So, why I am stressing this point is to tell you that: "If any human being thinks he has a choice in his personal evolution, let him think over it a hundred times." Like your child cannot say, "Papa, I don't wish to grow. Let me remain three years old." You have no choice in the matter of growth, in the internal dimensions of spiritual growth. Your child cannot say, "I don't want education. I am happy as I am. Mother gives me sweets. You bring me presents. Everybody who comes into the house loves me, adores me, kisses me, pets me. Let me remain ever a child." You will say, "My dear son, this is not for which you were born. Look at the next door man. Look at Maruthi, look at Vikram. Yesterday they were children, today they are riding bicycles, in two years they will be riding Lunas (mopeds), and then they will be on the job, they will get married. Don't you want to be like them?" "No, no papa, I am happy as I am. This blissful state of childhood where will I get?" But as adults, we wish to remain foolish, we wish to remain arrogant, we wish to remain selfish, self-indulgent, attached to pleasures, attached to gratification of the senses, hoping that God will permit us to continue to enjoy our existence, at our will, not His Will, and we have a separate existence, and that we need not participate in our evolution.

I stress the word 'participation' because I deny that a human being has any possibility of growth by himself. Given the samskaras, given the awful burden of samskaras that we have brought with us, it is like expecting a stone to do something by itself. We are as immovable, as incapable of self-motion or movement as a stone is today, because our inner samskara is so awful in its gross tendencies, that any individual who thinks that he is free to do as he chooses, is blind. If he thinks he is moving, if he thinks he is speaking, if he thinks he is acting, yes–he is acting like a locomotive under the power of steam–our steam being the compulsion of the samskaras that are in us, which makes one become a scholar, he doesn't know why he becomes a scholar; another becomes an artist, he doesn't know why he becomes an artist; another becomes a doctor, he also doesn't know why. A man who becomes something and doesn't know why he became that, is under a compulsive existence. He is under the pressure of compulsive forces locked up in him—no better than a steam locomotive which goes on and on until the steam pressure is exhausted, and it can move us no more. But when the Almighty is given a seat in the heart, and the cleaning takes place and the samskaric burden is removed, the first traces of freedom begin. We can now take a positive hand in guiding our own evolution, we get into the mainstream of evolutionary existence, which God's will dominates, which His purpose guides, and the Destination which is Himself, is there. This is the aspect that I want to emphasize before you, that if anyone should think he has an opportunity—yes; if he has a choice—no. Never has it existed, never shall it exist, that I have a choice to stop my evolution.

But, I repeat, there are times when we can arrest that evolution, like keeping a packet of seeds locked up in a drawer for ten years. And you can say, "I am the master of the situation, because this seed cannot, dare not, mature and become a plant. This much I can do. I can do it not only to a packet of seeds, I can do it to myself." You can say, "What is this power of the Lord that you people are speaking about? He is the Ultimate, He is the Infinite. He has no power over me. I am the same fool, the same arrogant, prideful, lusty individual that I was, and He cannot change me." Then we find out, sometimes too late, that if He wishes to do it, like a stone cutter breaking open a stone, He can do it at the cost of our lives—I mean the temporal life here. But the yogic Masters however are not so unkind. Therefore, the concept is not of *videha mukti* but *sadeha mukti*. It is a blessing for us, because the grace, the charity, the mercy that we attribute to God—which in the *para-rupa* He does not possess, that is what the Shastras say—He assumes when He descends to take the form of a guru and deals with us mercifully, lovingly, kindly, when He says, "Yes, you want to remain what you are and yet you want to become what I want you to become, *thathastu*. I will permit you to do it. You can still retain your human form, you can still retain your human tendencies, but let me refine them, let me divert them to the right goal, divert them to the right orientation." It is like turning a car. I don't interfere with its speed, I change the direction. So the guru comes precisely to give us the love and the service which the Ultimate cannot give us. Of this, there are some references in the Puranas. I need not bore you with them. Siva and Parvati try to help a *bhakta*. Vishnu in his Purana tries to help a bhakta. The bhakta is going ahead without taking any notice of the blessings that are being showered upon him in material form; he says, "These are all nonsense."

So all that I am trying to tell you is that evolution cannot be denied, evolution cannot be stopped. There is no such thing as progress. Ideas of progress and regress, of day and night, of advance and return, these have given us the wrong ideas, misunderstandings, that there is a possibility of going in two directions. Yes, temporarily. I am fond of giving the example of a wheel which is in motion. The whole wheel is going forward. But at the bottom-most point it is momentarily moving backwards (otherwise it will not rotate). But at that point, if that part of the wheel should think in its arrogance "I am moving backwards, how can the wheel move forwards?" It would be making the same mistake that human beings almost without exception are making–that they think they can stop evolution because they, with their tiny egos, tiny arrogances, tiny achievements, insignificant in this grand universe that we are facing–they also think that they can retard progress, that they can curb society, that they can take away Sita from Rama, things like that. History teaches us otherwise. Evolution teaches us otherwise. I can sit back, I cannot stop growth.

So, my prayer to you, friends, brothers and sisters, is–"Get into the mainstream. Remain in the mainstream of evolution. No choice is involved." I have just to give up 'myself' and float.

Evolution, II

Those who have heard the morning talk will recall that I said there is no choice in the matter of personal evolution. Only co-operation is there. All that we can do is to delay it a little here and there and suffer by the delay.

I gave the example of the packet of seeds, which you can keep without sowing even for years, and think we have prevented the course of Nature, but all that we achieve is to delay the process. What Nature cannot get from us by co-operation, it will somehow get by other ways. All those who have trained children, who have trained animals, know that there are two ways of training–the 'way of love' and the 'way of force'. The way of force is obnoxious, we don't like it. No parent likes to train his child by force. No animal trainer ever uses force–it is the way of love. Nature, too, does not use force on us.

It is a great misconception to think that God punishes or that God rewards. My Master has repeated over and over again that reward and punishment do not exist. Of course, religions have taught–it is not the speciality of any single religion–all religions have said again and again that good action is rewarded, bad action is punished. For virtue we go to heaven, for sins we go to hell. All these sorts of things are being propagated by religions. As my Master has said, the instruments of religion are sin and temptation. Religions have always tried to guide humanity into what the leaders of religion felt was the correct course of action, by tempting man with offers of heaven and salvation, and by trying to guide him with fears of hell and damnation. But Sahaj Marg, my Master's system, does not recognize the existence of either of these two. Man is not a child to be tempted or to be guided with fears. So, in every man and woman there reside childish tendencies and animal tendencies. So, if we suffer or if we enjoy, it is because our tendencies manifest, we behave like animals, perform animal-like actions, suffer the consequences of our own actions. There is no punishing agency. For the good tendencies, similarly we have good actions, feel self-satisfied, get the praise of our neighbours, of society, and feel consequently happy. We are rewarding ourselves. There is no God in heaven who is rewarding us or punishing us.

So, in Sahaj Marg these two things are absolutely unrecognized. Why? They don't exist first! We don't recognize the existence of virtue or vice. In Sahaj Marg the greatest teaching of the Master, which he says again and again, is: "Every thought that we think, every act that we indulge in, these leave impressions on our mind which subsequently form samskaras, and which guide our future actions and thoughts. So it is we who create our futures. If we suffer, it is because in the past we had acted in such a way, thought in such a way, that we have created certain samskaras which push us into certain tendencies, the consequences of which are inevitable."

So, my Master says: "From now you start moulding your thinking and your actions in such a way that you are able to live without the formation of impressions." A stage comes when we can think without forming impressions upon our minds, we can act without forming impressions. Because, one who is born, who is being born into this world, cannot live without thought and action.

This is one of the truths which is said by Lord Krishna in the Gita. He says, "Even I am not free of action, but the difference between you and me, Arjuna, is, whereas you are bound by action and thought and you are bound by the results of your actions, I am not bound either by my actions or the results of my actions." He does not explain why. He does not explain what is the difference that binds one and does not bind the other. That my Master has said. What the Lord does not reveal in the Gita, my Master has revealed, and has said, "It is precisely because a person can live without forming impressions that he has no more any sense of the future." Such a person can be said to live eternally in the present. The future is right in my present–or, if you like to think of it the other way, my present is in the future, both co-exist. I do not create anything for myself from such a moment.

So this is one of the greatest teachings of Sahaj Marg, that it liberates us—we are talking all the time of liberation—liberation from what? Liberation from myself, liberation from my thoughts, liberation from my actions, which have hitherto, through aeons of time, through many births and deaths, bound me to the slavery of my own self. I am the slave of myself, not of any God, not of Satan, not of hell, not of heaven. If anybody has imprisoned me, it is myself. If anybody is making me suffer, it is myself. This greatest truth, unrevealed hitherto—hinted at perhaps in Hindu literature but nowhere else—is that "Friend, you are your own salvation, or you are your own condemnation. Get rid of yourself, and there you are."

Many people ask us, somewhat naively, somewhat childishly, "Why do you want to participate in yoga abhyas? Why do you want to do meditation? Are you dissatisfied with life? Are you frightened of yourself? Are you frightened of the consequences of existence? Why are you seeking to escape?" I must tell you most emphatically that yoga is not a means of escape—from either this life or future life or anything. We are not escapists. If anybody thinks yoga is escapism, then they are equating yoga with things like drugs and drinks. We are not escapists. As I told you this morning, I wish to emphasize again, we are not participating in meditation and this process of Sahaj Marg to escape from life.

We are participating in it to make our life what it should really be—a Divine existence, free of temptations, free of problems, free of worries, free of sickness, all of which we have caused ourselves. Any child knows that if it eats something wrong or eats too much of something which may be very good, it suffers from its own misdeeds. Every drunkard knows that it is his drunkenness which is condemning him to headache, to liver problems, to cirrhosis, and ultimately, to death.

Do you mean to say that God has nothing better to do than to watch millions of humanity through aeons of time, looking at each one and seeing what he is doing and what she is doing, and then condemning us and punishing us? On the one side we say, "God is Love"! On the other side we say that He is condemning, He is punishing, and He is sending us to hell this way or to heaven this way. If you permit me to say it, if you pardon me for saying it, it is one of the most childish conceptions of God. And, unfortunately, no religion is free from it. All religions have been uttering this foolishness from the time man became conscious of himself. I cannot possibly conceive of a God who has no better business to do than to think of us, watch us, punish us, to condemn us and judge us! It is we who suffer, by our own actions, by our own thoughts.

Let this be clearly understood. If I am seeking to escape from anything, it is from the consequences of my own foolishness, of my own viciousness, of my own selfishness, knowing that these are the causes of my bondage, because they lead me into actions from the results of which I cannot escape. Once we indulge in a thought, action follows. Once action results from that thought, its result comes. Its result has its own consequence. It is a form of 'breeder reaction'. No external agency but myself is responsible for this. This is the most fundamental truth that we have got to recognize and understand. When we know the true import of this, it is no longer necessary to fear a God or approach a God in a slavish beggarly way, seeking benefits which He cannot give.

God does not want us either to demand from Him, or to slavishly beg of Him. Because, in His Ultimate mercy, charity, divine grace is flowing all the time everywhere. It is like praying to the sun, "Please give me illumination." Sitting in a dark room where we close the doors and windows, we pray to the Lord of the sun, "Oh Almighty Lord, bless me with sunshine!" Could the sun speak, it would only ask: "My dear boy, when did I ever stop shining? From the beginning of creation I am shining, and I am shining without prejudice. I know no caste, I know no colour, I do not know whether you are human or animal. I don't shine for you. I shine because it is my nature to shine." Similarly, God does not bless, knowing that He is blessing. If He were to do that, He is no better than a human being.

It is said in the great religions that, "Let not thy right hand know what thy left hand is doing." If that applies to man, human beings, how much more should it not apply to God Almighty Himself? Can He be ever conscious that He is punishing me, rewarding you, condemning her? Then, when God becomes conscious of what we in Hinduism call 'duality'–*dwandvas*–if He Himself is conscious of punishment, reward, sin and virtue, where is His Divinity? These are our conceptions! These are concepts created by man to judge himself, to evaluate his neighbours, and to evaluate the behaviour of society. God did not create good and evil. God did not teach that there is 'good and evil' or 'vice and virtue'. In fact He cannot teach because He cannot know what is good and what is bad. Because, as I said a little earlier, if He knows that two things are existing, He ceases to be God.

So, this is something–you know it is very shocking when we hear it first–it may be very troublesome to understand, it may be very difficult to understand, that God cannot be conscious of good, God cannot be conscious of evil, God cannot be conscious of darkness, God cannot be conscious of light.

It is all right, religions have said that God said, "Let there be light," and there was light. It was man who said "God said!" We have not heard God saying it! It was a man who said it, you see, that God said such and such a thing. Because it is the human endeavour to understand the mystery behind creation. It is the human mind which evolves a concept of God, which evolves an idea of God, because it requires something to aspire to, to aspire for, something to reach up to, something ultimately to achieve. And to that we ascribe the doership of everything that we see and hear and smell and taste and what not.

So, I may even venture to say–as some philosophers have also said before me–that God is a human creation. Because, for those of us who have not achieved the Divine state of existence, we do not know what God really is, who God is, whether such a thing exists. It is like a beggar talking of wealth. For him, instead of five paise, if he gets ten paise, it is wealth! What is the meaning of wealth? It is a comparative statement. One man gets ten rupees, another man gets fifteen rupees, the man who gets ten rupees envies the man who gets fifteen rupees! So, there are no absolute concepts. So, my Master says, "Wait till you reach That state. Then only can you know what Divinity is!" And, what is the way of knowing Divinity? To become divinised yourself! By knowing yourself at That level, you will know what He is! Till then God is an abstract entity, it is a mere concept about which we have no authority to speak, about which we have no knowledge at all which can enable us to speak, whom we have never experienced in our existence, either as a punisher or as a rewarder. So, let me say to all those who speak about God without having become divinised themselves–"Well, your statement is as good as mine!"

So, this is one of the most fundamental concepts of Sahaj Marg, in the teachings of my Master, that God is an abstract thing, a notion, that if He exists, we have to find out whether He exists by advancing on the path of divinisation by the help of a Master who comes to us in a human form and says, "My dear friend, now this is the state of God Himself! This is what we call the Divine state of existence! Now you know it by personal experience!"

Can we see God? No, because there is no physical form to see. He is nameless, you cannot call Him by any name. He is formless, you cannot see His form. He has no qualities, therefore you cannot describe Him by any quality. And, finally, my Master says, God can have no mind because when He has a mind He has consciousness. When He has consciousness the duality of existence is before Him–He ceases to be Divinity, the Ultimate Divinity. He may be the son of God, but He cannot be God Himself.

So, I wanted to amplify my morning talk by adding a few more facets about Sahaj Marg and dispel this ignorant idea that people who indulge in the participation in self-evolution, are running away from life. Let me assure you that in Sahaj Marg we do not run away from life. We are trying to break our way into real life, into eternal Life, into Divine Life–but leaving behind us, all those foolish miseries of a human existence, of a merely human existence, by throwing off our chains of bondage which are nothing but our own creation, created by our past thoughts, by our actions.

This is the first level of liberation: that I liberate myself from myself! Then follow subsequent liberations from so many things which I pray that our Master may bless us all with!

Thank you.

Time

This is a classical example of how in trying to avoid trouble today, we get into trouble tomorrow! I never thought that by not speaking yesterday I would be forced to speak today!

So, there is a hidden meaning in this. If at all you have to be in trouble, it is better to be in trouble today, when we can afford to do it, when we have the strength to do it, when we have the means to do it, when we have the time to do it! Whereas if we postpone it, you may find yourselves in a situation where you are too old, without the necessary capacity, without the necessary strength, and that the problem which you put off to solve on a later day, is beyond your capacity to resolve! This happens to all of us in school: "We don't want to study today, we will study tomorrow." So "today" is always being delayed, with the result the boy fails! Most people go to office–what they cannot solve, they put off: "We will look after it later. Let us solve all the easy problems first–easier files, easier papers." What happens is, the hard ones always remain at the table; tomorrow it becomes harder, the day after tomorrow it becomes almost impossible to do it!

So, "The same wisdom," Master says, "bring it to your sadhana." You see, when we get up in the morning, it is a common experience, most of us wake up sufficiently early to instinctively obey the first commandment. I mean it is part of the Indian way of life, that generally we are awake before the sun rises. But how many of us meditate? The Westerners find it impossible to get up! But Nature has made us, or trained us, in such a way that we cannot avoid waking up. But having woken up, we cover our heads, cover our feet, and "lie down," as we say, "a few minutes more," and we get up at half past seven!

Talk at Bangalore, 19 March 1985.

One morning is lost! We say, "What does it matter? There are umpteen mornings in my life! Let me meditate tomorrow morning! From tomorrow, I shall be regular!" If there is any truth that is revealed by this sort of attitude, it is that "tomorrow never comes"! Not for us!

So, what has to be done today, must be done today, **now**–performing the duty of the moment at that moment itself, and fulfilling the responsibility to that moment. It is not to society, it is not to people, it is to **time** itself we are fulfilling a responsibility! Time tells, "My dear friend, I am here. I am passing." Have you answered this appeal? Forget God, forget society, forget your friends. It is when the rain rains, the *vyavasayee* [farmer] must be ready with his field tilled, ready to sow the seed, ready to do the harvest. Otherwise he has to wait for the next rains. It may not come. Every vyavasayee knows this, that he must be fully prepared. "Time and tide wait for no man." And we also know ourselves the value of time.

Those of us who wish to make money say, "I have no time, Sir. I have an appointment here. I have to go to the bank. I have to file the income tax returns." They are rushing! "Rushing" means, in one way, trying to overcome the speed of time itself, by making more use of that time, than time would normally allow us! And, we have this experience in meditation, that either time is shortened, when we have a one hour sitting and it looks like five minutes; or we have the elongation of time, when we have meditated five minutes and it looks like one hour! So, this is an indication that if man would but make the requisite effort, time can be lengthened or shortened. It is not just a mere matter of a subjective experience, or a subjective consciousness, that we feel time is lengthened or shortened.

It is my personal experience that time **can be** expanded in such a way that you can put eternity into one moment of time! Otherwise, it is meaningless. If time is going to be like a footrule, the 'twelve inches' always a 'twelve inches', what is the fun in trying to do more in less time? Language also has a meaning. I mean, does the individual understand it when I say, that for one who works, time seems to be more than time itself? Like for one who wants to love or to be loved, love itself makes the way open for further love. It is the thing in which you participate that enables you to participate in that thing itself. It is like, you know, the classic occult symbolism of the snake swallowing its own tail! In some way, we have to make use of time to overcome time. And that is what we are doing in our spiritual sadhana!

When we talk of liberation, realisation, merger, and all these things, we are using time to gain time, to overcome time. It means a lift from time to eternity. And as regards eternity, the most foolish concept is that eternity is unlimited time! It is as silly as saying that enjoyment of food is in going on eating it forever and ever! The wise man knows that if he puts one drop of honey on his tongue, it is enough! He has enjoyed its taste! You don't have to swallow a bottle of honey and then purge! And, if you refer to the Gita where Krishna says, "I am time; *kalosmi*," God has to be used. And, if you cannot use God to achieve God, it is not possible to achieve Him in any other way! It is like fire fighting fire; like setting a thief to catch a thief; using a needle to prick out the thorn in your foot; we have to use that which is causing the trouble to overcome that trouble–use that which has been causing you that trouble. It looks very complicated when you put it to work. But it is really so easy, trying to overcome time to get out of the clutches of time to slip into Eternity! Because if God says, "I am time", you have to use God to overcome God Himself, look beyond Him into the Ultimate, where He does not (as God) exist any more! There He is no longer God! We call Him "It"! "That thou art." We don't say "Him thou art." We say, "That thou art." "*Tat twam asi.*"

So, now it becomes necessary that I know what time is. I know what God is, or at least I accept that there is something called God. If I know that this is a ladder which will enable me to climb to the first floor, and you say, "I don't accept this ladder"–well, you have to remain where you are! It is the beauty of ladders, that they can permit you to climb up, without themselves going up! It is a funny idea (you know sometimes I think I can be misunderstood as being disrespectful) when I say that every stone that is set across or set over in climbing to the temple and going into the *sannidhi* or the sanctum-sanctorum of the temple, is made of stone! We have still the consciousness of stepping on it! Yet without that stone we cannot step up! It is not necessary that something which is serving you should be higher than you! *Per contra*, there is no need to assume that it is lower than you! It is there at your service. The barber is there. We have to go to him for shaving. The old brahmins used to think that he is a *neecha jaathiwala* [lower caste]. They used to bathe when they came back! But bath or no bath, you have to go to him for a hair cut! Isn't it? The barber has his function!

It is a funny thing that most of those people whose services are absolutely essential were low caste people -- the barber, the *dhobis*, the *chamars*. And, ultimately when the body has to be disposed of, without the attendants at the burial ground, without their services, we cannot get the job done. And perhaps it is to prove this truth that, "My dear fellow, however great you are, you need this service!"–that Harischandra was made into a burning-ghat attendant himself. "Experience it, my dear friend! See what it is to consign your own son to the flames."

So, this is this concept of 'high and low'–that stupid concept, that vulgar concept, that inhuman concept, if you will permit me to say it! I think personally that every time we praise our Master, we are really insulting him: "He is beyond praise, he is beyond slander, he is beyond insult." And this is our stupidity, our ego, that we want a pat from him, his hands on our backs when we say, "Babuji, you are superior, you are beautiful." "*Haan, haan*, yes, yes." And in his heart he says, "Look at this fellow, trying to tell me what I am! Does he know what I am?" We are fools, presuming that he is too humble, he is too kind, too generous, too loving–but if you have been able to interpret his mind, his piercing glance, you would have kept your mouth shut for all time, after that!! "I dared not speak in his presence!" How can you tell him what he is, without knowing what he is? So, as I said in Tirupati about a month or two ago, we are liars, as shown by the fact that we are flattering him; 'flattering' being a description of a person of whom we know nothing! And if you say, "How dare you say such a thing?", I would quote the Master himself who said, "Everybody comes to see me, but nobody sees me." He need not have said it if it was not true!

So, what do we know of the Master that we think that we can evaluate him, much less his Master, Lalaji, or even his successor? This is all a futile exercise! What do we know of Masters? What do we know of mastery? We are here to receive the meanest, the lowest service the Master is offering us! Master has said that the service of the abhyasi in the heart region is like plunging into the gutters of humanity, the sink; the stink that we have to bear there! You should have seen his face when he said these things; the expression on his face! He used to say, you know ! This is service existing! His successor is nothing but a sweeper of gutters! And if you call him a Master, it is your fault. He is a sweeper, but a very necessary sweeper. Because we all know that if the water stops in the tank, we can exist; but if the latrine gets choked up, we are in deep trouble, because it is going to give disease. Gutters have to be cleaned. Water tanks need not be cleaned!

So, let us realise that it is not the time for judging. "Judge not that you be not judged," Christ said! Why? Because the man who dares not show his face before the mirror, achieves nothing by breaking the mirror! His face does not change! He may break a hundred mirrors; we are all doing it all the time. Every man vents his hatred for himself by throwing stones on buses, breaking structures, robbing coconuts. We are venting our hatred for ourselves on other people whom we see, on whom we have a hold, who are vulnerable!!

And if you look at it in one way, the Master is the most vulnerable person, poor fellow! My Master, I used to pity him for his plight. It is a blasphemous thing I am saying; but I have pitied him more than I have done anything else! Because when you have moved as intimately with the Master as I have moved with him; experienced the sorrow that was his eternal share; experienced the loneliness that was his permanent companion; experienced the misery of his failure in his work–when he could not mould an abhyasi because the abhyasi was foolish enough to resist his divine assistance–and seen him at night when he could not sleep, and said,

"These people come to me! I don't know why they come to me! They don't permit me to work on them. They don't listen to me. At least in their sleep let me do something." And he used to remain awake, and when they all are asleep, work on them!

So, ultimately, if the Master gets anything it is our pity! And my idea is, let us at least have that for him! So don't think that you know what a Master is. None of us can possibly know it. Because in the Puranas, it is said that Brahma and Vishnu wanted to see, to measure the height of Shiva. And one went down, and one went up. They could never find the limit. Because it has no limit!

Can you define a Master? It is said in the Vedas, that if you say this is God, it is no longer God! *"Neti, Neti."* It is much more so in the case of a Master, "If you say this is a Master, he ceases to be a Master." Because Mastery is as infinite, as unlimited in scope, in conception, in powers, as Divinity itself! One reason why we cannot know a Master, and why Master said, "Everybody comes to see me but nobody sees me," is because, in a sense, he was unknowable, he was unseeable, he was unperceivable. As we know an artist by his product, you can only judge a Master by his products, if you have the good fortune to be in that group.

So, you cannot judge the Master. But you can judge him by what he produces! You cannot judge a cook except by what he cooks! Isn't it? So, the only request that, ultimately, I desire to make to you is, whoever he may be, give him an opportunity to work, and then judge the result! Let us not prejudge. Pre-judgement is called prejudice. And it is the greatest sin in spirituality.

So, coming from the disillusionment of postponing today's work to tomorrow, I have in the end to request you, also, not to make the mistake of pre-judging what should not be judged hastily. When the brinjal vegetable is still cold in the pan, and you try to eat it, it is *katcha* [raw]! How can you taste it? Let it cook.

And who is to judge, and by what? Judge him by the effect he has on you, the result he produces on you! Because, ultimately, Master or no Master, he is nothing if he cannot change me! Because he exists for me, I exist for him. If a doctor cures you and kills me, for me he is a useless doctor! What does it matter to me if nine hundred and ninety nine cases are successful but my case is going to be a failure? Isn't it?

So, the test of my Master is: what he did for me, what he could do for me, what he shall continue to do for me. So, the test for each one of you is what he is able to do for you, in you, with you. Let me add one caution, that if it fails, it would not necessarily be his failure, it may be yours.

Thank you.

Reality Unveiled

As the old statement goes, "The truth is one," but we say so many things about it; describe it in so many ways. So, each one from the angle of his own experience tries to describe what he has felt, what he has experienced, and hopes that he is on the path progressing to a stage when he shall have nothing to describe.

There has been in the minds of most abhyasis, an undue emphasis on experience. In the beginning–yes! Many people have some experiences. I think most often it is granted deliberately by the Master to bring some sort of conviction into the minds of the newcomers that there is something here. Now, food can be entirely good without any taste; really good food should be tasteless! Taste has no special value to your nourishment or for your growth. Taste is something additionally imposed on food. This is something of a perversion, that things should have splendour; things which are to be eaten should have taste; things which are to be heard should be couched in beautiful language; and even deities in temples should be bedecked in suitably beautiful form so that we can appreciate them.

So we are in that tradition where we have not been trained to accept Reality as such. We have been conditioned to accept things either tastefully decorated, or couched in acceptable language, or dressed suitably and, in that way, from hoary ages of the past, Reality has been covered up; Reality has been occluded, as it were. And today we have to search for it in the mass of confusion, in the mass of beauty, in the confusion of language, so that our mind is no longer able to grasp Reality in its naked condition. Therefore, the need for speeches and, much more important, the need for cleaning.

Talk at the Founder's Day celebration of Tamil Nadu State, 11 August 1985, Salem.

Now, we have all been hearing so much about the spiritual cleaning that the Master is doing, the preceptors are doing, and that we ourselves are expected to do every day, in the evening. That is the internal cleaning of the samskaras which have already been formed. But we do not realise that we have to co-operate in a different way, in a continuous cleaning process, where we should try to rid ourselves of all these social and cultural conditionings of the past–that a thing must look beautiful to be really good, that food must taste well to be really good, that the language of the speaker must be brilliant for his thoughts to be good. All these small conditionings we have to reject.

I have come out of many lectures where many accepted speakers spoke brilliantly, but even as I came out of the hall and put on my *chappals*, I heard people asking each other, "What did he say?" and the reply was, "I don't know, but it was beautiful." I do not know how something can be beautiful when you do not even know what it was! It has long been my suspicion, and now I am convinced of it too, that the beauty of language is used deliberately to confuse people and to prevent them from knowing that there is nothing to say. Similarly, food is made attractive to look at because often it has no instrinsic value. You know all these tricks are being practised upon us to cheat us, to beguile us, and to continue to corrupt us–not without our knowledge, not without our co-operation, but with both our knowledge and our co-operation! These tricks of the trade are being practised upon us in hotels, from political platforms and, unfortunately, from religious platforms, too.

So this is a most unfortunate thing that in the name of Religion, the name of Divinity, we are allowing ourselves–we are allowing our children, we are training our children to allow themselves–to be cheated, to be lied to, to be corrupted, to be drawn further and further away from Reality, further and further away from the subtlety, from the utmost subtlety that Divinity is. You must forgive me if I appear to speak in very strong terms but this is the truth. The truth is always unpalatable particularly for those who claim to be orthodox. I don't know what the real meaning of orthodoxy is, but apparently those who are fooling themselves and fooling the public are the orthodox people. Well, let them have their orthodoxy. Let them cling to their illusions and artificial embellishments. If there is one person here who says he is not familiar with the corruption that is going on, left, right and centre, he is a liar. So if you want to be corrupt and a liar on top of it, it is your privilege. Human beings are free, and nobody can compel them to accept the truth, nobody can compel them to be even truthful.

Today there is a growing awareness, appreciation, recognition of the fact that people seem to think that only if they are untruthful, only if they are corrupt, they can succeed. And even children are told, "Don't be a fool. If you behave this way, this way and this way you can be like pappa, who is a multi-millionaire with seventeen properties here and others in the making in other cities; but if you are going to be truthful, well, you will be pulling a rickshaw on the street." So, from the cradle we are training our children to be liars, so that they can be what we hope they will be–successful citizens! Not good citizens, but successful citizens. And to these are added slogans which are imported from the West like, 'Nothing succeeds like success,' 'That is true, which is believed by all.' You see, truth is not truth any more, but that which you believe to be true is the truth! That which most people repeat again and again becomes the truth, because we are in an age when the more the people that say something, the more truthful it becomes. The only answer I can give to this meaning of truth is a statement from Rudyard Kipling, where monkeys say, "We all say so, so it must be true."

So all this talk about Reality, about realisation, is a waste! As Kannan pointed out, we are supposed to be some sort of fanatics or Nastikas because we don't worship in temples. That shows that not only are people corrupt, but they are unwilling to recognize how gross they have become, how self-deluded they have become; nobody is deluding us, we are allowing ourselves to be deluded; we prefer to be deluded. It is nice and comfortable to be deluded and lulled into a state of almost narcotic sleep where, instead of my being one with God–having God within me so that He is looking at my every thought, action, and every moment of my existence–I can be relaxed if I go to a temple somewhere. I go there once in two or three years, put in twenty rupees if I am poor, two and a half lakhs if I am rich, and thus try to salve my conscience. But you cannot cheat God. You can cheat yourselves. The greatest ignorance, the greatest foolishness, the greatest stupidity that we exhibit is in thinking that if we throw some money in the *hundi* of a temple, we have got away with it. Got away with what? Can we ever cheat God? I believe what we need is more exposure to truth, more reality thrown at us, not palliatives as in allopathy, not pain-killers, not drugs to make us sleep. This is all that the religion of modern day is giving us!

So to this extent, my dear brothers and sisters, we have fallen. Now my Master Shri Ram Chandraji Maharaj of Shahjahanpur, and His Master before Him, Lalaji Maharaj, have stated all these truths quite forcibly. Master has exposed in his book *Reality at Dawn* the most profound truths about religion, about gods, in absolutely unambiguous language. If somebody reads it and says he is confused, that confusion is deliberate. He does not want to understand.

So whether you accept the truth or not, the truth remains what it is. The truth does not depend on your acceptance, does not need your acceptance. But we need the truth in our lives. That is why when people tell us lies we become so annoyed. But when we lie to others we think it is an achievement. Lying is a two-way transaction. How can you expect not to be lied to if you are telling lies all your life? Can you consider it a prerogative of your existence that you can lie but you should not be lied to? There is no law which says that. On the contrary, the Christian precept says, "Do unto others as thou wouldst be done by." If you want others to tell you the truth, start by telling the truth. If you want others to be charitable towards you, towards your mistakes, to your sins, be charitable first. If you want God to redeem you, start by redeeming others. Because what we broadcast from our hearts comes back to us as gifts from the Infinite.

There is nothing that the Infinite can give us which we cannot give ourselves. It is a travesty of truth to say that God bestows blessings on us, or that God gives punishment. It is not God who punishes or blesses, in that sense. I would venture to say that He is far too busy to bother about each and every individual human being, and his actions! God has no time, He has no interest. He has created us and it is for us to evolve up to Him.

I cannot imagine a God who will stoop to punish us. As our elder brother, Shri C. S. Ramakrishnan, said, even rebirth is a gift. We think of it as a sin, as a result of sin, as a curse upon us; but it is God's magnificent charity, His benevolence that says, "Have another chance." No lawgiver on earth has ever given a second chance. The law punishes us exactly and it punishes us immediately. But as the old saying goes, "The mills of God grind slowly but surely." The word 'slowly' here applies to His mercifulness which gives us aeons of time to redeem ourselves, to correct ourselves, to connect ourselves back to Him again. The word 'surely' means, that in the end there will come a time when we shall have to suffer the consequences of our own sins, of our own viciousness, of our corruption, not as a punishment from Him, but as an act of self-condemnation imposed by ourselves upon ourselves.

So let us not just stop with hearing these lectures and talking about reality, and buying *Reality at Dawn*. We are not to be satisfied with reality just at dawn, but it should pervade all our twenty-four hour existence. Let us be willing to face reality–the first reality we have to face being, "What am I?" And then, you know, it applies to all of us, to me as much as to you. And when we are able to see what we are, and to recognize the filth that lies inside us, and we are unable to bear that sight–as we should be if we have seen it– let us rush to the Master and say, "Master, forgive me for all that I have done. I now hand my own self over to you so that you may do with my life something better than what I have done with it myself"! Anyone who is not willing to do this, is only interested in hearing about Reality, but not to achieve it; to speak about corruption perhaps, but not to correct it in himself; to talk about telling the truth, but not in telling the truth himself. And to my mind this has gone on for centuries and centuries. I say this because of slogans like '*Satyam vada*'. I have rarely come across these slogans, "Tell the truth," anywhere else in the world. Because when you are telling the truth, there is no need to tell you to tell the truth. So, other people may look up and cry "Satyam vada," but a society pervaded by truth doesn't need them.

The first liberation is from the idea that I am a good person. As Master pointed out, there is no such thing as good samskaras. As Babuji once said, "If you are in a golden cage it is no better than being in an iron cage or a bamboo cage or any sort of cage. A cage is a cage. The gold belongs to the owner who imprisoned you, and not to you. The bird doesn't enjoy the gold, it is still in the prison." So the first liberation is the liberation from the foolish idea that since I have donated so much to this temple, and I have done charity, and I am a good man, and I have not harmed anybody, I don't need anything else.

Most people, when we talk of Sahaj Marg, say "Sir, my conscience is clear." Well if it is **really clear**, I think he will be one in a hundred million people perhaps born once in a hundred thousand years. Let us give up all these ideas first. Let us understand that right action alone is what matters. Sahaj Marg does not recognize good action or bad action, whatever philosophy may say about it, whatever religion may say about it. There is no such thing as good action. There is only right action. And while it is right to feed a beggar who is at your door, you are no more entitled to any merit than he is in allowing you to feed him at your door. We should recognize that they do us a service by accepting what we think of as charity, which my Master says is nothing more than a human duty towards a suffering human being.

So, dear friends, more than duty you have nothing else to do. Sahaj Marg doesn't say, "Do good." Sahaj Marg says, "Do what is necessary." Sahaj Marg doesn't say, "Be virtuous." Sahaj Marg says, "Live such a life in which there is no creation of samskaras, good or bad." Sahaj Marg does not say, "Be a saint." Sahaj Marg says, "Live this life as it should be lived, and this life will lead you inexorably to the path on which the goal can be achieved without even your consciousness that it is being achieved."

So let us not confuse Sahaj Marg with religious precepts, and with slogans like 'Satyam vada'. They are all right in their place. We are only concerned with working, thinking and acting in such a way that it proves us to be human beings who are interested in Divinisation, and who would go to that goal without swerving from the path.

Adhere To One Teaching, One Goal

I learn that the question of 'What happens after death?' is being discussed. I do not understand the question properly. But there seems to be some concern that, "If you are a liberated soul, can you come back again?" Is that correct? Something like that? Now, this question rises again and again. Because I have had this question asked in Europe also in some places. One boy asked me, "You are promising me a lot today! And, if I am to come back after *mahapralaya* again, what is the use? You may as well not have liberation and continue with this life!"

So harbouring such thoughts, you know—we seem to have *deergha darshan* in a very negative sort of way. It is like saying, "Suppose I am to become a criminal, and I am to go to jail, why not I go to jail today itself?" Because at some stage everybody is a criminal–if not in the past, at least in the future. It is like saying, "If I am to go on a holiday and come back to the house, I might as well not go on a holiday! If I am to eat, and become hungry again tomorrow, I might as well not eat!" Isn't it? And, "If I am to live and to die again, why should I live at all? Let me commit suicide!" So it is a very morbid thought, that I should not aspire to change this condition, because there is a possibility of that condition reverting to this condition again. So it is like saying, "Today is going to become 'tonight'; so let me close all the windows and make it dark, now itself!"

Human logic, human sensibility says, "Be in the sun when there is sunlight. Be in the dark when it is darkness. And make both the same." I am surprised people are talking today of Gita and all these things—make *siddha* and Buddha same; make this and that same; make wealth and poverty the same. But you do not want to make life and death the same! You do not want to make liberation and the state of non-liberation the same!

We should study Master's thoughts carefully without going into extraneous systems of philosophies. There is an unfortunate tendency in the educated people to mix philosophic systems, and confuse the whole issue. You know in the cinema world this is a very common practice, the face of an actress is merged with the voice of another person who is a good singer, and we get a composite woman, and we think that a beautiful woman should sing well. But rarely does a beautiful woman sing, or a good musician appear beautiful. That is a composite which the cinema people do, to exploit fools like us who are willing to get deceived again. In reality there is no such composition.

Reality is one. It cannot be mixed with anything else. It is so with every thought of Sahaj Marg and the Sahaj Marg philosophy and the truth that Master has placed before us. We should interpret Sahaj Marg by Master's teachings, not bringing other considerations, other philosophies, other saints; because all of us know that Babuji Maharaj never referred to another. He referred to some other philosophies very rarely. In fact, he has written that at the age of sixteen or seventeen, he called for the book Mill's *Utilitarianism*. He read a few pages and put it away. "Because," he said, "if I keep this, I will repeat these thoughts and my originality will be lost." So to that extent you have to be pure.

You see, sometimes we talk of chastity. We have certain conceptions of chastity. But the total conception of chastity is: the guru, his teachings, his goal–they **alone** are mine. I know there is a system of practice in South India, where, if you are listening to another guru's teachings, they say you are committing "adultery through ears"! That is another form of chastity: "Listen not to somebody else's teachings, lest your teachings be corrupted." That is why there used to be an old saying: "After being with your guru, go back straight home. Do not wander on the streets because you may be led astray somewhere on the way!" In our old Samskriti also, it is said "Go to the temple and get back home. Don't come via this street or that street. Who knows what is lurking in those streets to catch you?"

So it is a very dangerous thing, to make a *kichhdi* sort of philosophy by putting together all that you have learnt from the past, and trying to make a composite picture of a Reality that does not exist. You know, for example, in Sahaj Marg the concept of *mukti* does not exist. Babuji does not even refer to it because he has often said that liberation is a child's play. He says, "I can give it with the wink of an eye." Just wink, and the man is liberated; and he saw that Lalaji could do it; he studied it and he himself was able to do it. So where is this liberation? What is this condition, mukti, which you are all talking so much? It is a child's play. It is a toy in the hands of a spiritual saint. So we should not talk of mukti, *mumukshuthva*, etc.–that is all gone. We have surpassed all those philosophies, as we must. Evolution means surpassing previous conditions, acquiring more of wisdom, more of abilities! What is evolution, but the transcendence of the past into the present, and from there into the future!

So any man who has an unnecessary hold on the past, and has a need for this past to fulfil the present, is still living in the past. And he is afraid to give up the past because he does not know what the present contains. So it is fear which makes us hold to the past, the traditions of the past, the teachings of the past.

There is no disrespect in this statement. Because, why are there so many Vedas for instance? Why are there the six systems of philosophy? Should not one be enough? And most importantly, why should an *avatara* come again and again and again? Why not he once and for all be able to give one transmission, and change the whole universe, and then keep quiet in his home in heaven? Because there is the need. And you see the evolution in the avatara trend itself, from *mathsya* to *koorma* to the *varaha*, you know, on and on. It develops from the fish to the human form, and then to the Divine form. That is how we are developing. As we develop, the avataras come to match our level. Because you cannot be taught otherwise. A primary school teacher cannot teach a college student. You always need a teacher of a higher level than our own knowledge. Otherwise he cannot teach us. That is why an avatara comes, bringing with him a knowledge that is advanced far beyond our time.

Our own Babuji has said in Munich, "My books are not for today. The present generation will not understand it. They are for the future." Why? Because they come from a time far in advance of us. You teach every child things which he does not know so that he can understand it at some future time–few days later; few weeks later; few months later; sometimes it takes even sixty years to understand what the teacher taught in the school. So, if you are to learn, you must have a teacher who is an advanced person; and the more he is advanced, the better. And if it is Divinity itself, it means it is coming here from the Ultimate–the Ultimate in time, the Ultimate in space, the Ultimate in all potentialities itself.

So when you start limiting these concepts with foolish things, childish things like mukti, and wonder whether you have to come again, I say, "why not?" Suppose Babuji did not come to us, suppose Lalaji did not come to us, what will we be? Surely Lalaji did not need to come! Babuji has said that this is the first life in which he had taken the *sthoola sarira* [physical body]. He came because of his *karuna* for us.

So we must remember that there are two aspects involved in our coming here again and again: one is like us, who come because of the bondage of the samskar. We have no choice. We have to come; it is not a question of choice. We are pushed here. The other is the *divya swaroopis* [divine forms]; you can call them saints– Divinity itself, who, out of compassion for its own creation, takes on the form, suffers with us, laughs with us, enjoys with us, teaches us, and goes back. Now suppose Divinity did not have this compassionate aspect to descend again and again, to teach us and lift us up, where would we be? We would be wandering in the mire of ignorance and sin, all our lives, life after life!

So let us not be afraid of coming back. On the contrary, I would say, it is a matter of great sorrow. And, it would also reflect ingratitude, basest ingratitude, if a person who is an abhyasi has been given the highest by the Master, and later on says, "Babuji, I do not want to come back again to this world." You should be not only prepared, but you should be willing to come again and again. Babuji says, "Go to *bhooloka* [earth] and do this work." "Yes Master." Next instant I am there. You all see some cinema pictures, where Sage Narada comes from there, and where Lord Narayana Himself comes here, and we are praising: "Wah, wah! You see what Divine grace!" If Divine grace did not descend, where would we be? How would we ascend?

So please do not have this foolish idea that we do not like to come again. Babuji once asked me, "Will you be ever with me?" I said, "Babuji, **yes**." He said, "In hell, too?" I said, "What is there? When you are there how can it be hell?" It is like the lamp saying, "Will you go with me wherever I go?" "Yes." "Even in the darkness?" "Naturally!" Because when I go with the lamp itself, where can there be darkness? Can there be heaven where no God is, and can there be hell where God is? There is little difference.

So we do not want these funny ideas of coming back, of being afraid of coming back. Life is a glorious thing wherever we exist, if we live it well. There is no special glory in the Divine existence; there is no misery in the physical existence. They are both our creations. I can make this existence a Divine existence, and I can be a fool in the Divine world and drop back again. There are stories which have given proofs for these things, that one who ascended, descended again for some foolish act. All that we should seek is His true presence, His eternal presence within us, and to be with Him wherever He is. So this is the greatness of spirituality.

And second thing, about *divya shakti* [Divine power]: in our Master's teachings, there is no such thing as divya shakti–whatever the Shastras may say, whatever the philanthropists may say, whatever any one else may say. In the Ultimate, there is no shakti, there is no knowledge, there is nothing. So what is the inference? I remember once Babuji was talking about his own powers being distributed: "Who is going to take it from me?" This was, you know, in 1965 or 1966. And he was quite unhappy. He said, "For all the work that I have done in the South, I should have produced hundred Personalities in South! Unfortunately I have not been able to produce even one! And I am concerned what I would do with powers that are in me! When I leave this body I will ultimately have to leave it." I said, "Why? Can't you take it with you?" He said, "No; powers have to be left here. Nobody can take powers with him."

So, when even the liberated soul cannot take powers with him, where is the question of God having power? That is why He has to descend here as avatara, take the power that is here, and work on evil that is here; destroy the evil, re-establish the *dharma*, protect the *dhaarmics* [righteous] and go back leaving the powers until the next avatara comes. Like the rich man has to leave his money and his property behind, even the elevated souls at the highest level have to leave their powers behind. They cannot take powers with them. So there is no power, except at the human level. This is the secret as to why God has to descend, because, where there is no power He cannot work! Here He comes down, accepts the power, accepts a form, accepts the job, performs it, and goes back. This is a proof that power is only here, not there! That is why even power politics is on earth, not in heaven–fortunately for us!

The whole object of my speaking to you is not to explain the questions. They are irrelevant. Because sometimes you understand them yourself. It is to emphasize the need to speak through one teaching, and not bring in the other considerations, however great their relevance to the past may have been. We are not concerned with it. Because the Vedas were written twenty-five thousand years back, they are not more important than Sahaj Marg, which is today's teaching. The new one is not bad, the old one is not good, just by virtue of their newness or the oldness. As Kabir said, "If the old things have to be taken care of by God first, then all the mountains would have been liberated long ago." "If the *Ganga-jal* [water of Ganga] is to give us mukti, every fish and crocodile in the river would have been liberated long ago!" "If stones have to be worshipped, it is better to worship the grinding stone which produces wheat flour which we use for cooking." This is what Kabir said!

So, the Ganga is useful to one who has achieved that point of liberation, that when he falls into the river he does not come out again. That can be achieved right in your own backyard–in your own pond or well water, if you have the capacity to do it. Unfortunately, with mythology to back us, with stories in our Puranas to back us, we have mystified all these things. We have given them a value beyond the truth that resides in them. For instance, the river Ganga is the same, but the water has not been the same ever since it started flowing. Every day the water is changing; every minute the water is changing; which water is it that is to give you mukti? And as my friend said, once I dip into the river, it is there and it is not there also; then why should not a bath in the sea give me mukti? Because, after all, the Ganga water is there also.

So it is like this spirit, the *atman*, which has no quality, no form, no name, nothing. When it enters a body it takes its attributes. So, similarly we have the various things, you know. It has its own powers. All these forms have their own powers. The Ultimate has no power, yet having no power, from there everything comes. This is the truth of Sahaj Marg as taught by Lalaji, and then perfected by Babuji. People hear this truth, but they cannot understand it. It is like saying, "Sir, how did this tree come from this seed? What is there in the seed?" Surely, the tree is not in the seed. But without the seed the tree cannot be there. Similarly the *paratatva*, as we call it, it has nothing in it–no power, no knowledge, no qualities, yet, the whole universe is its eternal presence. That presence we want to bring into ourselves in Sahaj Marg, by the Guru's grace, by His transmission.

So please stick to Sahaj Marg. Read Sahaj Marg books. Understand Sahaj Marg teachings. Comparisons are unnecessary. As I said (sometimes in the past too) Sahaj Marg stands on its own two legs. We do not need any authority from any other systems of philosophy, any other teachings, any other Puranas, even the Vedas. It is no disrespect; I bow in respect to all the past *acharyas*. They have themselves gone, and handed over things to us. You see it is like this baton that you get in the relay race. It has no power except that it symbolizes our position in the race. If you drop it, the race is finished. But the man who is carrying it is different. He comes with a different force. He comes from different systems. His powers are different; eternally they are changing.

Listen To The Heart

In the Christian tradition it is said, "You have eyes but you see not; you have ears but you hear not;" things like that. I used to think that Christ was very uncharitable when he said that. But after I listened to our speeches, in place after place, I am convinced it is true. The speeches are all predictable and are invariably on what is the *panthathi*, what is Sahaj Marg, what is cleaning, how to meditate, how to sit, etc. In my twenty-two years with Babuji Maharaj in this Mission, I must have heard this at least one thousand times! And I wonder what our listeners do when they sit in front of us! Because obviously they are listening to us–but do they hear anything? Christ said, "You have ears but you hear not."

He did not say, "You do not listen." We listen, but we do not hear anything. Because our attention is always somewhere else. A poet says, "My words fly up; my thoughts remain below. Words without thoughts never to heaven go."

So I suspect, like that, we bring our bodies to hear this lecture, but we leave our minds elsewhere. And further proof is that every time, there are some people asking questions. "What exactly is meditation?" And once Babuji was very upset when, in a preceptors' meeting, one who had been a preceptor for fifteen years wanted to know what is transmission! And of course, Babuji did not answer. He was very upset. One could see it in his face. He was so upset that he did not answer. He said, "Secretary saab, answer." And there again I had to, you know, sort of fill up the gap. And later on, when we were back in his room, he said, "I wonder what this preceptor has been doing for the last fifteen years, when he does not know what is transmission?" It is not a criticism on preceptors. It is a general criticism on human nature that we are never completely in one place; we are never wholly in one place. We go

Concluding talk at Nellore, 26 August 1985.

to the temple, our heart is in the house. We go to the school, our heart is in the playground. We go to the office, the heart is at home. And even people who recite the Vedas–you know, the *pujaris*, the *purohits*, they can go on reciting the Vedas hour after hour, day after day, without missing one word–they do not know the meaning.

I think we have become conditioned, in some way, to be able to listen without hearing, to be able to see without really seeing what is going on. Because, once I observed that when Babuji entered the hall, many people did not know that he had come. This was in Shahjahanpur–Basant Panchami day! And I had to bring Babuji on the dais, and in one corner, one section of people were still talking, chatting, and they did not even know that Master had arrived. We are all anxiously sitting, waiting for the Master's presence, but we are so inattentive that when he actually comes before us, we do not know that he is there. And then somebody has to get up and make an announcement: "Babuji Maharaj has come. Please be quiet. He is going to start meditation in a few minutes." And then occasionally people are also upset, "Why I was not told in advance that Babuji is coming; I would have been more attentive."

This is nothing new, because Babuji himself has said that in Lalaji's times, when he would go to the *bhandara* and sit right at the back–often Lalaji would sit down and start transmitting without saying anything, and he was the only person who became alert and sat in meditation. And Lalaji Saheb used to tell him, "Ramchander, you are the only person who knows what I am doing and when I am doing. All are sitting like this and they know nothing." So this is nothing new. So, we need not be too unhappy. It is not unique to today's people or today's society. But at the same time, it is tragic that humanity can go on for hundreds of thousands of years, developing, if anything, greater and greater ability to be not alert, greater ability to not listen, greater ability to not see!

I think our qualities are being developed in negative directions. And in one way, it is called callousness. We are callous, when we see somebody brutally beaten on the street and we can just cover our eyes and walk away, pretending we have not seen anything. We see a man's pocket being picked by another man; still ignore it and walk away pretending we have not seen it. Because we do not want to be involved. If you see a man beating his wife on the street, and if you try to stop him doing it, you have to be involved in that; the man might beat you; or if there is a police complaint, you have to go to the station, give a *panchanama* and so on. So it is easier to pretend that we have not heard or seen these things, and keep moving!

This training seems to have permeated into our spiritual life, where because perhaps one half of me says that I have to reach the destination, my goal, the other half says, "Well, what is wrong with this life? It is so beautiful; there are so many things to be enjoyed, so many pleasures not yet tasted. What is wrong with this life?"

So it seems that there is this dichotomy in our make-up, so that even though we come to listen, we choose not to listen. And by an act of deliberate will, or by some sort of closing the window of awareness on one side, we register our presence, without anything registered inside us. Our presence is registered, nothing more. We neither listen nor do; because I think, I suspect, the cause is the same, that if you were to really listen to the Master or the people who are speaking to you, and if you are really to register these things in your heart, you become committed to follow it.

So here again, it is very useful and very helpful to see without seeing, to hear without hearing, so that we can satisfy the conscience that, "as an abhyasi I was present at the meeting; as discipline demanded, I sat through the lectures, whether I understood them or not; and thus, having fulfilled my duty, my Master is bound to take me to the destination, even though I have done all this without any sense of commitment, either to Him, or to the teachings, or to the Mission, or to myself." So, if you are not willing to commit yourselves, I have a suspicion that the Master is not going to commit himself to us; because as Babuji has said very very clearly, that one who commits himself to the sadhana–to him the Master has to commit; to his progress the Master is committed; to his welfare the Master is committed. But if we just come and register our presence, I do not think that the Master has any commitment to us, in the way that he is bound to lift us up to this highest goal of human evolution.

So, I am just telling you this to suggest very humbly, that we can commit the Master to our progress, to our welfare, to our spiritual evolution, only by our committing ourselves to His teachings. This sort of superficial listening and hearing, like we have done all our lives, in *Kathakalakshepams*, *Pravachanams*–when we come out, we do not know what had happened–that will not do. It will not do for those people who want to progress. For the others, of course, it is all right, you see, because there are many people who wish to pass time for lack of anything better to do; or, out of fear of doing something worse, they come to such places and listen to some things and are happy that they did not do any mischief. Because, after all, much mischief can be done in half an hour!

That is one aspect. Now the second aspect is, even for those who are committed, few seem to know what is the goal. I mean, few have even enquired what exactly are we here for. "Yes, I know what is meditation. I sincerely listened to what is being said. I have read the books. I know how to sit; how to ignore unnecessary thoughts. I know what to do during cleaning. My preceptors tell me, the Master tells me that my condition is good. But what is this all about?" Even after many years, people are confused. They say, "What is Divinisation?" Now, I think it was one of our speakers this morning who said that we do not become Gods. But we become God-like. Now, what is "God-like"? Unless you know what is a God, you do not know what is 'God-like'. Isn't it? It is like saying, "It is like halwa", when I have never eaten halwa! So, is a man who is telling you what is your goal competent to tell you what is that goal? He can do so only by knowing for himself what that goal is, or by having achieved it. So I would suggest that the Master is the only person competent in that sense, to speak about the Goal. For the rest of us, it is something in the future. It is something in the future, in time; it may not be tomorrow; it may not be the day after; it may be this minute, too. Future does not mean an unspecified future. What that Goal is, the Master knows. He has achieved it. He is in relation with that Ultimate. He is in permanent contact with it. He is part of it; or maybe he is the whole of it, whatever it be. So, we have to adopt a trusting nature as far as the goal is concerned, without asking to be told in advance what that goal is.

You know, I have often wondered about, say, education. We tell a child, "It is necessary to be educated;" and then we bribe it to study. Most of the educative processes are achieved by bribery, whether it be with a biscuit, or with the promise of a wristwatch if you pass the exam–or a holiday in Ooty if you come first–it is bribery. It is not corruption; it is bribery. Why do we do it? We don't do it with any ulterior or *male fide* motives; but we are sincerely interested in the welfare of that child who is our responsibility. So we have to tell it slowly, make promises, give gifts, show resentment occasionally, to encourage it on the path of education; so that one day it will realise, as it grows up, that this is what education was for! You see, you have to be educated before you know the value of education! Can a man on the street who has no education tell you what is the value of education? It takes a rich man to know what riches can buy! A rickshaw puller cannot tell you what wealth can buy. He can imagine so many things, but he does not know. It is a rich man who knows what money **can** buy, and unfortunately, tragically, what all it cannot buy, too! Similarly, the educated man, if he is really wise, knows what education can achieve, and the immense things that education cannot achieve. It takes a really wise man to know what wisdom cannot penetrate! The BSc's and MSc's are no use in these things, you see! Because he is not wise; he has only got facts, he has only mugged up facts to get a degree, a degree on the wall! It is as good as the preceptor's certificate, if it is not backed by that wisdom which says, "Go ahead! This is not the end."

So, real wealth tells you the limitations of wealth. Real education shows you what it can do, and the limitations of that education, or the limitations of that wisdom. Similarly, you have to be a *sadhak* first, before you can know what can be achieved and what cannot be achieved! Babuji put it very simply: He said, "You want an MA degree, and then you want to start learning A-B-C. Start learning A-B-C; and automatically, you will get the degree!" So practice comes first, achievement comes as a result of that practice.

Now we all want to be divinised, without knowing what is divinisation. You see, I will tell you a small story–at one stage, Babuji forbade me from telling it. Somebody very close to him [Babuji] was passing away; an extreme case as they say. And he was called. He was sitting in his room, he was called out to see whether he could do something. And when he came, he found this, what we call *Yama paasam*, you know, the noose of Lord Yama, around the neck of this person whom he loved very much. And he was enraged! He said, "My people, and this Yama paasam around the neck of that fellow!" And he shattered it with one transmission! He just said, "I disintegrated the paasam." And then he was adjusting himself to destroy Yama himself! And then, voice came from Lalaji: "Yes, you can do it! Not one Yama, you can destroy anything in creation you like! But beware, you have to take over the duties of Yama." Then Babuji laughed, you know, in his own inimitable way, and said, "Which fool will accept that dirty job?" I said, "Babuji, he is supposed to be a god." He said, "Yes, but he is a sweeper among gods! Because he takes away all the filth of humanity." Yama does not come to the *punya athmas*! He comes to the *papa athmas*! And for the ordinary *papathmas*, he sends his *dhoothas* [messengers], you see! For the real *papi* [sinner], for the great papis only, he comes. So it is a signal honour, if Yama comes to us personally!

You see, it is like the income tax fellow coming to raid our house! Or the bootlegger who comes to our house to collect the bribe, and being followed by the prohibition man to arrest us. You see, one way, it is an honour! You find today people whose houses have been raided become more popular: "Raid *ayee poyindee*, Sir! Seventeen and a half lakhs!"–the implication being that there are other seventeen and a half lakhs, or thirty-five lakhs not yet recovered! So he is really a rich man. So, if a man can get raided and lose seventeen and a half lakhs to the police, or the revenue officials or the customs authorities, and still have his three cars and air conditioners and his refrigerators and everything, it is a sign of signal wealth. Similarly, if Yama comes personally, I mean it must be something about which even the gods must be wondering! "Aha, Yama going himself personally today on his buffalo. There must be some great guy who is there on earth. Let us go and see!"

So, you see, a god has responsibilities. High responsibilities, like you say Saraswathi is for knowledge, Lakshmi for wealth! Or the lowest, or the gutter type of responsibility as that of poor Yama! Which do we want? Obviously we don't want responsibilities! Most of us, I suspect, are in the spiritual field so that we can bask in the guru's grace, without having to do anything. We don't want to work, we don't want to–I mean, most of us are here as an escape from responsibilities, from duties. And then, when we find that here also there are duties and responsibilities, in some way we feel hurt and cheated! Some people feel cheated, you know, "Why didn't that old man tell me there are duties and responsibilities here? I thought this is free! We can do what we like, we can behave as we like! Well, half an hour in the morning, ten minutes in the evening, two minutes at night, well, I am prepared for that, you see. But I didn't know that my commitment to honesty has to be total, my commitment to morality has to be total, my commitment to the Master has to be total. And, I have to give Him my heart! Who told me these in the beginning?"

So these questions are asked. I am not telling something from imagination. People are asking these questions: "Sir, why didn't you say when we first came to you that this is a total commitment?" I said, "Nice. To whom?" They said, "To the Master!" I said, "Nonsense. What has Master to do with you and your wonderful heart? Have you a heart at all first? Look for it!" Then they get more upset. I said, "I mean it. Do you have a heart? Because, in society I know how you are represented. You are being called a heartless fellow. You have been called a victimizer. Your wife questions your heart. Your children don't think you have a heart! Where is your heart? And, the man with no heart, what does he do here? Where is the possibility of committing when you have nothing to lose?" Then they say, "No, no, Sir, I assure you I have a heart." I said, "Physically, yes! Perhaps you had a heart attack, so you know it better than I do." Still coming back to the same question, "To whom are you committed?" Then he is bewildered. He says, "No, no, but everybody says I have to be committed to the Master. I have to be committed to the practice." Then I said, "Friend, you are committed to yourself, to your progress. It is not for his sake that the Master asks for your heart. It is not for his sake that the Master asks you to commit yourself to this practice. It is not for his sake that he wants you to commit yourself totally to honesty, ethics, morality. It is for **your** sake!" Therefore, the commitment is to yourself.

You see, the idea of commitment, and to whom that commitment is made, and the degree to which that commitment is made, nobody has understood! And when they understand also, they get frightened: "What is this commitment? Does it mean I cannot do this, I cannot enjoy that?" You know, in our country (to go off the track a little) the family planning programmes have been great failures, because our only commitment is to pleasure! Any technique that is advertised by the government, this fellow will come with his demand, head-scratching–and very very delicately pose a question; and it generally has to do with pleasure. So our commitment is only to pleasure! And here, when we come and we are told, "Rise before dawn, eat from pious earnings," and these sort of things, the ten maxims you see. He says, "What happens to my commitments to myself?"–not knowing that it is for a higher commitment to yourself which you are seeking, and not your lower commitment which was an animal commitment, for animal fulfilment, for animal pleasures.

And even after you tell him, he has this idea, "A bird in hand is worth two in the bush. Let me enjoy something here! Who knows about the hereafter, you see! A good fling at life here! Well, let us see what the future holds! People say there is another *janma*, people say there is *naraka*, there is *swarga*, who has seen these things?" When you tell them, "My dear friend, it is not the future or the next life! You get drunk today, you have a headache tomorrow; you have cirrhosis of the liver next year. It is within your foreseeable future which you can see yourself. You don't need a god to come and prove it to you. You don't need Yama to come and prove it to you. It is there for you to see. Or, if you cannot or don't want to see it in yourself, look at your neighbour! Look at your cousin! Look at your so-and-so, you see."

So in some way, there is an unwillingness to see what is truth, there is an unwillingness to commit to the truth, because the truth is often unpalatable. All because, there is a fear that, "In the aspiration for something which is promised, maybe we will lose that which we have now. Bird in the hand is worth two in the bush."

These ideas of Divinisation we hear, and we say, "Yes, one more speaker we have listened to today! And, of course, he spoke beautifully, you see. There is no question about it." That is a grudging sort of remark, to satisfy the speaker! But no speaker is useful until his speech, or his talk, the things contained therein, have been practised and translated into reality in our own lives! As Master has said so often, "People come to see me but nobody sees me." He does not add, "People come to hear me, but nobody hears me." He should have added that, too! Because many people used to go to him and ask, "Babuji, what should I do in such and such a situation?" And even before he answers, they are talking to the friend who had just come with them.

Babuji, you know, is about to answer; then he looks at him and starts smoking his hookah, because there is no use! People want to ask questions, but don't want to receive the answers, because they know the answers! It is not as if we don't know the answer when we ask questions. We know the answer. Because we don't like the answer given by our heart, we ask somebody else, hoping that he will give a different answer. But when you go to the Master, you know he can give you only one possible answer; so, you talk to your neighbour and avoid getting the answer. You have asked the questions, your duty is done. You have not received the answer, your interests are fulfilled. You can go back home, self-satisfied, with a *laddu* or something which you buy in the market, and which has been offered as *prasad*. So, our sadhana remains! And the years that we have spent in sadhana (I mean mostly, I won't say by all, but by most of us, most of the time) are frittered away like this in foolish fantasies, in self-delusion; thinking that the Master is happy with us because we have paid three visits to him, we have had the prasad offered to Lalaji, we have asked him the proper question. Our interest is satisfied because we have not heard the answers; therefore, we are not committed to listen to anything; to doing anything. He is there, we are here. The whole thing is being ritualized into another idol *puja*, idol worship, temples!

I want to tell once again what I have been telling everywhere– that temple worship is popular not because we are *bhakthas*. It is popular because there we have a form of God, who is fixed, who is immovable, and who is where He is. He can be left there conveniently, to be visited occasionally at our choice, when the need is there, bribe Him with a coconut and two bananas, conscience salved, come back home and start writing your black accounts or doing your misdeeds all over again–in the hope, sometimes with the conviction, that "My duty to God is fulfilled, so He cannot possibly harm me!"

So, the tendency to make an idol out of the Master and a temple out of his residence continues, not because we don't know what we are doing, but because it is the most useful way in which we have to attack religion. "Leave him where he is; to be called up, to be called upon, when we need"–with minimum expense to him, with minimum expense to ourselves. No commitments on either side. Society is satisfied. Relations are happy. "My husband is a God-fearer. He goes to the temple every morning." Friends say, "You have not seen him, Sir! He does nothing without going to the temple." And we hope God is satisfied with these explanations that, "he is a true bhaktha; because, all said and done, he does visit me once in a way!" Because Krishna says very conveniently in the Gita, "Even if you think of Me, I am there." One Telugu speaker once told me, "When you say Rama, even when you say 'Ra', He comes because in Telugu, 'Ra' means come!" You see how convenient we have made these languages, and these names, to fool ourselves. No God is fooled.

We have become adepts at fooling ourselves, cheating ourselves, deluding ourselves. And these *Sampradayas* of the past, these traditions of our society, have been inculcated in us, which we accept longingly, willingly, because they are beneficial to us to continue our life of corruption, of ease, without doing anything about it ; and yet having a conscience!

Today even black marketeers say, you know, "I have done no harm, Sir! Why does this thing come to me?" I don't know what exactly they mean by 'doing no harm', when a man sells rice at twenty-five rupees a kilo in times of famine and considers it 'no harm', but genuine and legitimate profit. You see, we have perverted even the idea of morality, that "when I do something with my money and it earns me a profit, however high, it is legitimate!"

So, we have twisted our ideas of morality, to suit our morals. We are not living by moral principles. We have twisted moral principles to suit the standard of life that we are living. If somebody says, "Why are you drinking?" "Sir, everybody is doing it today. Who is not drinking?" "Why are you cheating?" "Who is not cheating?" "Why did you bribe the minister?" "Sir, today nothing can be done without bribery, you try it!" You see how easy, how facile this is–that 'everybody is doing it, and so I am also doing it.' I mean, when you say everybody is going to hell, you are also to be prepared. You have lost your breath. There is a wailing on your back, and also on your front. Then he says, "But what have I done that everybody else is not doing?" They are genuinely bewildered, you see. "How can I be singled out for punishment?" But they don't understand that all the others also are being similarly punished–not by any Deity, but by themselves–because you have your conscience which you have to answer; this is God.

So, that brings me to the concluding aspect of spirituality, "What is God? Where is God?" It is not as if there is somebody sitting in heaven, you know, waiting to say, "This you did–it is wrong. This you did; it is right!" That God who is going to be answered by me, and whom I have to answer without fail, whom even death cannot escape, is here, in my heart, my conscience; which, when it develops we call the higher Self, the Divine Self; which is the Master seated in the heart. Him I cannot escape, because He is within me! I need not go to a temple, or I can go deliberately at one o'clock when I know it is closed and say, "Sir, I made every effort to go there; but the temple was closed. What can

I do?" But this temple is never closed! And here, the God who lives, resides in me, is my Self, as He should be. This is what I am, as I am now.

So, we have the two ends, an enormous stick of life–the Divine end coiled up within my corrupt human self, telling me from inside, "This is what you have to become. Don't do this. Don't do that!" And we coolly say, "Shut up! My priest says I can do this because I have given him a hundred rupees donation. My doctor says, 'No harm in drinking, the cirrhosis of the liver is far away.' Who the hell are you to tell me from here? Shut up!"

So, we have shut our hearts up, and because our hearts are closed, we have become incapable of love, we are incapable of honesty, we are incapable of charity, mercy, all the values associated with human life. Therefore, a Master has to come to open the hearts up, with his first transmission. And then come all these problems. People who come genuinely, they stop after some time, because they now find the heart is open. It is a terrible thing, you see. It says, "Love," and he doesn't want to love! It says, "Give," and he doesn't want to give! It says, "Be honest," and he doesn't want to be honest! And some of them come and ask us, "Sir, what shall I do? You know, so long I have done this and this and this and it has given me so much profit. I also made a donation when I went to Babuji, you see. But this year what shall I do, because I feel that this is wrong?" And, if you tell him, "It is wrong," he says, "I didn't come to you for that answer! If you had told me 'Double the donation, multiply it ten times, a hundred times,' I would have been willing to do it." He would like me to say, "Go ahead. This is after all a worldly thing. See, there is no God in judgement." But how can I tell him that, when his heart is telling him that he is wrong, though I may be willing to co-operate with him.

Suppose a big businessman says, "Sir, I am willing to give you ten lakhs this year out of my profits, if you will permit me to do black marketing". Even supposing I am prepared to say "Yes," his heart does not permit him. Therefore, he dies of heart attack after two years! The heart just stops! It says, "My dear friend, I have co-operated with you for forty-eight years. Last three years, I have been telling you again and again, 'Don't do this, don't do this, don't do this.' You have not listened to my voice! I might as well not work, not be with you." It stops and the man is dead. Hearts don't stop for nothing. They stop when we allow them to speak, and we don't listen. It is like an advice, you know; you go to a friend repeatedly and ask, "What should I do?" And he tells you the advice and you don't listen to him. Next time when you go, and he says, "Well, you see, what is the use of this coming to me again and again? I have told you so many times that you should know it. It is better our relationship is not spoiled. Better you don't ask me!" Our friendship is gone. Now, this friendship, the most intimate friendship on which my life depends, on which my future eternal life depends, that stops! Because I don't listen to this voice which is my most intimate friend, who is my real lover, who is my real God; and one day He goes to sleep. And He goes to sleep eternally!

So, if we want to be spiritual, let us learn to listen, let us learn to hear what is being said, translate it into practice fearlessly! Because you know, this is the only path which is fearless. Everywhere else, it is a fear. "When I do something wrong, I have got to be afraid not of somebody else, but of myself, that I should not repeat it in a bigger way, you see!" A man who has committed a murder once does not bother about a second murder. It becomes very easy. His sin, his capacity to sin, his capacity to do vicious things, increases. And concurrently, the voice of the conscience decreases, so that one day he becomes the utmost, the absolute sinner, and the conscience is totally silent. There are no allowances made any more. And at that stage, forgive me if I say it, I beg to differ from all the spiritual leaders who have said, "At any moment a man can be redeemed." I believe when a man is a total sinner and he has no conscience at all, it is my conviction that he is beyond redemption. So, at least let us stop before we reach that limit!

I would also be pardoned for saying that our satsangh is not composed of saints. I mean, saints have no business here. If they are saints, they should not be here. It is precisely because we are not saints, we are here, hoping that some day we will achieve that level; but we have to work for it; we have to start listening carefully, we have to start practising carefully; set all fears aside, of what will happen to this beautiful life of mine, my bungalows, my cars, all these things, you see. Everything has to go, if it has to go! If Master is benevolent, benevolent enough to say, "Well, keep it; I shall allow you to keep it and yet progress," that is our good fortune! If not, we have to be prepared to let all these things go.

That utmost sacrifice has to be made, that "I am prepared to sacrifice all the comfort, all the joys, all the pleasures of this life, for that one thing which is Eternal, Immutable, Absolute." So if this conviction is not there, spiritual value has no meaning, spiritual life has no meaning.

Thank you.

Glossary

ABHIMANYU: Arjuna's son.
ABHYAS: Practice.
ABHYASI: Aspirant; one who practises yoga in order to achieve union with God.
ACHARYA: Guru, teacher, usually spiritual.
ADHARMA: Unrighteousness, opposite of dharma.
ADHIKARI: One who has authority.
ADI GURU: Original Guru; Lalaji, in Sahaj Marg.
ADI-SESHA: The Lord of Serpents upon which Vishnu reclines.
ADITYA: Sun-god. One of the powers of Nature.
ADVAITA (ADWAITA): State of unity (non-duality).
ADVAITA PHILOSOPHY: The Philosophy of Non-dualism i.e. all creation is manifestation of ONE truth.?
AGAMI: A body of spiritual literature dealing with temple rituals, temple architecture, etc.
AGASTHYA: Ancient eminent sage or rishi of India.
AGASTYA MUNI: Celebrated saint of ancient India.
AGNI: Fire, the fire element or principle.
AGYA CHAKRA (or AGNYA CHAKRA): The fire point located between the eyebrows. Trikuti.
AHAM BRAHMASMI: I am Brahma.
AHANKAR/A: Ego, or sense of "I", "I-ness".
AHIMSA: Non-violence.
AJAPA: Meditation without utterance of any mantra.
AKASHA: Space, sky. The space element or principle.
AKBAR: Moghul Emperor who ruled in the 16th century.
ANADI: Without beginning.
ANANDA: Bliss.
ANAHAT/A: Sound which cannot be heard. Literally, 'not hit.'
ANIRUDDHA: Grandson of Lord Krishna.

ANTARYAMIN: The God within; the In-Dweller.

ANUBHAVA: Intuitional perception or personal experience in the realm of Nature or God.

ARCHA: The external form of the deity as we worship Him in temples, churches, and so on.

ARJUNA: One of the five Pandava princes in the Indian epic Mahabharata and to whom Krishna gave the lessons of Gita before the war.

ASAN/A: Posture, usually yogic.

ASHRAM/A: A place of spiritual retreat.

AULIA: A saint in the Islamic tradition.

ATMAN: Soul.

ASHTANGA YOGA: Patanjali's system of Raja Yoga, having eight limbs: yama, niyama, asana, pranayama, pratyahara, dharana, dhyana and samadhi.

AVADHOOTA: Generally revered as elevated souls, but are really persons with spiritual aspirations who have become 'fixed' at a certain level because their development has been arrested.

AVADHOOTA-GATI: Stage or condition of avadhoota.

AVARANA: Layers of grossness; coverings.

AVATAR: Incarnation of a Divine soul.

AVATARA PURUSHA: Referred to a person having qualities of an Avatar.

AVIDYA: Ignorance.

AVYAKTA GATI: Indifferent state. State where one is completely liberated from Maya limitations. Inexpressible condition.

AYODHYA: Birthplace of Lord Rama.

BADAAM: Almond.

BAITHAK: A seat; sitting place; an assembly.

BANASURA: A demon whose daughter married Aniruddha, and who was killed by Krishna.

BAQA: Spiritual state given by guru to disciple in which the two become very close. See SAYUJYATA.

BASANT PANCHAMI: Birthday of Lalaji Maharaj; fifth day of spring in the lunar calendar.

BHAGAT ROOP: Devotional form.

BHAGAVAD GITA: "Song of God". An essential scripture of Hinduism, containing the portion of the Mahabharata in which Lord Krishna transmits divine knowledge to the warrior Arjuna on the battlefield just before the start of the Mahabharata war.

BHAGAWATAM: Scriptures of Ancient India, containing stories of Lord Krishna.

BHAGWATI: Wife of Babuji Maharaj.

BHAJAN: Chanted prayer.

BHAKTI: Devotion.

BHAKTI YOGA: The Yoga of Devotion, according to which, "Oneness" can be achieved through love and devotion to God.

BHANDARA: A spiritual gathering or celebration.

BHARATA: Half-brother of Rama, in the Ramayana.

BHARAT VARSHA: India.

BHAVAN: Abode.

BHIMA: One of the five Pandava princes in the Mahabharata.

BHINDI: Okra or ladies-finger vegetable.

BHISHMA: Grand-uncle of the Pandavas and the Kauravas in the Mahabharata.

BHOG/A/AM: Process of undergoing effects of impressions; experience; enjoyment.

BHUMI : Land or this world.

BHUTAS: See PANCHA BHUTAS.

BIJ DAGDHA: Literally, 'burnt seed.' Refers to a spiritual condition in which root causes have been removed ('fried') by the guru's grace so that the same responses will not germinate when old situations or temptations are encountered.

BRAHMA/N: God as Creator or Centre; God; Ultimate.

BRAHMANA: In this context, one who is Brahmin by caste.

BRAHMACHARYA/S: Student phase of life; celibacy, literally "like Brahman".

BRAHMANANDA: An Indian saint, contemporary of Vivekananda.

BRAHMANDA: Brahmanda Mandal, or Cosmic Region in Sahaj Marg.

BRAHMANDA MANDAL (or BRAHMANDA DESH): Mental sphere, supramaterial sphere, cosmic region; sphere where everything manifests under a subtle shape before taking place in the material world.

BRAHMARANDHRA: A point or opening in the crown of the head.

BRAHMASTRA: Brahma's weapon.

BRAHMA LOKA: World or realm of the Divine.

BRAHMA SUTRAS: Divine Scriptures

BRAHMA VIDYA: Knowledge of or about the Brahman.

BRAHMIN: One of the castes of Indian social system—the learned people (usually learned in the scriptures).

BRINDAVAN: City in U.P. where Lord Krishna spent his childhood.

BUDDHA GAYA: Place in Bihar, India, where Buddha obtained enlightenment.

BUDDHI: Intellect.

CHAITANYA MAHAPRABHU: A Vaishnavite saint from East Bengal who lived in the 15th Century A.D. Also, one who preached and practiced Bhakti Yoga.

CHAKRA: Centre of super-vital forces located in different parts of the body, figuratively called lotus.

CHAKRA TIRTHA TANK: Name of pond in Neemsar where pilgrims take holy bath.

CHAKRA VYOOHA: Military formation in the form of a wheel. From the Mahabharata.

CHANDRAMA: Moon.

CHELA: Student or disciple.

CHINTAK: Thinker; thinking or reflecting upon.

CHINTAK VASTU: Object of thought.

CHIT/TA: Consciousness.

CHIT LAKE: Another name for Brahmanda Mandal.

CHITRAGUPTA: An Indian Emperor.

CRORE: Ten million.

DAKSHINA: South. Also the offering by disciple to guru for training received. (Guru dakshina.)

DAKSHINAYANA: The six months of the sun's southern path.
DARSHANA: Vision of someone's inner Reality or vision of God.
DASARATHA: Father of Lord Rama; great king of the solar dynasty.
DASAVATARA: Ten Incarnations of Lord Vishnu, namely, Matsya, Kurma, Varaha, Narashimha, Vamana, Parasurama, Rama, Balarama, Krishna and Kalki.
DAYALROOP: Embodiment of compassion; a form of God.
DAYAL SHAKTI: Power of compassion.
DEVA/TA: A god. Also, refers to Divinity, or Cosmic personality.
DEVA VANI: Divine voice.
DHANUSHKOTI: An island in the southernmost part of India near Rameswaram, now submerged in the sea. A holy place.
DHANVANTARIJI: The physician of the gods. Said to have sprung from the ocean when the gods and demons churned it.
DHARANA: Mental focus, determination; sixth limb of Patanjali's yoga.
DHARMA: A term with many applications, depending on the context: duty; righteousness; destined way; truth; virtue; duty, that which upholds.
DHARMA SHASTRA: Dharmic literature; specifically, scriptures dealing with codes of conduct.
DHARMAPUTRA: Eldest of the five Pandava brothers in the Maha Bharata. (Also called Yudhisthira.)
DHOBI-GHAT: place on riverbanks where clothes are washed.
DHOTI: A long cloth worn by men, tucked around the waste.
DHRUVA (DHRUV PAD): Highly evolved soul. First or lowest level of cosmic functionary. Below the Dhruvadhipati.
DHRUVADHIPATI: Godly functionary of great calibre who directs the work of the Dhruvas. Below the Parishad.
DHYANA: Meditation; seventh limb of Patanjali's yoga.
DRAUPADI: In the Mahabharata, wife of the five Pandava brothers.
DURVASA: An ancient saint noted for his sharp temper.
DURYODHANA: In the Mahabharata, eldest of the 100 Kaurava brothers. His refusal to compromise with the Pandavas led to war.

DVAITA: Duality. Also refers to certain schools of philosophy that do not believe in the Supreme Oneness, but in the co-existence of Positve and Negative, Good and Bad etc.

DVANDAS (DWANDWAS): Dualities. The pairs of opposites (e.g., good-bad, pleasure-pain, etc.).

DWAPARA: Third of the four yugas or ages of the worlds, which generally represent a slow degradation from original purity into darkness. The first yuga is the Satya Yuga, in which wisdom and virtue reign. The second is the Treta Yuga, followed by the Dwapara Yuga. Our time occurs within the Kali Yuga, mythically the final and most depraved age, characterized by passion and cruelty, which will bring on the end of the entire universe and give rise to the next Mahayuga, or cycle of yugas.

DWARAKADHISH: Lord Krishna at Dwaraka in Gujarat.

EKAGRA VRITTI: Tendency to fix our attention on one thing at a time.

EKKA: Horsecart with single seat (one seater).

FAKIR: In Islamic tradition, a saint. One who has renounced the world, like the sannyasi of the Hindu tradition.

FAKIRI: Spritual state or condition of the fakir.

FATEHGANJ: District in Fatehgarh.

FATEHGARH: Birthplace of Lalaji Maharaj. City in Uttar Pradesh about sixty kilometres from Shahjahanpur.

GANDEEVA: The Divine bow of Arjuna.

GANDHIJI: Mahatma Gandhi.

GANGA: The holy river Ganges; the goddess embodied as the Ganges.

GANGA YAMUNI: A level of transmission from Lord Krishna.

GARHI: Hindu astrological unit of time, equivalent to about 2.5 seconds.

GAYA: Place in Bihar where Buddha attained enlightenment under the Bo tree.

Glossary

GAYATHRI: Shri P. Rajagopalachari's home in Madras, named after the Gayathri mantra.

GHAT: Steps and bathing place along rivers in India.

GHAZAL: An Urdu poetic form, a poem of love.

GITA (GEETA): Song. Usually a shorthand reference to the Bhagavad Gita, or "Song of God". (See above.)

GNANI: See JNANI.

GNANA YOGA: See JNANA YOGA.

GOPIS: Milkmaids or cowherds of Brindavan devoted to Lord Krishna.

GOTRA: Persons belonging to the same Gotra have common ancestery. There are only sixteen Gotras in India.

GOVARDHAN: A hill near Mathura. This hill was lifted by one finger of Lord Krishna to provide protection to the cowherds from severe rains.

GRANTHI: Knot.

GRIHASTH/A: One who leads a worldly life, a householder.

GRIHASTHA ASHRAMA: Conditions of a household life.

GUNAS: Qualities. In Hindu philosophy, the three qualities of nature: *sattava, rajas* and *tamas.*

GURU: Spiritual teacher. Master who transmits light, knowledge.

GURUDAKSHINA: See DAKSHINA.

GURUDOM: As used by Babuji, this pejorative term refers to the ancient guru-disciple tradition in its imitative or degenerate form, in which the "guru" claims privileges and honours and fees from his followers, who must in turn become sycophants or dependent children, not independently loving devotees.

GURU NANAK SAHIB: Great saint who founded Sikhism.

GURU PASHU: One who is attached to the guru's physical form, almost to the point of addiction.

GYANAKANDA: The Chapter of Knowledge.

GYANI: See JNANI.

HAJIS: In Islam, devotees who have visited Mecca.

HAKIM: Physician, medical doctor.

HANUMANJI MAHARAJ: Hanuman, monkey devotee of Lord Rama; a god in the Hindu pantheon.
HARIDWAR: Religious pilgrimage site in foothills of Himalayas.
HARDA: See ANTARYAMIN.
HATHA YOGA: The first four steps of Patanjali's Ashtanga yoga. The practice of yoga concerning the body.
HATHAYOGI: One who practises and/or has mastered hatha yoga.
HAZRAT BAQI BILLAH: Muslim saint.
HAZRAT MOHAMMED: The Prophet. ("Hazrat" is an honourific title of great respect.)
HOLI: Hindu festival of colours celebrated annually each March. Symbolic of end of evil and also beginning of spring.
HOOKAH/HUKKA: A water-pipe or hubble-bubble. Babuji's favorite smoking device.
HRIDYA CHAKRA: Heart plexus.

INDRA: Ruler of Devas, or powers of nature.
INDRIYAS: Ten sense organs of Indian philosophy: Jnana indriyas¾the five senses pertaining to perception, knowledge or wisdom; and karma indriyas¾the five senses pertaining mainly to action.
INVERTENDO: Term coined by Shri Ram Chandra (Babuji) to describe the apparent inversion Truth undergoes as it moves through higher levels of abstraction.
ISHA: God, as Ruler.
ISHAANA: God who rules over the northeast; northeast direction.
ISHTA-DEVATA: A God who is worshipped.
ISHWARA (ISHVARA): Determinate Absolute. God as Existence endowed with all the most subtle attributes.

JAGIR: Ancestral property; estate by government granted for meritorious service.
JAINISM: A religious sect, initiated by Mahavira, known for non-violence and disciplined life.
JAMUNA: The holy river Yamuna.

JANAKA (RAJA JANAK): A raja rishi, a king who excelled in yogic discipline, considered to be the greatest example of the idea of human living, where the material and spiritual excellence meet. He was the father of Seeta, wife of Lord Rama.

JANMA: Birth.

JANMASHTAMI: Birthday of Lord Krishna.

JAPA: Repetition of a mantra.

JEEVAN MUKTI (also JIVAN MOKSHA): liberation while one is still living, or more precisely, incarnated in a human body.

JIVA: Individual incarnated soul; life.

JIVATMA: Soul embodied in body.

JNANA: Supreme wisdom or knowledge leading to Realisation.

JNANA YOGA: Attainment of liberation through the path of divine knowledge.

JNANI: Gnostic; one who has Divine knowledge.

KAAL: Time.

KAAL-CHAKRA: Time wheel, said to be the original source from which avatars descend.

KAAL ROOP: Destructive form of avatars.

KAAL SHAKTI: Destructive power.

KABIR: Saint Kabir, the great poet and sage claimed by both Hindus and Muslims. Kabir lived in Varanasi (Benares).

KABIRI: Spiritual condition, pertaining to Kabir.

KALI YUGA: The present yuga, last of the four yugas. See Dwapara.

KALPA: Age or eon.

KALYANA PURUSHA: A person who rectifies a degraded society.

KAMA: Desire.

KANTHA CHAKRA: Throat plexus (vishuddha chakra).

KARANA SHARIR: Causal body.

KARMA: Action, deeds.

KARMA BHOOMI: World of action.

KARMA KANDA: Ritualistic practice of the Vedas.

KARMA-PHALA: Fruits or rewards or results of action.

KAYASTHA: A Hindu sub-caste of clerks and scribes to which both Lalaji and Babuji belonged.

KOSHA: Sheath. The five sheaths that contain the essence and together comprise a human being are the food-sheath, breath-sheath, mind-sheath, knowledge-sheath and bliss-sheath.

KOTHI: Building or dwelling.

KRISHNA: Lord Krishna; most recent incarnation of Vishnu; divine personality in the Mahabharata.

KRISHNA CHAKRA: A Divine weapon used in the Mahabharata; Krishna's wheel.

KRIYA: Action or procedure, usually ritualistic.

KRODHA: Anger.

KSHATRIYA: One of the four major castes of India. The warrior caste. The others are: Brahmin (priest), Vaishya (merchant), and Sudra (worker).

KSHOB: The original impetus which upset the equilibrium and caused the creation of the universe; original "stir" caused by the will of God to effect creation.

KUBERA: Mythic Lord of wealth; one of the powers of nature.

KUBJA: A pilgrimage site near Brindavan; literally 'hump-backed'.

KULA-DEVA: Family god.

KUMBHA MELA: Religious fair held once every twelve years in Allahabad.

KUNDALINI: A coiled knot, which if uncoiled, awakens divine knowledge.

KURTA: Indian dress, long shirt almost upto the knees.

KURUKSHETRA: The battlefield where the war between the Pandavas and the Kurus took place, in the Mahabharata.

LAILA: Beloved of Majnu in Persian poems and tales; Majnu represents the devotee and Laila the Divine.

LAKH: Hundred thousand.

LAKSHMAN JHOOLA: A bridge across the Ganges in Rishikesh; a holy site.

LAKSHMI: Lord Vishnu's consort; Goddess of Wealth.

LAKSHMI KUND: Round hole in the ground for receiving and preserving water; here named for Lakshmi, it is a holy place located near Rameswaram.

LANKA: Previously called Ceylon, now known by its ancient name of Sri Lanka.

LAYA: Mergence, dissolution; hence, release or liberation.

LAYA AVASTHA: The state of complete mergence whereby two become One.

LOBHA: Greed.

LOKA: A world or region.

MAHABHARATA: Great moral and philosophical epic of Indian culture and world literature, it tells of the dynastic struggle between the Kurus and the Pandavas, two branches of a single ruling family.

MAHA-KAAL: Original source from which avatars descend.

MAHAMAYA: Subtle energy used by the Divine—Great Maya or great illusion. The spiritual sphere from which avatars come.

MAHA PARISHAD: The highest cosmic functionary; Ruler of the Universe.

MAHA PRALAYA: State of complete dissolution when everything in existence merges with the Centre. The complete dissolution of the whole universe.

MAHARAJ: Literally, 'great king.' Term used to express respect for an elevated soul.

MAHASAMADHI: The final samadhi when a saint renounces his body and enters the brighter world.

MAHATMA: Great soul, saint.

MAHAVAKYAS: Great sayings.

MAHAYUGA: The four Yugas—Satya, Treta, Dwapar and Kali together make a Mahayuga (4.32 million years).

MAHESH: Lord Shiva.

MAJNU: Lover of Laila (see LAILA).

MANAS: Psyche, mind.

MANASA LAKE: The lake of the mind; Manasarovar; another name for the Brahmanda Mandal.

MANOMAYA KOSHA: Mind-sheath. The realm of the mind.

MANTRA: Sacred sound, word, or phrase.

MANU: Mythological father of the human race. There are supposed to be fourteen Manus, and the seventh is said to be the founder of the present race of living beings and also the founder of the solar race of kings.

MAYA: Phenomenal appearance. It is really a power of God. All manifestation or expansion which seems illusory is the play of Maya. Illusion.

MECCA: City in Arabia, birthplace of Lord Mohammed, and place of pilgrimage for all devout Muslims.

MEERA BAI: Female saint and great devotee of Lord Krishna. She accepted poison and drank it as prasad to her beloved Lord.

MOHA: Attachment; hence, delusion.

MOKSHA: Enlightenment.

MOORTHI (MURTHI): An idol.

MUKTI: Liberation from the physical plane of existence or in other words, freedom from the bondage of rebirth.

MUNI: See RISHI.

MUNSARIM: Title of record-keeper in a court.

MUNSIF: Magistrate in a court.

NACHIKETAS: An Indian saint whose name appears in the Upanishads.

NAKULA: One of the five Pandavas of the Mahabharata.

NARADA: A celestial sage; devotee of Narayan (Shiva).

NARAKA: Hell.

NARAYANA: Another term for the Supreme God.

NARENDRA: Vivekananda's given name. Literally God of People.

NETI, NETI: "Not this, not this" (from Keno Upanishad). A formulaic expression indicating that one cannot place boundaries or definitions around the Absolute.

NIRGUNA: Without attributes or qualities.

NIRVANA: Illuminated state.

NIRVIKALPA: Samadhi in which there is loss of world-consciousness.

NISHKAM KARMA: Work without attachment to the result; desireless action.

GLOSSARY 437

OM (or AUM): Sacred syllable, untranslatable fundamental universal sound, basis of many mantrams.

PAATAAL: Netherworld. The region of Sesha (serpents).
PAL: A minute of astrological time.
PANCHA BHUTAS: The five elements or principles in Hindu cosmology: earth, water, fire, air and space.
PANDAS: Priests at religious festivals.
PANDAVAS: The five sons of King Pandu in the Mahabharata.
PANDIT: Learned person, traditionally well versed in the scriptures, lately, well versed in any subject.
PANDIT NEHRU: Jawaharlal Nehru, became first Prime Minister of India in 1947.
PARA: Transcendental; beyond.
PARA BRAHMAN: Indeterminate Absolute; God as the Ultimate Cause of Existence.
PARABRAHMANDA: Supra-cosmic consciousness.
PARALOKA: The other world; heaven.
PARAMANANDA: One of the swamis of India who preached yoga.
PARAMANUS: Subtle particles.
PARAMARTH: The highest knowledge.
PARAMATMAN: The Supreme Soul; God.
PARISHAD: Cosmic functionary below the Maha Parishad who directs the work of the Dhrubadipatis.
PASHU: Animal; one enslaved to animalistic tendencies.
PATANJALI: Composer of Yoga Sutras and explicator of Ashtanga Yoga.
PINDA (PIND): Material or gross existence, that which exists in the gross or material state.
PIND DESH (or PINDA PRADESH): Material sphere; the heart region.
PIPAL: A species of fig tree in India, considered one of the holy trees.
PRAKRITI: Nature or creation.
PRALAYA: State of dissolution, applied not to the whole universe but only to a part of it.

PRANA: Life, breath.

PRANAHUTI: Process of yogic transmission by a realized Master. Derived from *prana* meaning life and *ahuti* which means offering. Offering of the life force by the Guru into the disciple's heart.

PRANAMAYA KOSHA: Breath sheath.

PRANASYA PRANA: Life of life.

PRANAYAMA: The regulation of prana (breath). Derived from *prana*–life, vital breath, and *ayama*–to restrain.

PRASAD: Divinized food, usually sweet; an offering to Master or God.

PRASTHANA TRAYEE: The three orthodox scriptural books of the hindus; viz., the Upanishads, the Bhagavad Gita and the Brahma Sutras.

PRATYAHARA: The inner withdrawal of the mind; the fifth branch of Patanjali's yoga

PUJA: Religious traditional practice (in Sahaj Marg, the meditation practice).

PUJYA: Revered, respected; used as an honourific before a great man's name.

PURANAS: Ancient Indian scriptures.

PURUSHA: Male; personality or entity. In this sense, God is the adi-purusha or Original Personality, and an avatar is a yuga-purusha or personality of the age. Unlike atma or soul, which has no subtle substance and is never born and never dies, purusha has substance and is made and can come to termination.

RABI'A: A major saint in the Sufi tradition, living in the seventh century B.C.

RADHA: Lord Krishna's beloved consort and primary devotee.

RADHA KUND: See LAKSHMI KUND. This Kund is located in Brindavan.

RAJA: King.

RAJA YOGA: Another name for Ashtanga Yoga. Ancient system or science followed by the great rishis and saints which helped them to realise the Self or God. Hatha yoga is considered a subset of Raj Yoga. Hatha yoga prepares one for the higher steps of Raja Yoga, i.e., meditation and samadhi. Sahaj Marg is considered Modified Raja Yoga, wherein meditation is treated as the first step.

RAJA YOGI: One who practises Raja Yoga.

RAJAS: One of the three gunas - the quality of action and passion.

RAJPUTANA: Old name for Rajasthan, a state in India.

RAMA: An incarnation of Lord Vishnu, who destroyed the demon Ravana. Also, the husband of Seeta in the Indian epic story Ramayana.

RAMAKRISHNA: Saint who lived in Calcutta in the nineteenth century. Credited with revivifying spirituality in India. He was the teacher of Swami Vivekananda.

RAMANUJA: One of the three acharyas; founder of the Vashishtadvaita system of Vedanta philosophy.

RAMAYANA: One of the two great epics of India (the other being the Mahabharata), in which is recounted the life of Rama, prince of righteousness. Also considered a religious epic about Rama as avatar.

RAMESWARAM: Pilgimage place in southern India.

RAM KUND: See LASKMI KUND. This is located near Rameswaram.

RAMZAN: Month in Muslim calendar in which the Ramadan observance occurs.

RAS-LILA: Divine dance of Lord Krishna with his gopis in which each felt He was dancing only with her, when Krishna was dancing really only with Radha.

RAVANA: Demon in the Ramayana who carries off Sita to Lanka. The Ramayana is the tale of Rama's quest to rescue Sita and conquer Ravana.

RISHI: Saint; seer; one who has realised Self.

RISHIKESH: Holy city in Himalayan section of Uttar Pradesh.

RUDRA: Name for the aspect of Shiva as Destructor.

SADHAKA: Disciple who practises a sadhana.

SADHANA: Spiritual practice.

SADHU: Religious or spiritual person.

SAGUNA BRAHMAN: God as Existence endowed with all the most subtle attributes. Determinate Absolute.

SAHAJ MARG: Natural path.

SAHAJ SAMADHI: Natural samadhi, considered the highest samadhi: simultaneity of total awareness with total inner emptiness of absorption.

SAMADHI: Original balance. State in which we stay attached to Reality. In Sahaj Marg, the return to the original condition, which reigned in the beginning. Babuji split the word into *sama*, meaning balance, and *adhi*, meaning original or ancient.

SAMARTH GURU: A perfect guru, who possesses all the qualities. A perfectly balanced guru.

SAMPATTI: A type of human realisation. In Sahaj Marg it is also the depth of the spiritual realisation.

SAMSKARAS: Impressions; grossness. In Sahaj Marg philosophy, believed to be the cause of all experience (good or bad) in the physical world. Removal of Samskaras is considered a goal of the Sahaj Marg practice.

SANATANA DHARMA: Universal Religion, i.e., not specific to a particular God or Master.

SANDHYA: Meeting point between day and night.

SANKALPA: An impetus of will.

SANKIRTANS: Congregational chants.

SANJAYA: Sage who reported the progress of the war between the Pandavas and the Kurus to the blind king Dhritarashtra, father of the hundred Kaurava brothers.

SANNYASA: Renunciation, vows of sannyasis.

SANNYASI: One who has renounced the world and leads a solitary life of celibacy and asceticism.

SANSTHA: Spiritual tradition, organisation, group.

SARUPYA: Identicality of form.

SARVAMUKTI: Simultaneous universal emancipation.

SAT: Being, Reality, Existence.

SATGATI: State of mergence in Sat, Reality.

SATPAD (SATYAPAD): Literally, The Path of Truth. In Sahaj Marg, state which is neither lightness nor darkness. It is a reflection of the Reality which itself is still further.

SATSANGH: Spiritual assembly; being with reality. In Sahaj Marg, group meditation.

SATSANGHI: One who attends satsangh.

SATYA YUGA: First yuga of a cycle, the yuga of truth and righteousness (see DWAPARA).

SAYUJYATA: Union with the divine, mergence of two into One.

SEETAKUND: Religious place near Rameswaram.

SHABDA (or AJAPA): Sound, inner vibration within, as opposed to japa.

SHAHJAHANPUR: City in Uttar Pradesh; birthplace and lifelong home of Babuji.

SHAIVAITE: Believers and worshippers of Lord Shiva.

SHANKARA: Great saint and scholar, an accomplished yogi who founded a new darshana, or school of thought, within the Sanatana Dharma, or Hinduism. (Also Shankaracharya.)

SHANTI: Peace.

SHASTRAS: Holy books, scriptures.

SHIVA: In the trinity of Hinduism, Shiva represents the destructive aspect of the Godhead.

SHLOKA: A verse.

SHRADDHA: Faith; devotion with faith.

SHREYAS: Spiritual practice.

SIDDHIS: Capacity to do miracles; powers.

SITA (SEETA): Wife of Rama, carried off by Ravana, in the Ramayana.

SMRITHI: Memory

SOODRA (SUDRA): The lowest caste.

SRAVAN: Hindu lunar month.

SRUTIS: Revelations of Vedas and all divine scriptures through direct communications from the Absolute to very high saints.

STHULA: Concrete existence; physical universe.

SUDARSHANA CHAKRA: Divine weapon of Lord Krishna. See KRISHNA CHAKRA.

SUFISM: The mystic science of the Moslems.
SWADHARMA: Duty as per hereditary affiliations.
SWADHISTANA CHAKRA: Second plexus or chakra.

TAM: The actual state we were in when the world was born. Real state of being.
TAMAS: One of the three gunas. Inertness. Leads to inactivity, sloth or procrastination.
TAPASYA: Ascetic practices to purify the soul and attract Divine grace. Literally means "heat", and indicates the heat generated by the friction of intense spiritual practice.
TAT: Literally "That". A neuter pronoun expressing the Indescribable Absolute.
TATTVAS: Elements or principles, essences of things, according to Hindu cosmology. (See PANCHA BHUTAS.)
TEJAS: Spiritual brilliance (outer or manifesting in contrast to the inner splendor termed *ojas*).
TIRIYA PASHU: One who is a slave of his own mind.
TONGA: A two-wheeled horse-drawn wagon.
TRIKUTI: Outer intersection of 'three points' formed by the bridge of the nose and two eyebrows where the inner ajna chakra is located.
TULSI: Basil; in India a plant of medical and religious value.
TULSIDAS: Sage who wrote the story of the Ramayana in Hindi, or Ram Charat Manas.
TURIYA: Fourth state of consciousness, the other three being: 1. Jagrat, the waking state; 2. Svapna, the dreaming state; and 3. Sushupti, deep sleep.
TURIYA AVASTHA: Fourth state of the soul, when it becomes one with God.

UPASANA: Devotional practice.
UPADESH: Sermon, instruction.
UPANISHAD: Portion of the Vedas which deals with knowledge of God. Said to be divine revelation.
UTSAV: Religious celebration.

Glossary

UTTAR PRADESH: State in Northern India where Babuji and Lalaji lived.

UTTARAYANA: Six months of the sun's northern path.

VAIRAGYA: Renunciation, detachment.

VALMIKI: Said to be the composer of the Ramayana in Sanskrit.

VARUNA: Mythic Lord of water; rivers, oceans, etc. A power of Nature.

VASISHTHA: Lord Rama and his brothers were sent for training under Sage Vasishtha.

VASISTH-ADVAITA: Advaita philosophy as propounded by Sage Vasishtha

VASU: Another name for Krishna. Also refers to cosmic functionary below the Dhruva, an elevated person who performs the lowest level of godly work entrusted to him.

VASUDEVA: Father of Lord Krishna.

VEDA PASHU: One who is addicted to the Vedas.

VEDAS: Ancient Indian sacred scriptures, in which a superior knowledge is revealed. Regarded by Hindus as the highest authority for all aspects of life—physical, mental and spiritual. Believed to be a synthesis of work done by rishis over hundreds of years. There is no particular author or these texts.

VIJNANMAYAKOSHA: Sheath of knowledge.

VIKARAS: Gross desires, impediments.

VIRAT: Cosmic.

VIRAT SHARIR: Cosmic Body.

VISHNU: One of the Hindu trinity¾God in his aspect of preserver and protector.

VISHVAMITRA: An ancient Indian sage.

VISHVAROOPA DARSHANA: Vision of the Lord's Cosmic form.

VIVEKA: Discernment or ability to discriminate between right and wrong.

VIVEKANANDA: (Swami Vivekananda.) Great saint of India who lived in the late nineteenth and early twentieth century, the first to bring Vedantism to the western world. Foremost disciple of Ramakrishna and a contemporary of Lalaji

VRITTIS: Outflow of mind; subtle desires or stimuli coming up in the mind causing action; mental tendencies.

VYASA: Compiler of the Vedas. Also gave the Mahabharata to mankind.

YAGNYAVALKYAJI: A rishi who is frequently quoted in the Upanishads.

YAMA: 1. As first step of Ashtanga Yoga - Self interdiction. Vow of abstinence of violence, falsity, robbery, unchastity, and tendency to acquire. 2. Lord of Death.

YATRA: Inner spiritual journey. Literally, voyage, journey, pilgrimage.

YOGA: A system of Hindu philosophy showing means of emancipation of the soul from further migration. From the word "yoke" meaning "connect" or "union". The state of yoga is the state of union of the soul with the ultimate divine soul. Any practice or sadhana that leads to the state of Yoga is also termed Yoga.

YOGASHRAM: A place where yoga is practised.

YOGI/N: One who practises yoga; one who achieves union with the Absolute. Yogi is masculin while Yogin feminine.

YUDHISHTIRA: See DHARMAPUTRA.

YUGA: Age or period, e.g., Satya Yuga, Kali Yuga. See DWAPARA.

ZAMINDARI: System of fiefdoms and land-holding in historical India.

Index

abhyas, 292
abhyasis, 126
achievement/s, 128, 369
action/s, 324, 338, 383, 385, 387
adharma, 334
admiration, 294
adoration, 237
advanced souls, 371-2
Archa, 23
Arjuna, 105, 204, 318
artificiality, 236
asana/s, 31, 54
asceticism, 19
Ashtanga Yoga, 14
aspirant, 88
aspiration, 250
atma/soul, 308
atmosphere, 135
attachment/s, 128, 172, 209
attention, 40, 52
attitude, 145
attributes, 292-3
  opposing, 321
Avaranas, 282
avarice, 111
avatar/a, 163, 405
awareness, 412

Babuji. *See* Ram Chandra of Shahjahanpur
balance, 75, 102, 108, 111, 112, 266, 329
barrier/s, 324, 332
beauty, 212

begging, 66
behaviour, 310, 350-2, 361
  pattern, 352
Bhagavad Gita, 97, 171, 318, 320
bhajan, 103, 104
bhakti yoga, 160
books, 277
brahmalaya, 308
brahmachari, 98
bribery, 414
brotherhood, 272-3, 350

callousness, 411
celibacy, 17
ceremony/shraddha, 303
change, 91, 277, 286, 298, 312-3, 362, 364-5, 376
  of humanity, 134
  in society, 134
chaos, 367
Chariji. *See* Rajagopalachari, Parthasarathi
chastity, 404
childhood, 245
children, 137, 313
choice, 378, 380, 382
civilization, 232
cleaning, 52, 55, 60, 63, 92, 93, 113, 121, 122, 178
cleanliness, 74
commitment, 299, 413, 416-7
compassion, 253
composite, 404
concentration, 52, 77, 85

concepts, 386-7
condition, 158, 274
conditioning, 397
conduit, 290
conscience, 41, 422
consciousness, 38, 41
constant remembrance, 299
co-operation, 51, 343, 364-5, 397
corruption, 355
craving, 234
creation, 280
   His, 281
criticism, 342

darshan, 202, 258, 260
death, 211
dedication, 299
demands, 133, 139
dependence, 87, 216, 218, 247
   total, 179
dependency, 215
desire/s, 59, 275, 320, 371
dharma, 317
differences, 272
direction, 109, 380
disciple, 180
discipline, 235, 350, 365-6
divine grace, 234
divinisation, seed of, 339
divinity, 277-8, 289, 317, 387, 406
divya shakti, 407
divya swaroopis, 406
double standard, 313
doubt, 168
duty/duties, 61, 209, 321, 373-4, 416

education, 68, 280, 333-4
ego/-ism, 89, 182
emotional sustenance, 28
energy, conservation of, 75

enjoyment of life, 102
escapism, 384
essence, 82, 308
eternal present, 61
eternity, 289, 390
eternity of the Master, 289
ethics, 41
evolution, 12, 68, 69, 378-81, 405
example, 351, 354
   setting an, 279
excess, 230, 231, 232
existence, 276, 372-5, 380, 407
experience/s, 116, 118, 119, 178, 396
external, 352-3

failure, 338
faith, 48, 168, 338, 340
   lack of, 274
false values, 321
father, 186, 187
fear/s, 5, 40, 146, 382, 422
fig tree, 370
five methods, 20
flattery, 327
force/s, 322, 382
   categories of, 322
form/s, 318, 332
   bound by, 332
   divine, 406
   divine manifestation, of, 163
   ultimate, 333
freedom, 131, 134, 215, 217, 356
friend/-ship, 248, 422
future, 383, 413

Ganga, 409
gaze/vision, 283
Gita. *See* Bhagavad Gita
gnana/wisdom, 284
goal, 20, 62, 78, 88, 90, 92, 100,

INDEX

157, 167, 207, 210, 276-8, 298, 374-5, 413, 414
God, 7, 20, 23, 30, 36, 41, 81, 97, 104, 160, 161, 164, 201, 223, 247, 248, 280, 315, 318, 337, 380, 382, 384-6, 391, 399-400, 408, 420, 422
   forms of, 4, 23, 82
   house of, 22
   like, 413
   seeking, 167
   will of, 380
gossip, 135
grace, 265
grossness, 75, 120, 127
growth, 133, 138
guru/s, 76, 94, 223, 252, 308, 309, 337, 380
gutter, 393

happiness, 174, 175
Harda, 23
hatha yoga, 14, 32
health, 341
heart, 7, 16, 43, 54, 104, 138, 334, 411, 416, 421
   of Master, 135
Hindu culture, 353
Hinduism, 353
hope, 298
humility, 89

ignorance, 38
illness, 342
impressions, 47, 51, 52, 53, 60, 61, 75, 76, 114, 121
India/-n, 353
   life, 353
   problem, 354
indiscipline, 349, 362
individual, 374

infinite, 73
infinity, 81, 86
inner, 351-2
   change, 361
   transformation, 353
instruments of the Master, 294
intellectuality, 127

Jesus Christ, 410
jhambavan, 290
journey, divine, 297
judge, 295, 394

Kabir, 408
Kant, 133
karma yoga, 14
Karna (in Mahabharata), 317, 319
Kasturi, Sister, 229
kindness, 321
knowledge, 116, 117, 118, 231, 280
Krishna, Lord, 39, 105, 165, 177, 204, 290, 317-8, 321, 332, 335
kundalini yoga, 14

Lalaji. *See* Ram Chandra of Fatehgarh
law of nature, 377
laya, 203
less-ness, 279
liberation, 384, 388
life, 253, 320, 407
light, 16, 78, 120
limitations, 414
Lord of the Universe, 320
loss, 340
love, 6, 29, 40, 41, 71, 97, 99, 100, 101, 118, 177, 187, 188, 189, 198, 205, 206, 210, 260, 272, 299, 313, 322, 328, 338, 371-2, 382

letter, 342
for Master, 159, 160

Mahabharata, 104
man, 25, 422
Master, 34, 88, 92, 94, 100, 114, 121, 123, 158, 159, 169, 180, 183, 185, 188, 207, 214, 215, 217, 226, 248, 253, 274, 316, 320, 325-7, 329, 393-4, 412, 419-21
  acceptance of, 278
  advice from, 139
  cooperation with, 158, 159
  divinity, 289
  health of, 135
  His life, 269, 272, 274
  knowing/understanding, 177
  love, 236
  need for, 53, 91
  physical form, 344
  praise, 392
  presence, 201, 202, 411
  reliance on, 10
  work, 221
Masters, type of, 46
mastery, 394
material
  existence, 108
  half, 265
  life, 19, 58, 109, 110, 112, 113
meditation, 15, 16, 23, 24, 32, 43, 53, 54, 62, 63, 71, 72, 77, 78, 84, 85, 154, 157, 158, 161, 162, 165, 208, 220, 264
  objects for, 120
  preparation for, 44
  purpose of, 53
  technique of, 46
mental development, 28
merger, 203

message
  of His Existence, 268
  of the Gita, 319
method, 184, 185
middle age, 247
mind, 42, 43, 44, 50, 84
  of the Hindu, 352
  powers of, 84
misconception, 271
miseries, 343
Mission, 184, 185
morality, 131
mukti, 405, 409
mysticism, 6, 23, 38, 154
mystics, 9, 81

Nature, 92, 167, 204, 382
  beauty of, 211, 212, 213
need/s, 25, 26, 27, 65, 371
non-attachment attachment, 61
normalisation
  of functions, 17

obedience, 99, 179, 366
old people, 314
opposites/dvandvas, 45, 171, 175
  pairs of, 173
organisation, spiritual, 291
outer, 351
  change, 361

pain, 342
papam/vice, 317
Para, 23
paratatva, 409
participation, 379
perception, 272, 283
perfection, 62, 212, 214
performance, 373
personality, 76, 143
  changes, 148

problems, 144
pleasures, 417
possession/s, 98, 184, 373
  material, 182, 183
poverty, 342
power/s, 126, 193, 287, 407-9
  of love, 336
practice, 265
praise, 328
prana prathishta, 155, 164
pranahuti, 55, 70, 86, 94, 308
pranasya prana, 33
prayer, 66, 153, 355
  aversion to, 65
  meaning of, 66
preaching, 354
preceptor/s, 72, 115, 225, 226, 227, 338, 410
  duty of, 125
prejudgement, 394
prejudice, 287
presence, 332, 409
present, 384
problem/s, 144, 263, 265
programme, erasing the, 276
progress, 274, 286, 323, 343, 369-70, 374, 381
promise, Master's, 339
punishing, 383
punishment, 382
punyam/virtue, 317, 319
purity, 98
purpose
  His, 284-5
  of life, 19

raja yoga, 15, 31, 42, 119, 161
Rajagopalachari, Parthasarathi
  fear, 147, 150, 151, 152
  incident, 151
  spiritual error, 226

Ram Chandra of Fatehgarh, 10, 160, 294, 406, 411
  associate of, 292
Ram Chandra of Shahjahanpur, 250, 304, 410-2, 415, 418
realisation, 104
reality, 236, 396, 400
Reality at Dawn, 277
reason, 168
religion/s, 5, 6, 8, 22, 29, 36, 80, 146, 162, 304, 306, 310, 382
  failure of, 8
  fear, 9
religious
  expression, 3
  laws, 37
  sentiment, 4
renunciation, 43, 45, 171
representative, 291, 293
research, 127
responsibility/ies, 390, 416
restlessness, 279
result/s, 212, 338
revelation, 318
reward/-ing, 190, 191, 382, 383
rich people, 358
ritual worship, 7

sacred inheritance, 300
sadhak, 414
sadhana, 158, 178, 191, 241, 255, 265, 335
Sahadeva, 335
Sahaj Marg, 10, 15, 18, 19, 55, 58, 120, 161, 162, 172, 180, 204, 209, 213, 214, 297, 308, 331, 383, 387, 401, 404, 409
  simplicity, 88
sahaj samadhi, 17
saints, 270, 422
samadhi, 17

samskara/s, 69, 126, 277, 281, 317, 379, 383
sankalpa, 83
Sarnadji, 376
scheme, 365
science, 124
search, 7
seeker, 89
self, aspect of, 347
self-deception, 265
selfishness, 136
service, 234, 254, 255, 326
  lowest, 393
  to Master, 240
shock/s, 303, 304-6
simplicity, 203, 220, 263-4
sin, 139
slavery, 217
sorrows, 269
souls, 372
Special Personality, 163, 297
spirit, 59
spiritual cleaning, 397
spiritual
  consciousness, 66
  evolution, 70
  growth, 339
  half, 265
  life, 108, 109, 110, 111, 112, 113
  mirrors, 277
  person, 284
spirituality, 6, 7, 9, 35, 36, 306-7, 309
Sri Krishna. *See* Krishna, Lord
stick, 360
struggle, 243, 244
suffering, 26, 174, 269, 271
superstition, 149, 150
support, 338
surrender, 42, 70, 168, 169, 198, 199, 215, 216, 218, 256, 257, 305, 345
sweeper, 393

taste, 396
teacher, 406
teachings
  His, 413
  of Guru, 404
  of Master, 136, 300
temple/s, 154, 155, 306, 419, 421
  worship, 419
temptation, 5, 329
ten commandments, 281
tendencies, 383
test of my Master, 395
texts, yogic/religious, 13
theories, 127
thirst for knowledge, 319
thought/s, 46, 62, 72, 83, 84, 121, 324, 383, 385, 387, 403-4
thoughtessness, 85
time, 390-1
tolerance, 102
Towards Infinity, 278
tragedy, 140
transformation, 44, 359
transmission, 10, 18, 33, 46, 47, 70, 71, 78, 86, 114, 122, 164, 218, 278-9, 308-9, 322
trust, 48, 300
truth/-s, 316, 328, 370, 397-9, 401

Ultimate, 9, 409
unbalanced living, 57
unhappiness, 174
Universal Prayer, 63
Universe, animate/inanimate, 377
unwillingness, 418
Upanishads, 33

vacuum, 93

values, 314, 317
Varadachari, Dr. K.C., 325
Viswaroopa Darsana, 317-8

wants, 26, 27
Western minds, 34
will, 83, 362
  power, 83, 109, 140
willingness, 190
wisdom, 292
women of India, 271
work, 190, 191, 192, 193, 194, 220, 221, 337
  for reward, 286

worship, 23, 153, 162, 212
  abstract form, 162
  external, 38, 164
  forms of, 4
  temple/idol, 38, 164, 223, 224, 419
  traditional, 154

Yama, 415
Yama paasam, 415
yoga, 14, 31, 38, 43, 50, 62, 89, 194, 203, 204, 205, 384
  factors in, 88
Yuga Purusha, 32